The Molecular Basis of Human Cancer

Edited by

Benjamin G. Neel, M.D., Ph.D.
Assistant Professor
Harvard Medical School
Beth Israel Hospital
Boston, Massachusetts

and

Ramesh Kumar, Ph.D.
Director
Hemoglobin Research Program
DNX Corporation
Princeton, New Jersey

**Futura Publishing
Company, Inc.**
Mount Kisco, NY

Library of Congress Cataloging-in-Publication Data

The molecular basis of human cancer / edited by Benjamin G. Neel and
    Ramesh Kumar.
        p.   cm.
    Includes bibliographical references and index.
    ISBN 0-87993-554-5
    1. Carcinogenesis.   2. Cancer—Molecular aspects.   I. Neel,
Benjamin G.   II. Kumar, Ramesh.
    [DNLM: 1. Neoplasms—physiopathology.   2. Signal
Transduction.   3. Growth Substances—physiology.   4. Recep-
tors, Endogenous Substances.   5. Cell Transformation, Neoplastic.
QZ 202 M71805 1993]
RC268.5.M633   1993
616.99'407—dc20
DNLM/DLC
for Library of Congress   93-23819
                                                                          CIP

Copyright 1993
Futura Publishing Company, Inc.

Published by
Futura Publishing Company, Inc.
2 Bedford Ridge Road
Mount Kisco, New York 10549

LC #: 93-23819
ISBN #: 0-87993-554-5

Printed in the United States of America.

This book is printed on acid-free paper.

Dedication

To our mentors and other discoverers of
the molecular basis of cancer.

Contributors

Ramesh Kumar, Ph.D. *Director, Hemoglobin Research Program, DNX Corporation, Princeton, New Jersey*

Veeraswamy Manne, Ph.D. *Senior Scientific Investigator, Department of Molecular Drug Mechanisms, Division of Oncology, Bristol-Myers Squibb Pharmaceutical Research Institute, Princeton, New Jersey*

Ximena Montano, Ph.D. *Research Scientist, Imperial Cancer Research Fund, Skin Tumour Laboratory, London Hospital Medical College, London, England*

Benjamin G. Neel, M.D., Ph.D. *Assistant Professor, Harvard Medical School, Beth Israel Hospital, Boston, Massachusetts*

Greg D. Plowman, M.D., Ph.D. *Oncology Drug Discovery, Bristol-Myers Squibb Pharmaceutical Research Institute, Seattle, Washington*

Friedrich Propst, Ph.D. *Institute of Biochemistry and Molecular Cell Biology, University of Vienna, Vienna Biocenter, Vienna, Austria; Formerly, Senior Scientist, Ludwig Institute for Cancer Research, St. Mary's Hospital Medical School, London, England*

Diego Pulido, Ph.D. *Staff Investigator CSIC, Centro de Biología Molecular (CSIC-UAM), Consejo Superior de Investigaciones Científicas, Universidad Autónoma de Madrid, Madrid, Spain*

Anthony F. Purchio, Ph.D. *Director of Molecular Biology, Bristol-Myers Squibb Pharmaceutical Research Institute, Seattle, Washington*

Ulf R. Rapp, M.D. *Chief, Laboratory of Viral Carcinogenesis, National Cancer Institute, Frederick Cancer Research and Development Center, Frederick, Maryland*

Michael P. Rosenberg, Ph.D. *Section Head, Department of Pharmacology, Glaxo Research Institute, Research Triangle Park, North Carolina*

Stephen M. Storm, B.S., Ph.D. (Cand.) *Biological Carcinogenesis and Development Program, PRI/DynCorp, Frederick Cancer Research and Development Center, Frederick, Maryland*

Kiranur N. Subramanian, Ph.D. *Professor, Department of Genetics, University of Illinois College of Medicine at Chicago, Chicago, Illinois*

Marius Sudol, Ph.D. *Assistant Professor, Laboratory of Molecular Oncology, The Rockefeller University, New York, New York*

Pramod Sutrave, Ph.D. *Associate Scientist, ABL-Basic Research Program, NCI-Frederick Cancer Research and Development Center, Frederick, Maryland*

Foreword

The accomplishments and discoveries in cancer research during the past 20 years have surpassed all the expectations of the planners and participants. No one predicted there would be a fusion of the traditional cancer research disciplines, much less that all of basic research in biology could be joined through molecular biology and molecular genetics. Aside from creating an identity crisis for certain academic departments, we could not have asked for a better outcome. What were considered to be unrelated research objectives a few years ago have converged to provide unlimited opportunities for exploring and understanding the molecular basis of human disease. Moreover, for most of this century, cancer research was dependent on avian and rodent model systems for the study of neoplastic transformation; but, during the past decade, the advances in research and technology have permitted an extraordinary and substantial shift in focus to direct human-based studies. This astonishing accomplishment results from technological advances that allow qualitative and quantitative measurements that are highly accurate and fundamentally noninvasive. Although cancer may well become the leading cause of death in the United States by the 21st century,[1] we can fully expect during the next decade revolutionary changes in cancer diagnosis and treatment.

By now we have discarded all prospects for identifying a single causative agent responsible for cancer. Yet, just when it appears that there are more genes responsible for neoplastic disease than we can ever possibly understand or control, is it possible that there may be a unified explanation for the malignant process? For many years, we have suspected that oncogenes influence the regulation of the cell cycle (couched in terms like "in the hierarchy of genes that regulate the cell cycle"). With the spectacular discoveries of the past several years revealing how the major cell cycle regulators, cyclins, and p34^{cdc2} kinase (and their related family members) are regulated, and

---

[1]Currently, each year more than 400,000 cancer-related deaths occur and one million new cases are diagnosed. The number of cancer-related deaths are likely to increase as the age of the population increases, especially if the number of deaths due to heart and circulatory diseases continues to decrease.

regulate progression through the cell cycle, the connection with oncogenes has become more apparent. For example, the *mos* proto-oncogene product was shown to function in the activation of p34^{cdc2} kinase as M-phase promoting factor (MPF) during meiosis, and the ras oncoprotein, p21, can substitute for the *mos* product to activate MPF. Thus, oncoproteins can, directly or indirectly, regulate MPF activity. Is this related to their transforming phenotype? Recently, a direct connection between an oncogene and a cell cycle gene has been discovered: a G1 cyclin has been implicated in several human malignancies as a potential oncogene. We have proposed that the major effects of the products of oncogenes and tumor suppressor genes are to influence the cell cycle by regulating entry into S phase or by expressing M-phase activities during interphase.[2] The former would be equivalent to rescuing cells from senescence, while the latter can explain the phenotypes of morphological transformation. We have also proposed that oncogenes and tumor suppressor genes compromise checkpoint function by promoting progression through the cell cycle.[2] This occurrence would reduce the ability of tumor cells to repair damage and could account for their adaptability and genetic instability. It can also provide an explanation for the sensitivity of tumor cells to antineoplastic drugs.

While the above is mostly hypothesis, with the wealth of new information on the molecular basis of cancer, it is now possible to construct unifying models. Experiments that disprove any or all aspects of such models can only improve our understanding of the mechanisms of transformation. In any case, the exciting discoveries in cancer research, many described in this book, will provide the means for significant improvements in diagnosis and prognosis and lead to the development of new approaches in therapy.

George F. Vande Woude
Director
ABL-Basic Research Program
NCI-Frederick Cancer Research
    and Development Center
Frederick, Maryland

---

[2]Vande Woude GF, et al. 1990 Views of Cancer Research, General Motors Cancer Research Foundation, 1990, pp. 128–143.

Preface

The knowledge of the etiology and pathogenesis of a disease greatly accelerates the development of effective therapeutic strategies. In this regard, neoplastic syndromes have suffered for the lack of any understanding of their molecular or physiological basis. Consequently, surgery and relatively nonselective phamacother- apeutic agents, such a chemotherapeutics and radiation, have been employed for various forms of cancer. The effectiveness of sur- gical intervention has been variable depending on the timing and precision of the procedure. Moreover, since the diagnosis of cancer has relied on end-stage symptoms, early treatment has not been feasible.

The quest for a molecular basis of cancer has been motivated by both diagnostic and therapeutic benefits expected to accrue from such information. Whereas the sum of all information acquired before 1960 pertaining to the cause of cancer can be summarized in one brief chapter, the summary of the most prominent discoveries in this area over the past 30 years will require not one, but many, complete books. This book is a condensation of a portion of the knowledge that is known today.

We decided that this book should be aimed at a general, rather than a specialist, audience, hopefully comprised of both clinical and research professionals. In keeping with the molecular themes in recent discoveries, we agreed to divide chapters among classes of genes involved in cancer, rather than divide the discussion among afflicted organs or types of tumors. We then decided to turn to young investigators actively involved in various areas for contributions to this book. Although writing a chapter for a book aimed at a general audience is usually low on the list of priorities for young and active researchers, we have been pleasantly and gratefully surprised by the enthusiasm of the contributors and the timeliness and quality of their valuable contributions.

We are very fortunate that Dr. George Vande Woude kindly agreed to write a thought-provoking foreword, which greatly enhances the book. Finally, this book is the result of the persistence and hard work of our publisher Steve Korn and his associates. We thank them for their valuable contributions.

Benjamin G. Neel, M.D., Ph.D.
Ramesh Kumar, Ph.D.

Contents

Chapter 1

The Discovery of the Molecular Basis of Cancer

Ramesh Kumar

Identification of Oncogenes

The determination of the etiology of cancer has long been a prominent and frustrating quest for the physicians who encountered and attempted to manage patients carrying tumors. The reported number of definitive cures or survival from cancer were limited, and most of the early knowledge of this disease was based on pathology and epidemiology. These studies have provided the foundation for the establishment of the molecular basis of cancer. Comparative studies highlighted important differences between the cancer cell and the normal cell. It was also apparent that cancer could result in many different cell types and that most tissues were susceptible. These studies, although illuminating, failed to reveal either the cause or the mechanism of transmission of this disease. Early epidemiologic studies, most notably one pertaining to scrotal cancer in chimney sweeps, pointed to a cause and effect relationship between an environmental factor and cancer. In this instance, it was hypothesized that pollutants in the smoke tar and soot to which chimney sweeps are exposed was an occupational hazard that contributed to the high incidence of scrotal cancer. These compounds are now recognized as the source of chemical carcinogens. The nature of the series of steps leading from exposure to these damaging chemicals to the appearance of a tumor has been slowly revealed in the past three decades.

From *The Molecular Basis of Human Cancer:* edited by B. Neel, M.D., Ph.D., R. Kumar, Ph.D. © 1993, Futura Publishing Co. Inc., Mount Kisco, NY.

A second major causative factor in cancer was discovered through efforts of veterinary science. Tumors in chicken and mice were both shown to be caused by viruses. These viruses, it was later revealed, belonged to a unique group of viruses, now called retroviruses, that contain and propagate an RNA genome. Ironically, although very few definitive cause and effect linkages of viruses and human cancer exist today, the bulk of our knowledge of the molecular biology of cancer summarized in the following chapters was distilled and derived from the studies in retrovirology. The most prominent discovery in this field remains the recognition that single genes carried by retrovirus were responsible for the transmission of cancer. Moreover, these cancer causing "oncogenes" were related to and derived from their cellular counterparts (proto-oncogenes) that were part of the genomic complement in every cell and whose expression and function was critically important to the growth, survival, and propagation of these cells. Later discoveries have pointed out that proto-oncogenes carry out functions that are cell type-specific and are involved in developmental, temporal, or spatial regulation of cellular functions.

Proto-oncogenes, in most instances, have been shown to encode proteins that have essential functions. These proteins are represented in each of the known classes of regulatory proteins and include growth factors and hormones, receptors for various ligands, enzymes of macromolecular modification, cell contact-related proteins, enzymes involved in intracellular communication, transcription, translation, and replication regulatory proteins. The largest number of these genes encode proteins that modify other proteins and are therefore believed to influence critical steps in the cascade of regulation.

The ability to isolate oncogenes relied on the emergence of the powerful tools of molecular biology. Three methods, gene transfer, polymerase chain reaction (PCR), and somatic cell hybrids were instrumental in the recovery and analysis of these genes. The first two methodologies became established less than 12 and 5 years ago, respectively, and have been responsible for most of the discoveries relating to the structure and incidence of oncogenes in tumors. Somatic cell hybrids played a critical role in the discovery of tumor-suppressor genes and will be discussed in Chapter 2. In addition to these methods, approaches based on transgenic animals have been very fruitful for dissecting mechanisms of carcinogenesis. The methods and applications of transgenic techniques are detailed in Chapter 10.

Isolation of Oncogenes

The concepts and experiments that have led to the discovery of the molecular basis of cancer originate from microbiological studies. The microbial etiologic agents of infectious diseases were identified through bacterial culture and established by satisfying Koch's postulates. These postulates, in part, required that a causative infectious agent must be transmissible from a diseased individual (or animal) to a healthy one, and that such transmission would infect and inflict the disease on the new victim. A crude parallel to such experiments in cancer research was achieved by the transfer of mammary tumors in mice through viruses found in milk. However, for many other tumors (and to date, most human tumors) infectious agents could not be identified. In the late 1970s, several molecular biologists attempted to invoke and test yet another concept of microbiology to address the question of transmission in cancer. In what constitutes a milestone in biology, in 1945, microbiologists were able to transmit a somatic trait from one bacterial type to another by means of transfer of genes (or DNA). Such gene transfer experiments proved that certain traits (in this instance, a capsule on the surface of infectious pneumoccocus) could be transmitted by the transfer of genes. In the late 1970s, a similar experiment could be carried out to test whether unique transmissible genes in tumors could convert normal cells into cancerous cells. The availability of cultured tumor cells and nontumor (normal) cells was crucial to this test. For various reasons, both historic and technical, one of the first successful experiments involved the use of a human tumor cell-line and a mouse normal cell-line. After the transfer of DNA from tumor cells, striking change in the morphology of the recipient normal (mouse NIH3T3) cells was observed (Fig. 1). Whereas the normal cell appeared, in a tissue culture plate, flat and undistinguished, tumor DNA carrying cells were converted (transformed) to a more refractile, disordered type. The transformed cells have distinct properties that are used to distinguish them from the untransformed ("normal") cells. These include loss of contact inhibition, ability to grow as tumors when injected into syngeneic or nude mice, the ability to grow in clumps in semisoft medium, and growth factor independence.

The transformed cells harboring transforming (onco) genes could then be utilized for the identification and isolation of these genes. The process of gene transfer and the isolation of the transferred gene is shown in Figure 2. Earlier attempts at oncogene isolation exploited the

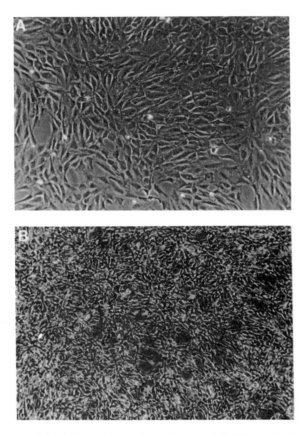

Figure 1. *Morphological transformation of mouse NIH3T3 cells by oncogenes introduced by DNA transfection. See Figure 2 and text for details. A: Normal NIH3T3 cells. B: NIH3T3 cells transformed with H-ras oncogene.*

different repetitive sequences found in human and mouse cells. "Alu" repeats are highly repeated (10^5 copies per genome) sequences interspersed in the human genome and are present within and near most protein coding genes. During DNA transfection, at least 10 kb of genomic DNA from the human tumor is often transferred and integrated into the genome of the recipient cells. On average, these genomic DNA fragments should carry (at random) several "Alu" elements. This property of the transfected DNA permits the identification and cloning of human DNA contained in the transformed cell. The detection of "Alu" repeated sequences in the transformed cells

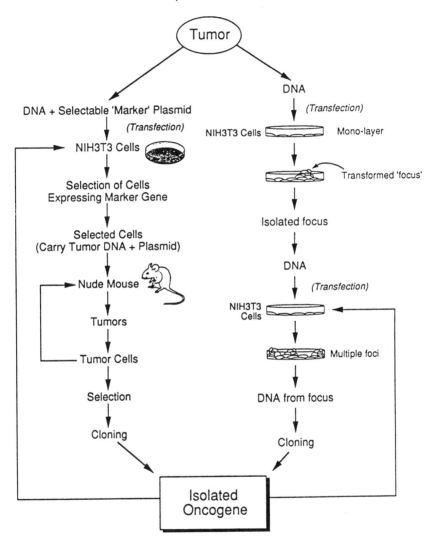

Figure 2. *Isolation of oncogenes from tumors. Genomic DNA isolated from tumors can be introduced into normal NIH3T3 cells. The successful uptake and incorporation of the DNA (transfection) can cause morphological changes (transformation) in the recipient cells. A group of transformed cells among normal cells is recognized as a "focus" which can be isolated and used to derive DNA for subsequent rounds of transfection and transformation. After the final step, DNA is isolated and cloned into bacteriophage vectors. The specific oncogene sequences can then be identified by molecular hybridization. Transformation assay can also be carried out using nude mice as recipients. Here, tumors can be isolated from the mice and used as a source of the oncogene.*

therefore indirectly indicates that human sequences contributed to the transformed phenotype. The DNA isolated from the transformed cells containing human DNA can be used to transform more NIH3T3 cells in a process called second-cycle transfection. In general, multiple rounds of transfection and isolation of transformed cells and detection of "Alu" sequences leads to the enrichment of human sequences required for the transformation of NIH3T3 cells. After enrichment, the genomic sequences containing the oncogene can be cloned by standard recombinant DNA methods. This method of oncogene isolation was the first to be successful and has been used for the identification of several oncogenes from different types of tumors. This method, however, suffers from the following disadvantages:

1. Only relatively small genes (<30 kb) can be isolated, the size of the gene being limited by the fragility of genomic DNA.
2. Certain oncogenes do not cause morphological transformation of NIH3T3 cells and therefore cannot be scored in this assay system.
3. Some oncogenes isolated by this procedure may represent results of in vitro manipulation and rearrangements of the transfected DNA rather than a replica of the oncogene present in the tumor.
4. Some oncogenes may not be isolated by the "Alu" hybridization method because of the lack of these repetitive sequences in the genomic span of these oncogenes.
5. Certain genes transferred into NIH3T3 cells by this procedure cannot be expressed in these cells and, therefore, cannot be detected by this functional assay.

A modification of the NIH3T3 transfection method, involving the use of an in vivo testing system has expanded the range of detection of this methodology (Fig. 1). In this method, after transfection, the cells containing oncogene sequences are transferred into a nude mouse where they can develop into tumors. The lack of an immune system and, therefore, immunological surveillance in nude mice prevents the rejection of the transplanted cells. The tumor that is derived from the oncogene transfected cell can be used as a source of genomic DNA for the isolation of the oncogene. Gene transfer methods have been instrumental in the discovery of nearly a dozen different oncogenes, including those of the *ras* gene family.

The seminal discovery that retroviral oncogenes have closely related cellular homologs (proto-oncogenes) opened the door for the identification of these genes. Since viral genomes were rapidly cloned by recombinant DNA methods, several DNA probes could be identified from these viral isolates. Each probe was then used to identify the cellular proto-oncogene that was the source of the viral oncogene. So far, over two dozen retroviral oncogenes have been shown to have cellular counterparts which represent structural predecessors of the transforming gene. In some cases, the search for oncogene related sequences has yielded multiple related homologs of a single viral gene, thus expanding the catalog of proto-oncogenes.

Another approach, based on cytogenetics, has been fruitfully applied to the detection of oncogenes in several leukemias. In these malignancies, pathologists have observed consistent alterations in the structure of the chromosomal complement of the tumor cells. These karyotypic aberrations are often the result of the transfer of a part of one chromosome to another, a process termed translocation. Often such changes involve reciprocal translocation, i.e., two chromosomes exchange parts with one another. Many of these exchanges result in the creation of a novel gene at the junction of the DNA sequences between the two chromosomal segments. In addition, such break and splice can also activate previously dormant genes at the rearranged chromosomal locus. In either case, the identification of genes at the site of translocation is useful for the understanding of the mechanism of transformation. Several oncogenes such as *myc* have been isolated by this approach. Clearly, this approach is limited to the isolation of only a small number of oncogenes.

Retroviruses have been exploited for the discovery of yet another class of oncogenes. These genes are not carried in the viral genome but instead are activated upon insertion of the viral genome in proximity to a cellular gene. Generally these proto-oncogenes are tightly regulated, either in terms of the specificity or the quantity of expression. Such insertionally activated genes have been found in both mice and chickens, but not yet in humans. Examples of such activated genes include those coding for the *wnt* growth factors and the *evi*-1 transcription factor.

Classification of Oncogenes

Comparison of the phenotype and growth rate of the normal NIH3T3 and the transformed cells indicates that oncogenes have a dramatic effect on critical steps in cell physiology. Cataloging of the properties of oncogenes and their products has revealed that proteins encoded by these genes exhibit a great diversity in their size, location, activity, and function. This variety can be interpreted to represent multiple checkpoints in the regulation of cell growth. Alternatively, the multiplicity of types of oncogenes may suggest specific pairing of tissues and oncogenes or tumor types and oncogenes. This latter explanation has not been proven correct. The same type of activated oncogene, e.g., H-*ras* can be isolated from tumors of lung, colon, and lymphocytes. Similarly one tissue type can generate tumors containing different oncogenes (e.g., multiple oncogenes such as *ras, trk,* etc., in tumors of the thyroid).

The simplest classification of oncogenes is based on the biochemical activity of their encoded proteins (Table 1), In general, most oncogene products are either enzymes or critical components of transcription, translation, and replication. The subcellular location of the oncoproteins is another basis for their classification (Table 2). Some proteins, such as receptors and cell adhesion molecules, are located in the cell membrane. Others are cytoplasmic or tethered to the inner side of the membrane.

TABLE 1.
Biochemical Classification of Oncoproteins

I. Enzymes
    A. Protein Kinases
        i. Serine-threonine Kinases
            Examples: *raf, mos, pim*
        ii. Tyrosine-kinases
            Examples: *src, abl, trk, met*
    B. GTPases
        Examples: *ras, gsp*
II. DNA-binding Proteins
    A. Transcriptional Regulators
        i. Activators
            Examples: myc, myb, jun, fos
        ii. Repressors
            Examples: *erb* A, *rel*
    B. Others
        i. Negative regulators of cell growth
            Examples: p53, Rb, WT-1
III. Ligands and Receptors
    A. Growth Factors
        Examples: *sis* (PDGF), TGFα
    B. Receptors
        Examples: *trk* (NGF receptor), *fms* (CSF-1 receptor)

TABLE 2.
Other Classifications of Oncoproteins

A. Based on Action
    i. Dominant (oncogenes) e.g., *ras, neu*
    ii. Recessive (anti-oncogenes) e.g., p53, Rb, NF-1
B. Based on Sub-cellular Location
    i. Integral membrane proteins: e.g., *trk*, erb-B2
    ii. Secreted proteins: e.g., *sis*
    iii. Cytoplasmic
        1. Attached to membranes: e.g., *src, ras*
        2. Free cytosolic: e.g., *raf, mos*
    iv. Nuclear: e.g., *myc, myb, ski, abl*
C. Based on Function
    i. Receptors: e.g., *mas*, erb-B2
    ii. Ligands: e.g., *int*-1 (Wnt)
    iii. Signal Transduction Molecules: e.g., *gip*
    iv. Transcription factors: e.g., WT-1
    v. Prevent programmed cell-death (apoptosis): e.g., *bcl*-2
D. Based on Sequence Homology
    i. *ras* family: H-*ras*, K-*ras*, N-*ras*, K-*rev*, etc.
    ii. *src* family: *lck, blk*, etc.
    iii. *erb*B family: *erb*B1, B2, B3
    iv. *trk* family: *trk, trk*B, *trk*C
    v. *fgf* family: *fgf* 1 thru 7

Many regulatory proteins encoded by oncogenes reside in the nucleus. Yet other proteins, typically growth factor-derived oncoproteins, can either be secreted from the cell or can be attached to the cell membrane. In some instances the subcellular location of the oncoprotein may be different from the location of the proto-oncogene product. Indeed, the altered location in the cell may be the molecular basis for different functions of the two proteins.

Oncogenes are dominant acting genes and the oncogenic activity is often the consequence of one or more mutations in the structure of the proto-oncogenes. As a result most oncoproteins have gained new functions not present in their proto-oncogene counterparts. In some instances, these changes may alter (either accelerate, retard, or modify) enzymatic activity. In addition, some oncogenic proteins exhibit altered specificity towards their substrates or targets. A distinct class of cancer related genes, the antioncogenes or tumor-suppressor genes, have been recently identified. These genes differ from dominant oncogenes in the way they are generated and in the mode of their action. By definition, these are recessive genes and their action is manifest only upon loss or silencing of both alleles of the gene. Often these genes encode proteins that negatively regulate cell growth or replication. Therefore, loss or inactivation of these genes results in the removal of normal controls that are exercised through their action in the cell. Many of these genes (actually gene-defects) are inherited, and the carriers are functionally hemizygous. A classic antioncogene is the Retinoblastoma (Rb) gene, so named because of the high incidence of tumors of the retina in young patients carrying an Rb mutation. Recessive oncogenes will be discussed in detail in Chapter 2.

Mechanism of Action of Oncogenes

A first step in the understanding of how oncoproteins act is to define the changes necessary to convert a proto-oncogene to an oncogene. These changes can affect either the activity of the protein (qualitative alterations) or the concentration of the protein (quantitative changes). Quantitative changes result from aberrant transcriptional regulation or alteration of the stability of the protein. Qualitatively a protein structure can be changed by point mutations (including nonsense mutations that can truncate a protein) or deletions, insertions, fusions, or other structural rearrangements (Fig. 3). Since many oncogenes are expressed specifically and in a programmed fashion, any disruption of this pattern, such as by ectopic expression in inappropriate environments, can also qualitatively alter oncogene activity.

The regulatory activity of many proto-oncogene products is reversible. In many cases, several proto-oncogene products regulate each other in a chain or cascade fashion. Similarly oncoprotein and products of recessive oncogenes can communicate in biochemical pathways. Oncogenic changes (mutations or deletions) can affect such fine-tuning by disconnecting the effect of ligand on the oncoprotein, resulting in their constitutive activation. This is illustrated by oncogenes such as *fms* which is derived from a growth factor receptor. Whereas the *fms* proto-oncogene encoded protein (the receptor for colony stimulating factor-1, CSF-1) is active upon binding its ligand, the oncogene product does not require such stimulation for its activation (see Chapter 5 for details). Some oncogenic changes can also affect enzymatic activity in a quantitative manner. For example the GTPase activity of the *ras* proteins is severely compromised in the oncogenic form. In addition, whereas the normal *ras* GTPase activity is

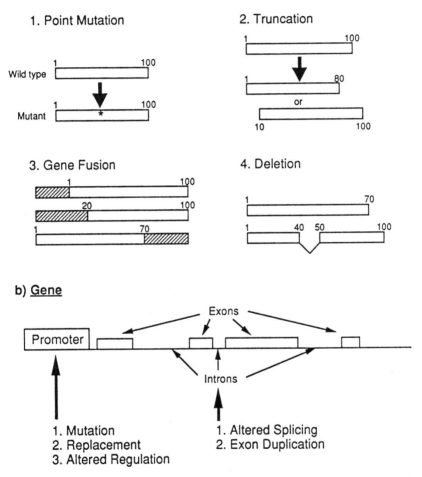

Figure 3. *Multiple mechanisms of oncogene activation. A proto-oncogene can be altered (activated) to make an oncogene. A: The changes in the gene sequence can result in the synthesis of proteins with point mutations, deletions, truncation, or additional sequences. B: Qualitative changes in the expression of a proto-oncogene can also be oncogenic. These changes may affect the promoter or the transcribed sequences.*

upregulated by an ancillary GTPase activating protein (GAP), the enzymatic activity of the oncoprotein is unaffected by GAP (see Chapter 3). This illustrates the fact that oncogenic alterations of a protein may have local effects (on the activity of the affected protein) as well as global effects by indirectly infringing on other proteins and pathways that interact with or may depend on the affected protein. The ultimate effect of oncogenic activity appears to be to liberate the cell from its usual stringent controls. Clearly, such regulatory oversight can result in unchecked growth, a hallmark of neoplasia. Cellular control pathways are comprised of multiple sequential steps and in many cases parallel or redundant circuits may be in place to prevent the effect of aberrations resulting from mutation. As a consequence no single change (affecting only one protein) can be expected to be sufficient to derail and deregulate cellular control. Multiple alterations are therefore necessary to convert normal cells into neoplastic cells. Very often, cancer cells contain a large number of mutations in several regulatory genes.

Molecular Events in Carcinogenesis

The definition of oncogenes and their molecular isolation have depended on the existence of dominant activated genes in retroviruses and tumors. It was fortuitous that the earliest assays (NIH3T3 transfection) permitted detection of single oncogenes present in tumor cell-lines and in solid human tumors. Studies of the incidence of cancer in human and experimental animals had suggested that more than one genetic change (or oncogene) may be required to generate tumors. This conclusion was based on the fact that tumors generally arise in old age. This fact was interpreted to indicate the requirement of accumulation of multiple alterations in genes for the manifestation of a tumor. For many types of tumors, it was possible to delineate several steps in the process of carcinogenesis. These steps often include the appearance of precancerous, usually hyperplastic lesions and, in some instances, the recognition of postmalignant stages involving metastasis. Once again retroviruses provided the first molecular proof that a combination of oncogenes rather than a single oncogene was required for the appearance of neoplasia. Several retroviruses were isolated that contained two different oncogenes in the same genome. Later, using recipient cell-lines other than the original NIH3T3 cells, it was possible to show that two oncogenes in combination, but not singly, could cause malignant transformation of these "normal" cells (such as Rat Embryo Fibroblasts [REF]).

These experimental findings have since been replicated in studies on human carcinogenesis. For example colon cancer, which has been recognized by pathologists as involving multiple sequential stages, results from the concerted action of multiple genetic insults involving both dominant acting oncogenes and tumor-suppressor recessive genes (Chapter 2). In some tumors, such as mammary and eye neoplasia, some of these molecular changes are inherited and others generated somatically. Where multiple events have been shown to be important, it is not yet established whether or not there is a requirement for a specific order in the way the mutated oncogenes are acquired. From the studies on colon cancer, it appears that the order of activation of these genes may be irrelevant, and only the sum of all changes may be significant. Similarly, it remains to be determined if there is a penultimate step of carcinogenesis and if the oncogenes capable of triggering this step have unique properties. This type of information could be of great value in devising therapies for cancer. The major types of human cancers and the suspected causative oncogenes are listed in Table 3.

TABLE 3.
Major Types of Human Cancer and Their Causes

Type[1]	Cause[2]	Activated or Deleted Genes[3]	
		Oncogenes	Suppressor
1. Lung	Smoking, Environmental	ras	p53
2. Colon	Dietary Factors	ras	p53
3. Breast	Hormones	neu	p53
4. Prostate & Bladder	Hormones, Smoking	?	?
5. Lymphoma	Retroviruses (?)	?	?
6. Oral	Tobacco	?	?
7. Pancreas	Smoking	ras	?
8. Leukemia	Radiations	ras, trans-locations	?
9. Melanoma	Radiations (UV)	ras, ?	p53
10. Kidney	Smoking	?	?

1. Listed in the order of incidence.
2. Only the leading (suspected) causal agents are listed.
3. Only those genes that have a significant incidence are listed.

Molecular Basis of Action of Environmental Carcinogens

The role of chemical agents found in chimney soot and cigarette smoke, and physical agents such as ultraviolet light and x-rays were originally suspected in the causation of human cancer through epidemiologic studies of various population groups at risk. Once oncogenes were identified in tumors, several attempts were made to test whether a cause and effect relationship existed between environmental factors and the molecular damage resulting in the activation of oncogenes. Many of these suspected carcinogens have in common the ability to interact with and damage DNA. Since oncogenes are generated by creating lesions in proto-oncogenes, chemical and physical agents that damage DNA can directly activate these genes. This provocative hypothesis has now been tested in an animal model system. Many chemical carcinogens have well-defined chemical activities, and it is possible to predict the molecular consequences (such as point mutations, deletions, etc.) of the interaction of the carcinogen with a target DNA sequence. A consistent mutagenic change in DNA associated with a specific type of chemical will then suggest a cause and effect relationship between the carcinogen and the mutation in the oncogene. In one recent study carried out using a rat model system, tumors of the mammary gland and the kidneys were induced upon exposure to the chemical carcinogen nitroso-methyl urea (NMU). In most of the tumors the same G to A mutation was observed in the 12th codon of the H-*ras* oncogene. This genetic change could be correlated with the chemical activity of the NMU, which is an alkylating agent and is expected to cause transition type mutations. The mutated oncogenes could be identified as early as two weeks after treatment with the carcinogen. These studies have also highlighted many other interacting features of carcinogenesis. Even though *ras* oncogenes were found to be activated early, mammary tumors developed only after sexual maturation and growth. In this instance, it was clear that hormone-induced cellular proliferation was required for the development of tumors from cells carrying activated oncogene. Although these studies have established oncogene activation as the initial step in cancer and highlighted the role of normal physiological growth signals in neoplasia, it is not yet clear what additional genetic changes were involved.

In most cases, only a few selective targets for mutation have been found in proto-oncogene sequences (e.g., 12th codon in *ras*). As suspected, these target regions also define the location of the critical parts of the protein. Some of these targets of mutation are favored over other, equally important, sites in a protein, and these favored targets are called "hot spots" of mutation. Hot spots have also been found in some antioncogenes. The choice of these preferred sites probably stems from the accessibility of these sequences to the mutagen or the inability of the cellular repair systems to correct the damage inflicted here. In addition to the hot spots in an oncogene, in some tumors only a specific oncogene may be activated by some but not all carcinogens and this specificity may not always be explained on the basis of the access of the mutagen to the DNA sequence. Another interesting finding to come to light is that the acquisition of a mutated oncogene does not directly earmark the afflicted cell for neoplasia. Instead, as discussed in the previous section, several different lesions may be required for the development of the tumor. It is also becoming increasingly clear that regulatory factors affecting cell physiology and, therefore, indirectly, oncogene activity, can be critical to the phenotypic expression of an activated oncogene.

Organization of the Book

The following chapters detail various aspects of our knowledge of the molecular basis of cancer. Several oncogenes are dealt with in chapters that deal either with a family of genes related by DNA sequence (such as the *ras* genes, Chapter 3) or with functional classes of oncogenes (e.g., growth factor receptors [Chapter 6], growth factors [Chapter 5], and transcription factors [Chapter 8]). Oncogenes encoding protein modification enzymes (such as protein kinases) are discussed in several different chapters (Chapters 4, 5, and 6). The causal association between human cancer and papilloma viruses is discussed in Chapter 9. The recent excitement in the area of tumor suppressor genes, including the methods leading to their discovery, are detailed in Chapter 2. Applications of transgenic mice in cancer research are described in Chapter 10. Therapeutic and diagnostic applications of oncogene research are summarized in Chapters 12 and 11, respectively.

Summary

A large number of cellular genes, representing many different functional classes of proteins, can be activated to become oncogenes. The proto-oncogene products carry out critical functions in the cell and are usually expressed at low levels in specific tissues under a strict temporal program. There is both redundancy and specificity in their function, and multiple proto-oncogene products can act in concert in a biochemical pathway. Oncogenes, which are altered forms of proto-oncogenes, encode proteins that have suffered changes in the rate, affinity, or specificity of action. Some genes involved in carcinogenesis are recessive and their oncogenic effect is manifested upon their loss by mutation or gene deletion. These genes, variously termed antioncogenes or suppressor genes, have been implicated in growth control. Oncogenic changes are brought about by environmental factors and can be inherited. A single oncogene can have a dominant effect, but it takes several different oncogenes to cause malignant transformation in vivo.

Chapter 2

Tumor Suppressors

Benjamin G. Neel

In his book, *The Structure of Scientific Revolutions*,[207] historian and philosopher of science Thomas Kuhn describes how the dominance of a particular scientific paradigm leads scientists to overlook results that are at variance with the paradigm but which, in retrospect, are quite obvious. Molecular oncology provides a compelling demonstration of Kuhn's thesis. Most work prior to the last five years focused on the identification and characterization of dominant cellular proto-oncogenes (c-*onc*) and their viral derivatives (v-*onc*). As amply discussed in other chapters of this book, c-*onc* genes, when mutated and/or expressed at abnormally high levels, confer various aspects of the malignant phenotype on appropriate target cells in a genetically dominant fashion. Technical advances spurred the rapid discovery of dominant oncogenes. This rapid progress led to confidence (perhaps better characterized as hubris) that all of the key target genes in cancer would soon be in hand.

Despite these dramatic successes, however, multiple lines of evidence, much of it antedating the discovery of dominant oncogenes, indicated that cancer resulted from the loss of specific genes. Such genes have been variously termed "negative oncogenes," "antioncogenes," "recessive oncogenes," or "tumor-suppressor genes." Almost by default, the term "tumor-suppressor gene" has gained the most currency and will be employed here. However, just as the purpose of oncogenes is not to cause cancer, the biological role of tumor-suppressor genes likely is not to prevent tumors—although many of them probably function to negatively control cell growth.

From *The Molecular Basis of Human Cancer:* edited by B. Neel, M.D., Ph.D., R. Kumar, Ph.D. © 1993, Futura Publishing Co. Inc., Mount Kisco, NY.

Progress towards the identification of tumor-suppressor genes was slow, owing mainly to methodological difficulties. Unlike the dominant oncogenes, which could be identified with relative ease, assaying directly for tumor-suppressor gene function was daunting. It is easy to identify a small number of transformed cells amidst a background of normal cells because the transformed cells have a growth advantage. The converse proposition, identifying a small number of (growth disadvantaged) normal (reverted) cells against a background of transformed cells, presents a formidable challenge. The cloning of the first tumor-suppressor gene, the retinoblastoma (Rb) gene, was achieved only through the laborious approach of screening tumors for homozygous regional chromosomal loss using restriction fragment length polymorphisms (RFLPs). Similar approaches, sometimes combined with educated guessing based on known genes within regions commonly deleted in tumors, have now been utilized to clone at least seven other tumor-suppressor genes.

In addition to verifying the existence of a new class of genes of perhaps even greater importance to human oncogenesis than the dominant oncogenes, studies of the products of two of these genes (Rb and p53) have led to exciting insights into the molecular mechanism of oncogenesis by DNA tumor viruses, and tantalizing connections between negative growth factor action, the cell cycle, and tumor-suppressor genes. Just as the discovery of c-*onc* genes led to a unification of the previously contentious fields of RNA tumor virology, chemical carcinogenesis, and growth factors and their receptors, it now appears that most (if not all) DNA tumor viruses cause cancer by inactivating the functions of tumor-suppressor genes, and that some (if not all) negative growth factors may signal via pathways containing tumor-suppressor gene products. If so, we may truly be close to the "holy grail" of molecular oncology—a unified theory of oncogenesis by diverse means such as RNA and DNA tumor viruses, chemicals, physical agents, and heredity, centered around a set of genes, the oncogenes and tumor-suppressor genes, whose alteration leads to cancer.

In this chapter, we will first briefly review the historical underpinnings of the tumor-suppressor gene field, focusing mainly on: (1) studies of somatic cell hybrids between normal and tumor cells; (2) familial cancer syndromes; and (3) evidence for loss of specific genes in cancer. We will then turn to a discussion of the cloning and characterization of the known tumor-suppressor genes and what is known about their mechanisms of action, including the exciting connections between tumor-suppressor genes, DNA tumor virus oncoproteins, negative growth factors, and the cell cycle. Using the elegant colon carcinoma system as a model, we will see how combinations of alterations in both dominant oncogenes and tumor-suppressor genes may account for multistep carcinogenesis. Finally, we will consider the current status of studies of several likely candidate tumor-suppressor genes. Several recent reviews have addressed many of these areas in some detail and will be cited where possible.

Cell Hybrid Suppression of Malignancy

An early approach to the molecular biology of cancer was to study the properties of hybrids formed between tumor and normal cells. The strategy of such experiments is illustrated in Figure 1. Pioneering studies by Barski and Ephrussi in the early 1960s[17,17a] demonstrated that somatic cell hybrids could reproducibly be formed, although at low frequency, between murine tumor cells of varying tumorigenicity. These rare hybrids, when expanded and injected into mice, were found to be tumorigenic. In the late 1960s, Harris and Klein reexamined the question of the tumorigenicity of rodent/rodent hybrids between tumorigenic and nontumorigenic cells.[145] Contrary to the results of Barski and Ephrussi, they found that the hybrids were nontumorigenic. However, hybrids passaged in culture for extended periods were tumorigenic. Careful studies documented that tumorigenic segregants arose during prolonged passage of initially nontumorigenic hybrids. This explained the earlier finding that tumor/normal hybrids were tumorigenic; due to the low efficiency of hybrid generation, longer in vitro culture had been required to obtain sufficient cells for tumorigenicity assays. During this period, tumorigenic segregants undoubtedly arose.

More importantly, reappearance of tumorigenicity was associated with the loss of chromosomes from the initial hybrids.[87,176] Painstaking cytogenetic comparisons between nontumorigenic hybrids and their tumorigenic segregants demonstrated that tumorigenicity was associated with the loss of a specific chromosome; in the original Harris hybrids, for example, loss of murine chromosome 4. Whenever a somatic cell hybrid contained even a single murine chromosome 4, it was nontumorigenic; if this chromosome was absent, a tumorigenic segregant arose.

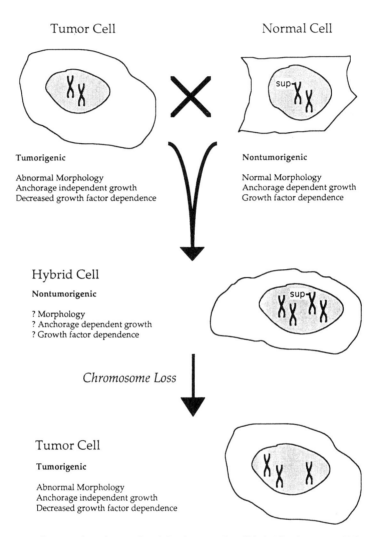

Tumor Cell

Normal Cell

Tumorigenic

Abnormal Morphology
Anchorage independent growth
Decreased growth factor dependence

Nontumorigenic

Normal Morphology
Anchorage dependent growth
Growth factor dependence

Hybrid Cell

Nontumorigenic

? Morphology
? Anchorage dependent growth
? Growth factor dependence

Chromosome Loss

Tumor Cell

Tumorigenic

Abnormal Morphology
Anchorage independent growth
Decreased growth factor dependence

Figure 1. *Suppression of tumorigenicity in somatic cell hybrids. Somatic cell fusions between normal (or nontumorigenic) cells and tumorigenic cells nearly always result in nontumorigenic cell hybrids. Other transformation parameters, e.g., morphology or anchorage dependence, may or may not be suppressed. Reversion of such suppressed somatic cell hybrids to the tumorigenic phenotype is always accompanied by specific chromosomal loss, presumably because these chromosomes contain the suppressor gene(s) required to block tumorigenicity. However, none of these genes has yet been identified (see text for details).*

These seminal studies of rodent/rodent hybrids were soon extended to hybrids between tumorigenic and nontumorigenic human cells, initially by Stanbridge[351] and later by Klinger.[196] Both groups found that when HeLa cells (derived from a cervical carcinoma) were fused with normal human primary fibroblasts, the resulting hybrids were nontumorigenic. As in the rodent system, tumorigenic segregants arose upon prolonged in vitro culture in association with specific chromosome loss. One advantage of the human system is the relative chromosomal stability of the hybrids. This facilitated the finding by Stanbridge and coworkers[353] and by Klinger[197] that loss of chromosome 11 was associated with tumorigenicity. Direct proof that chromosome 11 was sufficient to suppress HeLa tumorigenicity was later obtained using single chromosome transfer by microcell fusion.[329]

Multiple experiments by several investigators, utilizing a wide variety of tumor cell/normal cell combinations, have confirmed that tumorigenicity almost always behaves as a recessive trait in somatic cell hybrids.[144,195,323,325] Suppression is not limited to intraspecific hybrids; as long as stable hybrids can be formed, normal cells from one mammalian species can suppress the tumorigenicity of cancer cells from another. Human-rodent hybrids, from which human chromosomes are selectively lost, provide a vivid example of this phenomenom. As long as the normal cell is of rodent origin and the tumor cell is human, the hybrid is nontumorigenic. The converse is not always true, however, because the rapid rate of loss of human chromosomes often precludes the selection of stable, nontumorigenic hybrids. These results not only help establish the generality of hybrid suppression of malignancy, but also indicate that the gene(s) conferring suppression must be highly conserved across evolution. Similarly, the ability to suppress tumorigenicity is not limited to normal cells of a particular differentiation state. Although primary fibroblasts have been the normal cell donor in many hybrid suppression experiments, fibroblast-like immortal cell-lines, primary keratinocytes, and other nonmesenchymal cells can also suppress tumorigenicity (see above reviews). Suppression is also not limited to cancer cells derived from spontaneous tumors. Both chemically transformed and at least some dominant oncogene-transformed cell-lines are suppressed by fusion to normal cells; an extensive series of such experiments has been provided by Sager and colleagues in the Chinese hamster embryo fibroblast system.[323,324]

More than one gene is capable of suppressing tumorigenicity in somatic cell hybrids, since loss of different chromosomes has been correlated with the generation of tumorigenic segregants of initally suppressed hybrids. For example, human chromosome 11 suppresses HeLa tumorigenicity, but human chromosome 1 suppresses the tumorigenicity of transformed baby hamster kidney (BHK) cells.[357] Likewise, fusions between some different types of tumor cells result in nontumorigenic hybrids,[385] suggesting loss or inactivation of a different gene(s) in each transformed parent and complementation upon cell fusion.

The ability to form tumors is the sine qua non of cancer, but most cancer cells share several other derangements of normal cell physiology. These changes include altered cellular morphology, loss of contact inhibition of cell growth, ability to grow in soft agar or methylcellulose (loss of anchorage dependence), and increased glucose uptake; collectively, these abnormalities comprise the *transformed phenotype*. Although tumorigenicity is nearly always suppressed in tumor/normal hybrids, other transformation parameters often are not. For example, in HeLa x human fibroblast hybrids, tumorigenicity is suppressed, but the cells are not contact-inhibited, grow to high density, and in soft agar, and retain the abnormal morphology of the transformed parent.[350,351,354] Such findings suggested that tumorigenicity and other transformation parameters were under independent genetic control. They also suggested that multiple genetic derangements (hits) had occurred in the original tumor (or at least in the cell-line being used as a model for the original tumor). However, in other normal/tumor hybrids all transformation parameters are simultaneously suppressed.[144,323] It is not clear whether this is due to different types of suppressor genes, some with suppressing activity limited to tumorigenicity and some with more generalized suppressing effects, or whether some tumor cells have fewer genetic abnormalities to be suppressed.

Ironically, although suppression of tumorigenicity in normal/tumor hybrids provided the first evidence for tumor-suppressor genes, it is not at all clear whether the genes responsible for hybrid suppression are the same as—or are functionally related to—the bona fide tumor-suppressor genes that have been identified. In many tumor-hybrid pairs, the mechanism of tumorigenicity suppression appears to be induction of terminal differentiation.[352] For example, upon injection into nude mice, HeLa x human keratinocyte hybrids produce a small nodule of cells displaying keratinocyte differentiation. Similarly, HeLa x human fibroblast hybrids form a fibroblastic scar at their site of injection. Since HeLa cells are epithelial, induction of keratinocyte differentiation in hybrids could indicate the inactivation in HeLa cells of a gene normally required for terminal epithelial differentiation. However, the imposition of a fibroblastic differentiation program in HeLa x fibroblast hybrids cannot reflect the loss (or inactivation) of such a program during the genesis of the original HeLa tumor, since cervical epithelial cells do not normally display fibroblastic differentiation. Instead, a gene (or genes) actively expressed in human fibroblasts may be capable of "pharmacologically" suppressing tumorigenicity by inducing fibroblastic differentiation in an epithelial cell that would not normally be exposed to that gene product. Alternatively, even though terminal differentiation is induced in these normal/tumor hybrids, the mechanism of suppression need not be induction of differentiation directly. Instead, suppression could result from a gene that blocks proliferation. Terminal differentiation would then occur as a default pathway, and the type of differentiation observed would depend on the nature of the normal cell. At first glance, such a mechanism might seem incompatible with the observation that many hybrids, including the HeLa x fibroblast and HeLa x keratinocyte hybrids discussed above, have the same growth properties as the parental tumor cells in culture. It is possible, however, that a putative growth suppressor gene might only function in vivo, perhaps due to factors, soluble or matrix, missing from the tissue culture medium.

For at least some hybrids, suppression of tumorigenicity may occur via other mechanisms. In an elegant series of experiments, Noel Bouck and her colleagues have demonstrated that suppression of the tumorigenicity of transformed BHK cells is due to suppression of tumor angiogenesis (see Suppression of Angiogenesis and Metastasis).

At least some cases of hybrid suppression probably are due to bona fide tumor-suppressor genes. Wilms' tumor (WT) is often associated with deletions of the short arm of chromosome 11 (see: The Wilms' Tumor Gene). Stanbridge and coworkers transferred a single human chromosome 11 into a WT cell-line.[384] The resultant hybrids were nontumorigenic, although their culture properties remained largely unchanged. Again, if the transferred chromosome 11 was allowed to segregate by removing selection for the resistance marker, reappearance of tumorigenicity directly correlated with loss of chromosome 11. Although this experiment could not directly prove that the same gene(s) targeted by the 11p deletions is responsible for suppression in microcell fusions, it seems highly likely that this is the case. A similar result has been obtained in melanoma cells, in which introduction of a normal human chromosome 6 suppresses tumorigenicity.[371]

The phenomenon of hybrid suppression was clearly of great importance in establishing the concept of tumor-suppressor genes. However, none of the genes responsible for this phenomenon have yet been identified (with the possible exception of the WT gene; see below). Even given the ability to effect transfers of single chromosomes by microcell fusion, moving from a multimegabase chromosome to a single gene remains a substantial task. It seems likely that some clever approach to directly cloning the relevant genes—perhaps employing retroviral insertional mutagenesis—will be required to move such studies forward. Only when the genes responsible for suppression of tumorigenicity in somatic cell hybrids are in hand will it be possible to definitively address the molecular details of their actions, as well as their relationship to tumor-suppressor genes lost from human tumors.

Familial Cancer

The vast majority of human cancers do not display simple mendelian inheritance, although it has been argued that all forms of cancer occur in familial and sporadic forms.[139,199,201,228,297] However, there are several well-defined tumor syndromes which are inherited as simple autosomal dominant traits with high penetrance. Retinoblastoma, a rare pediatric eye tumor, is the prototype of this group. Several other examples are shown in Table 1. Moreover, although their inheritance is not strictly mendelian, many more common human malignancies show clear familial clustering. Thus, both genetic and environmental insults likely contribute to oncogenesis.

The autosomal dominant cancer syndromes share several features.[139,199,201,297] First, most are rare; in the aggregate, strictly mendelian human cancer accounts for but a fraction of total cancer incidence. Second, they often predispose to cancer of more than one organ. For example, as we shall see, patients with familial retinoblastoma also have subtantially increased risk of developing sarcomas, in particular osteogenic sarcoma, as well as several epithelial malignancies. Third, the tumors found as part of a dominantly-inherited cancer syndrome also can occur sporadically (without any inherited predisposition) in other individuals. However, tumors nearly always arise at an earlier age in patients with heritable cancer syndromes. This association is so strong that a familial cancer syndrome should always be suspected when a young patient presents with a tumor not usually seen at that age. The precocious presentation of familial cancers probably is in part responsible for their relative rarity. Unlike sporadic cancers, which usually occur in individuals beyond reproductive age, familial cancer often occurs before or coincident with reproductive maturity. This should result in selection against the cancer-predisposing gene.

Studies performed on the pathogenesis of retinoblastoma, and later extended to WT and other familial cancers, have established that autosomal dominant cancer results from mutations of tumor-suppressor genes, at least for all of the syndromes examined thus far. On the surface, this appears paradoxical, and is also a source of confusion to newcomers to the field: How does dominant inheritance result from loss-of-function mutations in tumor-suppressor genes? Or, stated another way, how does dominant inheritance result from mutations which, by definition, must be recessive at the cellular level (since loss of both alleles of a tumor-suppressor gene is necessary for oncogenesis)?

In 1971, following earlier suggestions by De Mars,[61] Alfred Knudson posed a theoretical solution to this seeming paradox based upon a quantitative analysis of the epidemiology of retinoblastoma.[200] Retinoblastoma is a rare pediatric eye tumor, with an incidence of about 1 in 20,000 live births. About 60% of retinoblastoma cases are sporadic, but the remaining 40% show autosomal dominant inheritance with high (approximately 90%) penetrance. The vast majority of these inherited cases appear to represent new germ-line mutations, since they occur in patients born to families without a prior history of the disease. Although all retinoblastomas occur before the age of five, the inherited and sporadic forms have clinically distinguishing features. Inherited retinoblastoma tends to occur at a much earlier age, usually before the age of two. It is not at all uncommon for inherited retinoblastoma patients to have tumors at birth. In addition, familial retinoblastoma patients usually have multiple tumors, often affecting both eyes. Although not all inherited cases show multiple tumors, multiple tumors always indicate inherited retinoblastoma. Familial retinoblastoma patients who either fail to develop retinoblastoma or who survive retinoblastoma have a substantially increased risk of developing other malignancies, especially osteogenic sarcoma. This increased risk is not due to prior cytotoxic therapy for retinoblastoma,

TABLE 1.
Familial Cancer Syndromes

Syndrome	Map Location	Cloned Gene
Retinoblastoma (secondary osteogenic sarcoma and other tumors)	13q14	Rb
Li-Fraumeni syndrome (multiple tumors)	17p13	p53
Wilms' Tumor syndromes WAGR (Wilms' tumor/aniridia/GU abnormalities/mental retardation) Denys-Drash (Wilms' tumor/severe GU defects)	11p13	WT-1
Familial Wilms' tumor*	ND	ND
Beckwith-Wiedemann syndrome (Wilms' tumor/heptoblastoma/ rhabdomyosarcoma/other tumors)	11p15-pter	ND
Neurofibromatosis NF-1 (multiple neurofibromas/cafe-au-lait spots/other CNS tumors)	17q	NF-1
NF-2 (acoustic neuromas/other tumors)	22q	ND
von-Hippel Lindau (renal carcinoma/cerebellar hemangioblastoma/other tumors)	3p25	ND
Familial Renal Cancer	3p14**	ND
Multiple Endocrine Neoplasia MEN-1 (islet cell tumors/pituitary adenoma/parathyroid adenoma)	11q	ND
MEN-2 (pheochromocytoma/ medullary thyroid carcinoma/ parathyroid adenoma)	10	ND
Familial colon cancer Familial adenomatous polyposis (may affect other tissues e.g., Gardner's syndrome)	5q21-22	APC
Hereditary non-polyposis colon cancer syndromes (Lynch I and II)	ND	ND
Familial breast/ovarian cancer	17q21	ND

but rather appears to reflect an intrinsic feature of the familial syndrome.[1] Sporadic tumors tend to occur later in life and are always single and unilateral. In contrast to familial retinoblastoma, patients with sporadic retinoblastama do not have an increased risk of developing secondary malignancies.

Knudson reviewed the case histories of a large number of patients with familial retinoblastoma. He found that the number of tumors per patient fit a Poisson distribution, with the mean number of tumors being three. Poisson distributions are consistent with single events occurring at low frequencies over time. The autosomal dominant inheritance pattern of familial retinoblastoma is consistent with one (pre-existing) hit, and the Poisson distribution of tumors in familial retinoblastoma patients implies another single hit, leading Knudson to argue that two hits are required to generate a retinoblastoma. In the familial form, one hit is acquired by germ-line transmission and the other acquired somatically. Since retinoblastoma is highly penetrant (approximately 90%), the frequency of the second event must be high enough so that most individuals would sustain a second mutation at the prevailing mutation rate. In sporadic retinoblastoma, both hits must be somatically acquired, so one would expect it to be rare (as it is). It should be emphasized that at the cellular level, inactivation of both copies of the retinoblastoma-predisposing gene must occur (i.e., the Rb gene is recessive at the cellular level). Predisposition to retinoblastoma is autosomal dominant because at typical mutation rates almost everyone who has inherited one defective Rb gene will sustain a second hit in at least one retinoblast.

Notes: Representative examples of inherited cancer syndromes likely due to mutations in tumor suppressor genes are shown, along with their most common associated tumors. The responsible gene, where known, is indicated.[16,138,228,224,297,298] See text for details. Not shown here are inherited syndromes that lead to increased cancer susceptibility but which show autosomal recessive inheritance, for example chromosome breakage syndromes such as Bloom's syndrome and Fanconi's anemia, or DNA-repair defects such as xeroderma pigmentosum and ataxia telangiectasia.

*Familial WT unassociated with WAGR or Denys-Drash syndrome has been shown by linkage analysis to be unlinked to either WT locus on chromosome 11 (see text). **Refers to a well-studied family with t(3;8) (p14;q22).[228]

Further data in support of his hypothesis was obtained when Knudson plotted the logarithm of the cases not yet diagnosed against time (i.e., the age of the patient). For familial retinoblastoma, this plot yielded a straight line, indicating a first-order or one-hit process. Conversely, for sporadic retinoblastoma, a curvilinear plot was obtained, consistent with a two-hit process. From the mean number of tumors, Knudson went on to estimate the mutation rates for the germ line and somatic mutations using Poisson statistics. These were found to be consistent with the estimated number of target cells in the retina, conventionally accepted mutation rates, and the incidence of retino-blastoma.

Molecular biology has largely substantiated Knudson's original hypothesis, which stands as a stalwart example of the power of critical thinking in science. Moreover, Knudson's hypothesis has provided the intellectual underpinning for thinking about tumor-suppressor genes in other forms of cancer. It is now clear that the genes responsible for at least two familial cancer syndromes, retinoblastoma and the Li-Fraumeni syndrome (see below), are also deranged in many sporadic tumors, including tumors not predicted from the spectrum of malignancies observed in the familial syndromes. This has sparked intense efforts both to identify and clone the genes responsible for other familial syndromes and to test the genes recently identified as the causes of WT/aniridia syndrome (WAGR) and neurofibromatosis (NF-1), respectively, for their involvement in other cancers.

Chromosomal Loss and Deletion in Familial and Sporadic Tumors

Knudson's model soon received experimental support from cytogenetic studies. As early as 1963, case reports had appeared describing deletions of the long arm of chromosome 13 (13q-) in the constitutional cells of some patients with familial retinoblastoma.[220] Larger studies soon validated these case reports.[104,107,406] Overall, about 3% to 5% of hereditary retinoblastoma cases were found to be associated with a gross chromosome 13 abnormality.[113] Some of the larger deletions were associated with craniofacial abnormalities and/or growth and developmental delays, presumably because of the involvement of genes adjacent to the Rb susceptibility gene. However, by the late 1970s, subsequent studies by several investigators, in particular Francke[104] and Yunis and coworkers,[406] uncovered retino-blastoma patients without growth or developmental abnormalities who had small interstitial deletions of 13q. In all cases studied, the deletion involved band 13q14; the finding of small deletions involving only 13q14, or part of 13q14, led to the suggestion that the putative Rb tumor-suppressor gene resided within 13q14. Concomitantly, advances in tumor cytogenetics permitted the analysis of retinoblastoma tumors. The finding that a small percentage (<5%) of sporadic retinoblastomas also had gross 13q deletions, always including 13q14,[10,116] supported the earlier studies and, furthermore, was consistent with the notion that familial and sporadic retinoblastoma involved alterations in the same chromosomal region.[113]

These findings of consistent regions of chromosomal deletion in retinoblastoma were initially greeted with much skepticism in many quarters. Nevertheless, specific chromosomal deletions were soon found by cytogenetic studies in other familial cancer syndromes, most notably the WAGR. A small but significant number of these patients were found to have gross constitutional deletions of band 11p13.[105,312] Specific and consistent chromosomal deletions were demonstrated in sporadic, nonfamilial tumors as well. The first such observation was the finding of visible 3p deletions in a subset of small cell carcinomas of the lung.[387] Many other reports, about many other tumors, followed. Far from being of questionable significance, specific deletions associated with a specific tumor type are now regarded as smoking guns pointing to the location of potential tumor-suppressor genes.

The rationale for this belief was provided by the development of molecular techniques for uncovering specific submicroscopic chromosomal deletions in tumors. Studies of retinoblastoma again played the central role in these developments. First, the enzyme esterase D was found to reside in the same chromosomal region as the gene for retinoblastoma.[349] Since esterase D isozymes existed, it was possible to use classic genetic analysis to demonstrate linkage of these two loci.[348] Moreover, patients with familial retinoblastoma and cytogenetically visible deletions displayed only 50% of normal esterase D activity in their constitutional cells.[349] Subsequent work comparing the pattern of esterase D isozyme expression in constitutional cells and retinoblastoma tumors indicated that a high percentage of patients constitutionally heterozygous for esterase D showed loss of one or the other esterase D isozyme in their tumors. This was interpreted as indicating regional somatic inactivation of the region around the esterase D locus.[125]

Studies involving the use of RFLPs provided the key evidence demonstrating that the observed inactivation of esterase D alleles was due to changes in chromosomal DNA in the esterase D region. Such studies soon showed that the true frequency of deletions in the region initially identified by cytogeneticists was much higher than the 3% to 5% noted above.

RFLPs represent variations in the restiction maps between individuals within a population. For example, at a given position within the genome, the two chromosomes of individual A might have an Eco R1 restriction site, whereas individual B might lack this site in both of his/her chromosomes (Fig. 2a). In the example illustrated in Figure 2a, if DNAs from A and B are digested to completion with Eco R1 and subjected to Southern analysis with a radioactive probe that hybridizes to part of this region (to the left of the extra Eco R1 site present in A's DNA), the blot of individual A's DNA will reveal a band of lower molecular weight (allele 1) than that of individual B (allele 2). Alternatively, if a probe spanning this entire region were used in the hybridization, A's DNA would show two bands, whereas B's DNA would show a single large band.

These variations in restriction pattern reflect evolutionary drift. Most RFLPs are found in noncoding regions of the genome, for obvious reasons: variations in noncoding sequences are unlikely to have phenotypic consequences. Other RFLPs do arise from sequence variation within coding regions. Again, the overwhelming majority of the time, these sequence changes either do not result in an altered protein (because they involve changes in a codon's degenerate third nucleotide), or result in protein variants without functional consequences. Rarely, an RFLP may mark an actual mutation within a coding sequence. Perhaps unfortunately, at least for pedagogic purposes, one of the first well-described examples of the medical use of RFLPs was the discovery of an RFLP that arises as a consequence of the sickle hemoglobin mutation. This has misled many into thinking that the major use of RFLPs is actually in the direct identification of mutations that result in the generation of a new RFLP.

Instead, the main utility of RFLPs is simply that they can serve as extremely useful genetic markers.[31] Since they represent discrete sequences in DNA, they are, of course, inherited in a mendelian fashion. For example, if individual A were to mate with individual B, their progeny should each have one copy of allele 1 and one copy of allele 2, i.e., they would be 1,2 heterozygotes. Prior to the advent of RFLPs, classic human genetic mapping required a phenotype to be scored. Such mapping is limited by the availability of discernible phenotypes, by phenotypic lag (the time taken for a particular genotype to be expressed as a phenotype), by the complex, multigenic origin of many phenotypes, and by incomplete penetrance. RFLPs allow direct mapping by genotype (the presence or absence of a given RFLP), thus greatly facilitating mapping studies.

RFLPs have been used in two distinct ways for studies of tumor-suppressor genes. First, RFLPs have been used to demonstrate regional chromosomal loss too small to be visualized cytogenetically. Initially used by Cavenee and his colleagues to demonstrate chromosomal loss in sporadic retinoblastoma tumors,[43] this approach relies on the demonstration of loss of heterozygosity (LOH) for RFLPs in tumors. Consider the patient in Figure 2b with sporadic retinoblastoma. Suppose that he/she is constitutionally heterozygous for six loci on chromosome 13, three on the long arm and three on the short arm. For the sake of illustration, all of the alleles on one chromosome will be indicated "1" and those on its homologue will be indicated "2"; however, for this type of analysis, it is not necessary that the actual phase of the alleles be known. It should be emphasized that these RFLPs are of no particular significance in and of themselves. Since their purpose is merely to serve as positional tags on chromosome 13, the only requirement is that their relative position on chromosome 13 be known. Suppose further that the retinoblastoma tumor suppressor gene (Rb) is located at the indicated position on 13q. According to Knudson's hypothesis, for retinoblastoma to develop, both alleles of Rb must be inactivated. One allele might be inactivated via a chromosomal event such as deletion (of an entire chromosome 13, the long arm of a chromosome 13, or an interstitial region of chromosome 13) or mitotic recombination. Chromosomal loss could occur with or without reduplication of the remaining chromosome. Smaller inactivating events are also possible. These include localized gene conversion, small (including intragenic) deletion, and point mutation.

The predicted effects of each of these events on the pattern of RFLPs in tumor tissue, compared with the constitutional pattern, is illustrated in Figure 2b. Loss of an entire chromosome 13, for example, the chromosome bearing all "1" alleles, would result in LOH at all chromosome 13 loci. A Southern blot of tumor tissue would reveal only allele 2 for each of the chromosome 13 RFLPs, whereas normal tissue (for example skin fibroblasts or white blood cells) from the same patients would show one copy of allele 1 and one copy of allele 2 for each locus. The intensity of the allele 2 bands in the tumor would be

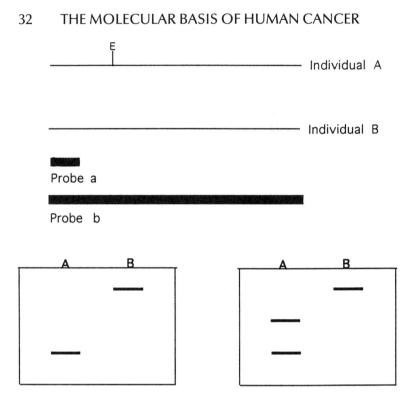

Figure 2A. *Restriction fragment length polymorphisms (RFLPs) in the study of tumor suppressor genes. Schematic illustration of an RFLP. The above cartoon depicts a random region of chromosomal DNA from two unrelated individuals (A and B). Individual A, but not individual B, has an EcoR1 site (E) within this stretch of DNA. Shown in the panels at the bottom of the figure are the expected results of Southern blots with two probes (a and b) whose extents are indicated by the solid bars. For details, see text.*

the same as the allele 2 band intensity in normal cells. Similarly, hemi-chromosomal loss would be visualized at the molecular level as LOH for all loci distal to the breakpoint of the deletion, whereas interstitial deletion would show LOH for interstitial RFLPs. Such results alone might not be that much more informative since chromosome loss, hemi-chromosomal loss, and/or large deletion can be seen by conventional cytogenetics.

The real advantage of RFLP mapping over cytogenetics is seen when one considers the other events that can cause LOH. For

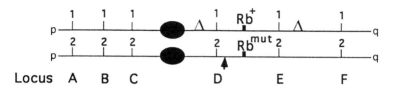

Locus   A   B   C   D   E   F

Southern Blot Patterns with probes to loci A-F:

	A	B	C	D	E	F
Somatic tissues	1— 2—	1— 2—	1— 2—	1— 2—	1— 2—	1— 2—
Tumor with:						
Chromosome loss w/o reduplication	2—	2—	2—	2—	2—	2—
Chromosome loss w/reduplication	2▬	2▬	2▬	2▬	2▬	2▬
Hemichromosome loss (q arm)	1— 2—	1— 2—	1— 2—	2—	2—	2—
Large deletion (Δ to Δ)	1— 2—	1— 2—	1— 2—	2—	2—	1— 2—
Mitotic recombination (at ▲)	1— 2—	1— 2—	1— 2—	1— 2—	2—	2—
Localized gene conversion	1— 2—	1— 2—	1— 2—	1— 2—	1— 2—	1— 2—

Figure 2B. *Use of RFLPs in loss of heterozygosity (LOH) analysis. A hypothetical individual carrying one mutant copy of the retinoblastoma gene (Rb^{MUT}) and one wild type allele (Rb^+) is indicated at the top of the figure. Such an individual would be phenotypically normal as long as he/she retained one normal RB allele. Also shown are several loci (A–F) at which this individual is constitutionally heterozygous (indicated by alleles "1" and "2" above each locus). For convenience, all of the "1" alleles have been placed in the same phase (i.e., on the same chromosomal homologue) as the Rb^+ allele; there is no need for this actually to be the case in vivo (see text). Shown in the bottom part of the figure are the expected Southern blot patterns with probes that detect the RFLPs at A–F in normal somatic tissues and in retinoblastoma tumors arising as a result of the normal Rb allele via the indicated mechanisms. D, endpoints of a hypothetical large deletion; Rb^{MUT}, mutant Rb allele; Rb^+, wild type Rb allele; p, short arm; q, long arm; filled circle, centromere.*

example, whole chromosome 13 loss is often accompanied by reduplication of the remaining chromosome. Cytogenetically, such an event would look perfectly normal, since there would be no way to distinguish the lost from the retained chromosome. However, consider the effect of this event on the RFLP pattern. Southern blotting of a tumor with loss of the "1" chromosome and reduplication of the "2" chromosome would reveal only "2" alleles, but at twice the intensity of the "2" alleles in normal tissue from the same patient. Similarly, a tumor in which mitotic recombination had occurred between the centromere and the first 13q RFLP would exhibit LOH for all loci distal to the site of recombination. Heterozygosity would be retained at all proximal loci. Such a tumor also would have two cytogenetically normal chromosome 13s. However, if a mutation too small to be seen cytogenetically had occurred prior to mitotic recombination or chromosomal loss with reduplication, the result would be homozygous mutation of the Rb gene. By using panels of RFLPs that map to different regions of a given chromosome, and studying LOH in enough tumors, a common region of deletion, often referred to as a minimal region of overlap, or MRO, can be identified. Based on the above reasoning, such a region might be expected to contain a tumor-suppressor gene. LOH studies can thus narrow the region to be examined by chromosomal walking techniques. This approach has been used successfully for nearly all of the tumor-suppressor genes thus far identified, as well as for defining the locations of putative tumor-suppressor genes in a wide variety of other tumors (see Table 2).

The sensitivity of RFLP analysis for detection of regions of chromosome loss depends on the number of informative RFLPs within the chromosomal region in question and on the types of chromosomal events that lead to tumor-suppressor gene inactivation. Some workers have attempted to supplement LOH studies with estimates of loss of copies of given loci in tumor tissue compared with normal tissue (dosage loss). Such studies are often difficult to interpret due to the variable ploidy of tumors. Polymorphisms arising from variable numbers of tandem repeats (VNTRs) are often highly heterogeneous in the population and therefore have a higher likelihood of being polymorphic than traditional RFLPs. Recently, length polymorphisms (polymerase chain reaction [PCR] polymorphisms or PCRPs) have been described which are detectable with the PCR and are not dependent on the presence or absence of a restriction site. These developments, along with the increasingly detailed human genetic map, are likely to substantially increase the ability of mapping techniques to define regions of consistent chromosome loss in tumors.

LOH studies are not capable of detecting deletions so small that their endpoints fall between the most closely linked RFLPs studied, for point mutations, or for localized gene conversion. Fortunately, at least for those tumors studied thus far, loss of at least one copy of a tumor-suppressor gene by a chromosomal mechanism that results in LOH has proven to be much more common than loss of both copies by small mutations that fail to result in LOH. Therefore, in any analysis of a significantly large number of tumors with a sufficiently large number of informative polymorphisms, one would expect to find frequent LOH in regions harboring tumor-suppressor genes—at least if that gene is behaving like previously described tumor-suppressor genes. This principle has been exploited to the maximum in the technique of "allelotyping," described by Bert Vogelstein and his colleagues.[378] Panels of RFLPs are used to examine matched tumor and normal DNAs and discern all regions in the genome in which significant LOH occurs. These regions are then viewed as potentially harboring tumor-suppressor genes.

The sensitivity of LOH analysis has proven to be substantially higher than cytogenetics. For example, using RFLPs that are fairly distant from the actual Rb gene, Cavenee and his colleagues were initially able to demonstrate LOH in over 50% of Rb tumors.[43] Note however, that LOH is not found in 100% of informative tumors. Even using RFLPs within the Rb gene itself, LOH is only found in 70% to 80% of retinoblastoma tumors.[113] Although this might at first glance seem contradictory (and at one point, was actually a source of some concern that the Rb gene had been incorrectly identified), it really is not. Those tumors that fail to display LOH within Rb simply have inactivated both copies by nonchromosomal mechanisms (such as point mutations or point mutation plus small deletion).

The second main use for RFLPs in studies of tumor-suppressor genes has been as genetic markers in linkage analysis of familial cancer. Again, the RFLP (or PCRP) is used simply as a positional tag for a given chromosomal location and is tracked through a pedigree of a patient with familial cancer. The RFLP is used here as if it were any standard genetic marker, such as isozyme type or blood group. If an RFLP (or more correctly, set of RFLPs) is linked to a tumor-suppressor gene, then it should not independently assort. Thus a specific RFLP allele will always be in phase with the familial cancer gene. For example, if allele 2 of an RFLP is tightly linked to the tumor-

TABLE 2.
Regional Chromosomal Loss in Human Tumors

Tumor	Chromosomal Region	Cloned Gene/Comments
Acoustic neuroma	22q	
Bladder carcinoma	1q21-23	
	9q	
	11p	?Beckwith-Wiedemann locus
	13q14	Rb
	17p13	p53
Breast carcinoma	1p11-13	
	1q; 3p; 11p;	
	3p11-24	
	3q11-13	
	11p15	Beckwith-Wiedemann locus
	13q14	Rb
	16q	
	17p13	p53
	17q21	?familial breast/ovarian Ca locus
	18q	(?DCC)
Colon carcinoma	1q	
	4p	
	6p	
	6q	
	8p	
	9q	
	5q21	APC, ?MCC
	17p13	p53
	18q	DCC
	22q	
Glioma/glioblastoma	1p32-36	
	6p15-q27	
	7q22-q34	
	8p21-23	
	9p24-p13	
	10q	
	17p13	p53; ?others*
Hepatoblastoma/Hepatocellular carcinoma	11p	?Beckwith-Wiedemann locus
Lung cancer**	3p13-14	
	3p21	
	3p25	?von-Hippel Lindau locus
	6q	
	9p	
	13q14	Rb***
	17p13	p53
	22q	
	Others	

(continued)

TABLE 2.
Regional Chromosomal Loss in Human Tumors *(continued)*

Tumor	Chromosomal Region	Cloned Gene/Comments
Mesothelioma	1p11-13	
	3p	
	9p	
	13q	?Rb
	17p	?p53
	22q	
Melanoma	1p11-22	
	6q11-27	
Meningioma	22q12-13	?NF-2 locus
Neuroblastoma	1p	
Osteogenic sarcoma	13q14	Rb
	17p13	p53
Ovarian adenocarcinoma	3p13-21	
	6q15-23	
	11p	
	17q	?familial breast/ovarian Ca locus
Phaeochromocytoma	1p	
	22	?NF-2 locus
Prostate carcinoma	7q22	
	10q24	
	13q14	Rb
	16	
Retinoblastoma	13q14	Rb
Renal cell carcinoma	3p13-21	familial 3;8 translocation; ? second locus distally (von Hippel-Lindau)
Wilms' tumor	11p13	WT-1
	11p15	?Beckwith-Wiedemann locus

Notes: A representative sampling of human tumors in which significant regional chromosomal loss has been detected (by loss of heterozygosity and/or large deletions) is presented. Those loci from which tumor suppressor genes have been cloned are indicated, as are those loci which may correspond to the map locations of inherited cancer syndromes (as defined by linkage analysis; see also Table 1) or to other interesting candidate genes. This table is compiled from various sources,[3,93,151,297,298,346] but should by no means be considered to be exhaustive. In many tumors, only a fraction of the genome has been assayed for chromosomal loss; hence the indicated regions likely represent an underestimate of the real frequency of chromosomal loss for such tumors.

*Although p53 mutations have been found in brain tumors, it is not yet clear that p53 is the only 17p gene targeted in these tumors. **Lung cancer is traditionally divided into small cell and non-small cell subtypes; for convenience, these are lumped together here. Most of the indicated changes probably occur in both histologic subtypes, although some (e.g., Rb) mutations are clearly more frequent in small-cell than in non-small cell. ***Rb mutations are found in virtually all cases of small-cell lung cancer, but are much less common in non-small cell carcinomas.

suppressor gene, then members of the family who develop cancer will almost always also have allele 2 in their genotype. As for any type of genetic analysis, the further away from the tumor-suppressor gene the RFLP is (i.e., the less tightly it is linked), the more likely a meiotic recombination event, and the less likely that cancer and allele 2 will be inherited together. Unless the RFLP itself actually arises as a consequence of mutation within a tumor-suppressor gene, and that mutation causes the familial cancer syndrome, whether allele 1 or allele 2 (or any other allele) is the one linked to the given familial cancer gene varies among different families; e.g., in family A, cancer may be inherited with allele 1 of a given RFLP, whereas in family B, it may be inherited with allele 2. The critical requirement for establishing linkage is that a given allele of a given RFLP (or given pattern of alleles of a set of RFLPs) is inherited coincident with the familial cancer gene at a rate greater than that expected for independently segregating loci (i.e., statistically more than 50% of the time).

Linkage analysis has been used to confirm the assignment of the Rb gene to 13q14, as well as to localize candidate tumor-suppressor genes for a number of familial cancer syndromes, including familial adenomatous polyposis (FAP), NF-1 and NF-2, and the von Hippel-Lindau syndrome.[139,297,298,344] The main limitations of linkage analysis in identifying tumor-suppressor genes are that it can only be used to study familial cancers and requires relatively large, well-defined pedigrees. Nevertheless, since sporadic forms exist for tumors that occur as part of familial cancer syndromes, the combination of LOH studies and linkage analysis can provide useful complementary data.

The Retinoblastoma Gene

The classic RFLP studies of Cavenee and his associates[43,44,140] led to several important conclusions. First, they unambiguously established that LOH of 13q markers was a frequent occurrence in sporadic and familial retinoblastoma.[43,44] Second, they revealed that the major molecular mechanism for generating LOH in retinoblastoma was mitotic recombination.[43] Third, and perhaps most importantly from the standpoint of validating the two hit hypothesis, they demonstrated that the retained chromosome in retinoblastoma tumors arising in familial Rb was inherited from the affected parent.[44] Fourth, as mentioned above, familial retinoblastoma patients have an increased risk of secondary malignancies, especially osteogenic sarcoma. LOH studies of secondary osteogenic sarcomas indicated that the same chromosomal region was rendered homo-or hemizygous in the genesis of these tumors, suggesting that the putative Rb gene (or a second, closely linked gene) was affected in osteosarcomas as well.[140]

Subsequent comparisons of 13q alleles retained in unilateral and bilateral retinoblastomas, as well as in osteogenic sarcomas, have revealed an interesting feature of the origin of mutations in the Rb gene. Initially, it was noted that for familial retinoblastomas with cytogenetically visible Rb deletions, the deletion was usually in the paternally-derived gene.[82] This prompted studies of familial cases without cytogenetically visible lesions, as well as sporadic cases. These studies indicated that the paternally-derived Rb allele (and therefore the presumed mutant allele) was retained in nearly all osteosarcomas (sporadic and germ-line),[368] as well as in nearly all bilateral retinoblastomas.[77,409] In contrast, unilateral retinoblastomas, the majority of which are sporadic, showed no such preference.[77,409] The reason for this parental preference is not clear. The Rb gene may be more susceptible to mutagenesis during spermatogenesis than oogenesis, perhaps because imprinting affects mutability. Alternatively, imprinting might affect susceptibility to chromosomal events such as mitotic recombination, such that an oocyte mutation is less likely to be "uncovered" by loss of a normal paternal chromosome.

With the recessive nature of the disease established, and the location of the presumptive gene narrowed to 13q14, the race began in earnest to identify and clone the Rb gene. One approach was to begin a bidirectional chromosomal walk from the esterase D gene.[218] Unfortunately, this was hampered by the presence of highly repetitive sequences in the direction later found to be "correct." The other approach, adopted by Thaddeus Dryja and his colleagues, was to use a flow-sorted chromosome 13-enriched library to search for probes that mapped within 13q14 and then to test these probes against a panel of Rb tumors, looking for deletions.[76] Although, in many ways, this approach is like looking for a needle in a haystack, it soon yielded a startling result. An anonymous probe, H3–8, detected a region that was homozygously deleted in the tumor DNA of two unrelated patients. Single copy subclones of overlapping phage clones generated by walking from H3–8 were also homozygously deleted in these tumors, indicating that the deletion spanned at least 25 kb. In addition, one of these single copy subclones identified a heterozygous deletion in a third unrelated retinoblastoma patient. Several other probes mapping to 13q14 were not deleted in these three tumors, and all three had normal levels of esterase D activity, suggesting that the deleted segment was relatively small.

Dryja's results suggested that the region around H3–8 was probably close (within a few hundred kb) to the Rb gene. Stephen Friend, Dryja, Robert Weinberg, and their colleagues quickly proceeded to identify a candidate gene.[111] Using chromosomal walking, they identified a single copy DNA fragment that was conserved in both mouse and human DNA, which suggested that it contained coding sequences. This fragment identified a 4.7 kb mRNA, which was present in adenovirus-immortalized retinal cells, but not in four retinoblastoma cell-lines. A full length cDNA was obtained and was used to study DNA and RNA from retinoblastomas and control tissues. Interestingly, the transcript was expressed at approximately the same level in all normal tissues studied, but was not detectable in the four retinoblastoma cell-lines or in an osteosarcoma line. More important were the results of Southern analysis. The cDNA for the 4.7 kb transcript, now renamed Rb (for retinoblastoma-predisposing gene), identified a large locus spanning more than 100 kb. In a survey of 40 retinoblastomas and 8 osteosarcomas, abnormalities in the Rb restriction pattern were found in about 30%. These included heterozygous and homozygous deletions with breakpoints outside the Rb locus itself. Since it was clear from Dryja's earlier mapping studies that the Rb gene was located in this general chromosomal region, this finding alone could merely have indicated that the gene specified by the Rb cDNA was highly susceptible to chromosomal breakage. More convincing were two internal deletions, one heterozygous deletion in a retinoblastoma, and a homozygous internal deletion in an osteosarcoma. Although RFLP studies had implicated the same chromosomal region in the genesis of retinoblastoma and osteosarcoma,[75,140] Friend et al. provided the first direct evidence that the Rb gene might be directly involved in the genesis of malignancies other than the extremely rare retinoblastoma.

The initial report describing the cloning of the Rb gene was both fortunate and misleading. The finding of such a high frequency of gross abnormalities in DNA (30%) and RNA (4/4) from Rb patients strongly supported the notion that the correct gene had been cloned. However, subsequent larger scale studies have shown that the true incidence of such gross abnormalities is substantially lower.[78,79,113,126,157] In fact, abnormalities detectable on Southern and Northern blots combined probably occur in no more than 20% to 30% of retinoblastoma tumors and cell-lines. In the vast majority of retinoblastoma cases, small deletions or point mutations inactivate one copy of the Rb gene (see below). The second copy is then lost, most often by mitotic recombination or some other large scale chromosomal event that does not impinge directly upon the Rb locus. This leads to a normal Southern blot pattern with an Rb probe. Similarly, unless the point mutation/deletion results in alteration of a splice donor/acceptor site or otherwise affects RNA processing or stability, the Northern blot pattern will also be unchanged.

Like Rb, other tumor-suppressor genes are usually inactivated by small genetic changes followed by chromosomal events that leave Southern and Northern blots unaffected. This has important implications for workers interested in identifying new tumor-suppressor genes. Even a low frequency of deletions in a candidate gene in the appropriate region, especially internal deletions, must be taken seriously. Conversely, failure to find gross changes on Southern and Northern blots cannot be taken as exclusionary evidence for a given gene, unless very large numbers of samples are studied. Graphic evidence of this point is provided by mutations of the p53 gene in colon cancer (see below). Perhaps the best approach would combine such analyses with early screens for point mutations/small deletions using one or more of several new techniques.

The initial findings of Friend et al. were soon verified and extended by the groups of Lee[218] and Fung.[112] These groups also used the H3–8 probe to walk to the correct gene. In addition, homozygous internal deletions of Rb were found in actual retinoblastomas, as well as in an osteosarcoma from a retinoblastoma patient, and comparison of the Rb gene in fibroblasts and tumor cells derived from the same patient gave a direct validation at the molecular level of Knudson's two-hit hypothesis.

Final proof was provided with the demonstration that retinoblastomas containing apparently normal Rb DNA and RNA have point mutations or other small deletions. Studies by Gallie's group using an RNAse mismatch assay first indicated the existence of small mutations in at least half of such tumors.[78] Subsequent work by this[79] and other groups,[157,158,400] using the PCR to amplify either Rb genomic DNA or cDNA, followed by DNA sequencing, has shown a wide variety of mutations in retinoblastoma tumors. These include point mutations and small deletions in the coding sequence, at splice donor or acceptor sites, and in the upstream regulatory region. It is now unambiguously clear that all retinoblastoma tumors are homozygously abnormal in the Rb gene.

The availability of Rb cDNA clones allowed characterization of the Rb gene and its gene product. First, Lee's group reported the nucleotide sequence of the retinoblastoma cDNA.[218] By itself, the sequence was unremarkable. There was no similarity to any protein in the database at the time, nor was there any clearly recognizable motif, although a potential leucine zipper domain was recognized later. Several groups reported the cloning of the entire Rb gene, which contains 27 exons and spans more than 200 kb.[26,102,156,365,391] It appears to have a simple upstream regulatory sequence, resembling a housekeeping gene. Intragenic RFLPs, potentially useful in genetic counseling, have been identified.[127,391] In addition, all intron-exon boundaries have been defined and sequenced, allowing direct molecular analysis of the most likely sites for mutations in retinoblastoma patients.[400]

The finding that Rb was expressed at comparable levels in all normal cells prompted a search for its possible involvement in other tumors. Perhaps surprisingly, given its primary association with a rare cancer syndrome, these studies soon showed that mutations in Rb occur in a variety of other neoplasms. In addition to osteosarcoma, which was already known to be clinically associated with retinoblastoma (and suspected to involve the same gene on the basis of RFLP studies) and related mesenchymal tumors, a high frequency of Rb mutations has been found in several epithelial tumors. First, Rb mutations were found in about 30% of human breast cancer cell-lines and tumors; these abnormalities included gross deletion, both homozygous and heterozygous, as well as more subtle abnormalities.[26,216,364] Other studies have reported a lower frequency of involvement of Rb in primary breast tumors.[19] These discrepancies may be due at least in part to variations in the extent of stromal contamination of primary breast carcinomas, a particular problem in these tumors. Subsequently, Rb abnormalities were demonstrated in an extremely high percentage of small cell carcinomas of the lung[141,157,405]; it is likely that nearly all such cancers have Rb mutations. Rb abnormalities have also occurred in nonsmall cell lung cancer, although at significantly lower frequency,[399] and in some bladder[157,158,366] and prostate carcinomas.[27,28] The finding of Rb mutations associated with diverse malignancies strongly suggested that the Rb gene product played an important general role in normal growth control.

However, the occurrence of Rb mutations is by no means a universal feature of carcinogenesis. For example, gastrointestinal tract malignancies, such as colonic and hepatocellular carcinomas, have not been associated with such mutations. The reason(s) why some cell types seem to be particularly susceptible to loss of the Rb gene product is not clear. The genetics of retinoblastoma suggests that, for early retinal cells, loss of Rb alone is sufficient to generate a retinoblastoma. For other cell types, such as bronchial or mammary epithelial cells, a number of additional mutations, both in other tumor-suppressor genes and in dominant oncogenes, seem to be required for tumorigenesis. It is possible that early retinal cells depend solely on the Rb gene product for negative growth control, whereas more mature cells have redundant growth inhibitory pathways. For example, it would be interesting to know whether the p53 tumor-suppressor gene, which appears to inhibit the growth of a wide variety of cell types and to be complementary to Rb's action (to be discussed in detail below), functions in fetal retinal cells. The lack of Rb mutations in certain tumor types need not imply that the Rb gene product plays no role in negative growth control in those tissues. After all, Rb is expressed ubiquitously,[111,112,218] so presumably it has a normal function in all cell types. The association of mutations in a given tumor-suppressor gene with certain tumor types, but not others, may be due to a variety of factors (see below).

Most importantly, the availability of the Rb cDNA allowed a direct test of the concept of tumor-suppressor genes. Several groups have attempted to restore Rb expression to tumor cell-lines lacking functional Rb, with varying results. In 1988, Lee's group generated an amphotropic retrovirus and used it to infect retinoblastoma and osteosarcoma cell-lines.[165] They reported that the Rb retrovirus, but not a control retrovirus containing the luciferase gene, led to substantial decreases in growth rate (both clonal growth rate and bulk population growth rate) and soft agar colony formation (a measure of anchorage-independent growth). The Rb virus also caused morphological changes compatible with the induction of cell senescence (flattening and marked enlargement of the cells). Interestingly, not all infected cells showed these effects; a rapidly growing population of small cells was found to lack Rb expression despite expression of the drug resistance marker. Upon prolonged culture, these Rb-cells became predominant, consistent with a selective advantage for loss of Rb expression. Moreover, in a different osteosarcoma cell-line, which had unmutated Rb alleles and expressed normal levels of apparently wild type Rb protein, the Rb virus had no apparent effect on any transformation parameter. Similarly, packaging lines expressing the Rb retrovirus cells apparently grew normally, suggesting that Rb expression was only growth inhibitory in Rb-cells.

Although the growth inhibitory effect on the osteosarcoma cell-line was so severe that not enough cells could be accumulated to test tumorigenicity in nude mice, tumorigenicity of the retinoblastoma cell-line infected with the Rb retrovirus was suppressed. Based on the relative in vitro growth rates of Rb virus-infected and luciferase virus-infected cells, Lee and coworkers argued that suppression of tumorigenicity was not simply due to the growth inhibitory effects of Rb, but rather, reflected an intrinsic tumor-suppressing function. They also argued that reexpression of Rb in retinoblastoma cell-lines was not invariably toxic to cells, since they were able to establish several clonal cell-lines that continued to express Rb when propagated for over a year in cell culture.

Klein's group has confirmed that expression of exogenous wild type Rb via Lee's Rb retrovirus can suppress tumorigenicity of retinoblastoma cells.[362,398] However, others have been unable to obtain any stable cell-lines from retinoblastoma or other cancer cells into which a variety of expression constructs have been introduced.[383] These results have been interpreted as indicating that the Rb gene product is a potent growth suppressor, and that its tumor-suppressing activity is indistinguishable from its growth suppressing activity.

Lee's group later used the same retroviral vector to introduce Rb into a prostate carcinoma cell-line that was homozygous for Rb mutation.[28] In contrast to the results with the retinoblastoma and osteosarcoma cell-lines, clonal cell-lines derived from the Rb virus infected prostate carcinoma cells displayed no significant differences in morphology, growth rate, or anchorage dependence compared with luciferase virus infected control cells. Nevertheless, these cells did display markedly reduced tumorigenicity in nude mice.

Recently, it has been reported that a plasmid construct expressing Rb under the control of the β-actin promoter can be stably expressed in a bladder carcinoma cell-line that lacks endogenous Rb.[366] Interestingly, however, clones from the initial transfection could not be expanded directly to mass culture. Instead, clonal cell-lines were only obtained after all of the drug resistant cells from the initial transfections with the Rb expression vector were first expanded into a mass culture and then re-plated at limiting dilution. The reason for this is not clear, but one possibility is that a second event had to occur in the original transfected cells to permit long-term stable expression of Rb. Furthermore, the stable transfectants expressed levels of Rb RNA and protein comparable to the low, endogenous level of Rb in normal human fibroblasts. This level of expression is particularly surprising in view of the strength of the β-actin promoter. Nevertheless, the Rb-expressing bladder carcinoma cells had interesting biological properties compared with control transfectants. Although their growth rate in 10% serum was identical to controls (or untransfected parental cells), they displayed markedly reduced growth in 3% serum. They also failed to form colonies in semisolid media. Most nude mice injected with these retinoblastoma protein-(RB-) expressing cells showed markedly reduced tumorigenicity compared with the parental carcinoma cells. However, they did invariably form small, nonprogressive tumors, which retained the histopathological features of bladder carcinoma. Interestingly, these tumors continued to express RB RNA and protein at levels comparable to the initial transfectants. Although these exogenous Rb alleles were not sequenced to exclude small mutations, it seems likely that, at least for this bladder carcinoma cell-line, RB replacement was not sufficient to eliminate tumorigenicity, although it did substantially impair it. A few rapidly growing, progressive tumors were also obtained; these tumors failed to express any RB.

The discrepancies between these various reports may be more apparent than real. All of these experiments indicate that normal Rb is a potent in vivo growth suppressive agent for Rb-tumor cells. Thus the predicted properties of tumor-suppressor genes have been confirmed in all aspects for the first cloned example of such a gene. The only difference of opinion concerns whether the growth suppressive activity is manifest in tissue culture and, if so, to what extent. Since all agree that Rb is growth suppressive, it seems likely that some levels of expression of Rb should totally inhibit cell growth. Given different promoter strength in different cell types, the ability of some groups to obtain apparent separation between in vitro and in vivo effects of Rb may reflect particular combinations of cell-lines and expression constructs, rather than some fundamental property of the Rb gene product. This suggestion is supported by a close analysis of the Lee group's initial report of Rb growth and tumorigenicity suppression. They noted that the level of expression of Rb in their *overexpressors* was comparable to the level of expression in the osteosarcoma cell-line that expressed *normal* levels of Rb. Since Rb is normally expressed at relatively low levels, their retroviral construct clearly was not being expressed very efficiently in the recipient cells. Perhaps this allowed them to attain just the "right" level of expression: enough to observe in vitro growth inhibition (and in vivo tumor suppression) without totally inhibiting cell growth. Similar reasoning may be applicable to the β-actin promoter-driven Rb replacement experiments in bladder carcinoma cells.

However, it is intriguing that the prostate and bladder carcinoma cell-lines showed less sensitivity to Rb replacement than retinoblastoma and osteosarcoma cell-lines. For the genesis of retinoblastoma, Rb mutation is both necessary and sufficient. For the genesis of at least some osteosarcomas, Rb mutations may be necessary, and perhaps only one additional mutation (in p53) is sufficient. Conversely, although Rb mutations clearly occur in at least some prostate and bladder carcinoma cell-lines and primary tumors, several other mutations are likely required for prostate and bladder carcinogenesis. It would be interesting if there were a strong correlation between the sensitivity of a particular type of tumor to Rb replacement and the frequency of naturally occurring Rb mutations in that type of tumor. Such a relationship would support the idea that the Rb gene product plays a more important (or perhaps less redundant) role in normal growth control in those cell types whose tumors display a high frequency of Rb mutations. A much larger study, examining the effects of Rb replacement on the growth properties of multiple Rb-cell-lines (or, better yet, fresh primary tumor cells cultured for brief periods) and controlling for levels of exogenous Rb expression, would be required to address this issue.

Despite their obvious limitations, the Rb replacement experiments offer a glimmer of hope clinically. Although it is now clear that most cancers, especially epithelial cancers, result from the accumulation of multiple mutations in both dominant oncogenes and tumor-suppressor genes, these experiments, and analogous experiments involving replacement of the p53 gene (see: Normal p53 is a Tumor-Suppressor Gene), suggest that in vivo correction of only one of the defects could result in tumor suppression, at least for some tumors. In vivo gene replacement into 10 to 100 billion tumor cells (the estimated tumor burden in a human cancer patient) poses a formidable, if not insurmountable, problem. It may, however, be possible to achieve the equivalent effect pharmacologically, if the molecular details of Rb (and other tumor-suppressor gene) function are understood. As we shall see in the next section, the flurry of recent progress in uncovering these details gives some reason for optimism.

The Rb Protein and its Function(s)

Lee's group identified the RB as a 110 kd phosphoprotein.[217] RB phosphorylation was found exclusively on serine and threonine. Both cell fractionation and immunofluorescence experiments indicated that RB was exclusively nuclear. Recent fine structure immunofluorescence localization experiments have suggested that RB is localized to at least two distinct nuclear compartments.[363] Some RB appears to be diffusely spread over the entire euchromatin as small granules, whereas the remainder exists in large nuclear granules. Whether these microanatomical differences reflect discrete functions for RB within the nucleus is not known. Fractionation on DNA cellulose columns established that RB had nonspecific DNA-binding activity.[217] These initial studies suggested that RB might play some role in controlling nuclear event(s) such as transcription or DNA replication.

A major advance then arrived from an unexpected direction. Ed Harlow and his colleagues have been studying the mechanism of transformation of adenoviruses. These DNA tumor viruses contain two genes, E1A and E1B, whose combined presence is necessary and sufficient for malignant transformation.[160,373] E1A alone is capable of immortalizing primary fibroblasts and is able to cooperate with *ras* oncogenes (or E1B) to fully transform such cells.[212,281,321] Harlow's group, along with the group of Phillip Branton, had been studying the E1A proteins. They had raised a series of monoclonal anti-E1A antibodies and shown that, even under stringent immunoprecipitation conditions, E1A coprecipitated with a number of cellular proteins.[142,143,402] Painstaking control experiments convincingly established that E1A formed complexes with these cellular proteins, which were initially known only by their apparent molecular weights on SDS-polyacrylamide gel electrophoresis. The most abundantly associated proteins were of molecular weight 105K, 107K, and 300K; others, of molecular weight 28K, 40K, 50K, 60K, 80K, 90K, and 130K are also found complexed with E1A under most conditions. Previous work indicating a strict correlation between the ability of E1A to form complexes with p105, p107, and p300, and its transforming ability, had led Harlow and his coworkers to suggest that E1A-mediated transformation might require formation of these complexes.[143] However, none of these E1A-associated proteins had yet been identified.

Lee's result establishing that RB was a 110 kd phosphoprotein suggested to Harlow the possibility that either the "105K" or "107K" proteins might be RB. Several lines of evidence then conclusively established that the E1A-associated 105K protein was, indeed, the RB gene product.[388] [Some confusion naturally arises from the apparent difference in molecular weight between the E1A-associated "105K" and RB, which was initially identified as a 110 kd protein. The confusion is increased by the SV40 large T-associated "110K" protein (which also turns out to be RB; see below), and "120K" protein (which turns out to be identical to the E1A-associated 107K). These discrepancies in molecular weight are due to differences in gel systems and molecular weight markers between different laboratories and, in some cases, to species differences. For example, the murine RB is slightly larger than primate RB. For the rest of our discussion we will refer directly to either RB or 107K, respectively, to indicate the appropriate E1A-associated protein.]

Harlow's remarkable result strongly suggested that E1A contributed to cellular transformation, at least in part, by binding to the Rb tumor-suppressor gene product. Moreover, since loss of both copies of Rb led to oncogenic transformation in retinoblastoma and other tumors, it seemed likely that the functional consequence of E1A-binding to Rb was inactivation of RB protein. The notion that a DNA tumor viral oncogene might act by binding to and functionally inactivating a tumor-suppressor gene provided a striking counterpoint to the mechanism of transformation of RNA tumor viruses, the overwhelming majority of which co-opt (and activate) the function of cellular proto-oncogenes. Furthermore, since E1A, like other viral oncogenes, presumably derived from some ancestral cellular gene, these results raised the intriguing possibility that cellular counterparts with E1A-like function(s) existed. The demonstration[98,302] that a small region of shared similar DNA sequence between E1A, the transforming genes of other DNA tumor viruses such as SV40 large T-antigen, and some cellular proteins, including the c-iMyc gene, lent credence to this notion (although there has been no clear demonstration for in vivo association of c-myc or its relatives with RB; see below). As we shall see, all of these predictions appear, at least in part, to hold true.

The first hint that inactivation of tumor-suppressor gene products might be a general strategy utilized by DNA tumor virus oncogenes followed rapidly on the heels of Harlow's initial discovery. David Livingston and his colleagues have been studying the mechanism of transformation by the papovavirus SV40. SV40 has a single transforming gene, large T-antigen, which is largely unrelated to E1A or any other known protein. However, as mentioned above, there is a very small region of large T (amino acid [aa] 101 to 118) that has weak sequence similarity to a region of E1A (conserved domain 2). Elegant experiments by Elizabeth Moran, reported at nearly the same time as Harlow's results, indicated that these regions of E1A and large T could be swapped and transforming activity retained, suggesting that this sequence similarity was functionally significant.[262] Livingston's group noticed that large T-antigen also coimmunoprecipitated with a small number of cellular proteins.[64] Notably, one of these was a "110K" protein and another a "120K" protein. Using an analogous approach to that used by Harlow for E1A, Livingston's group soon found that the 110K protein was RB.[64] Furthermore, a point mutation that eliminated T-antigen transforming ability also eliminated RB-binding, solidifying the correlation between T-antigen's ability to bind RB and its ability to transform cells. Subsequent work[80,88,89] established the identity of the E1A-associated "107K" and the large T-associated "120K."

Exhaustive mutational analyses of both E1A and large T have shown a complete correspondence between the ability (or inability) of E1A[229,230,262,263,334,345,389,390] or large T[49,64,183,262] to bind RB and ability (or inability) to contribute to transformation: any E1A or T mutant that loses its ability to bind RB also loses transforming ability. Similarly, several naturally occurring RB mutations (from retinoblastomas and other human tumors) have lost the ability to bind E1A and large T.[28,158,163,168,181,338,339] Together, these studies strongly imply that the region of RB required for binding to E1A and large T, which has been localized to the C-terminal half of RB,[163,168,181] is important for RB function. Since DNA tumor virus gene products can bind to this region, and presumably DNA tumor virus gene products were derived from normal cellular genes at some distant time in evolution, these studies further implied that RB should interact with other cellular proteins through this region. Indeed, recent studies (see below) suggest that this is the case. However, although ability to bind RB is necessary for E1A and T function, it is not sufficient, since E1A mutants exist that retain RB-binding but are transformation-defective by virtue of their failure to bind other E1A-associated proteins (see below).

Susequent studies have demonstrated that a wide range of DNA tumor virus-transforming genes, separated by millions of years in evolutionary time, bind to and presumably inactivate RB (Fig. 3). These include the human papillomavirus (HPV) E7 protein, and the large T-antigens of polyoma, BKV, and JCV.[81,244,267]; Close examination of the sequences of these transforming proteins indicates similar-

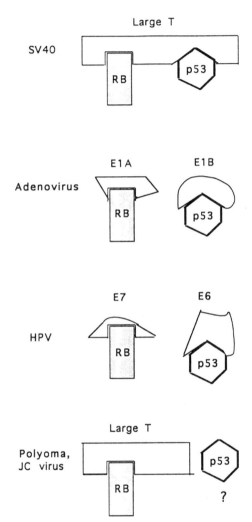

Figure 3. *Interaction of RB and p53 tumor-suppressor gene products with DNA tumor viral oncoproteins. Schematic diagram of the indicated interactions. The binding surface(s) on the oncoproteins for RB and p53, respectively, are rendered similarly to indicate likely conformational similarity. Although inactivation of RB appears to be achieved solely by its binding and sequestration, HPV E6 may inactivate p53 by promoting its degradation (see text). Likewise, it is not clear whether polyoma virus and JC virus contain oncoproteins that directly inactivate p53 (indicated by "?" in figure). Since middle T-antigens activate members of the* src *family of nontransmembrane PTKs, which would be expected to have a* ras-*like effect, they may bypass the need for direct inactivation of p53 (see text for details).*

ity to the homologous regions of E1A and large T discussed above. HPVs are of particular interest clinically and are the subject of another chapter in this book.

It is not clear why such apparently disparate viruses share a common ability to bind RB (and p107 and p53). Harlow's group[81,388,390] have suggested that the reason may be a common requirement of these viruses to parasitize the host cell's replication machinery to aid in viral DNA synthesis. Because the majority of potential target cells for viral infection in vivo are in G0 or G1, these viruses require some mechanism to prod the cells into S phase. Since RB likely helps control the G1 to S transition (see below), inactivation of RB may help achieve this goal. Whatever the reason, the common acquisition of RB-binding ability by a wide variety of tumor viruses attests to its functional importance.

The identification of RB as the E1A-associated 105K protein naturally focused attention on the other E1A-associated proteins as potential tumor-suppressor gene products. As mentioned above, the E1A-associated 107K is identical to the T-antigen-associated 120K, suggesting that oncoprotein-binding of this protein is also important for transformation by both viruses. None of the other E1A-associated proteins have been reported to complex with large T. Nevertheless, association of at least some of these other proteins with E1A appears to be required for transformation. The domains of E1A required for binding to 300K, RB and 107/120 have been mapped to discrete but overlapping regions of E1A. RB-binding requires amino acids 30 to 60 and 121 to 127, 107K-binding requires amino acids 121 to 127 alone, and 300K-binding requires amino acids 1 to 76.[389,390] These regions in E1A are conserved across various strains of adenovirus and mutation in any of these regions is sufficient to eliminate (or substantially reduce) E1A-induced transformation.[390] Studies of E1A deletion mutants indicate that inactivating 300K-binding without disrupting RB- (or 107K-) binding results in transformation defectiveness. Similarly, mutations that preserve 300K-binding but disrupt RB/107K-binding are nontransforming. The overlap between the binding sites for 300K and RB, and RB and 107K, has made it difficult to tell whether binding of all three proteins is necessary for transformation; however, it is clear that binding to 300K and at least RB or 107K is required. Since RB is clearly a tumor-suppressor gene and there is at least some evidence suggesting an independent requirement for 107K-binding for E1A transformation, it seems most likely that binding of all three cellular proteins (300K, 107K, and RB) is necessary for E1A transformation.

An analogous series of mutations in large T[64,88] indicates that RB-and 107K-(120K-) binding by large T is mediated by a common region, the region previously identified as sharing sequence similarity with E1A (and E7 and c-*myc*; see above). It is not clear why large T can transform cells without binding 300K, whereas 300K-binding appears essential for E1A-mediated transformation. One possibility is that large T does bind 300K under physiological conditions but with affinity too low to survive immunoprecipitation.

The 107K protein has recently been cloned and sequenced.[89] As predicted by its shared binding surface on E1A (aa 121 to 127), 107 shares a domain with approximately 40% sequence identity to RB. Interestingly, the chromosomal localization of 107 (20q) is in a region perturbed in some cases of myelodysplastic syndrome. The discrete E1A-binding specificity of 300K makes it likely that its sequence will be substantially different than RB. Whether this structural difference will also reflect a functional difference, of course, remains to be seen.

Although the most prominent proteins that bind to E1A (with the exception to RB) remain unidentified, the 60K E1A-associated protein has been identified as mammalian cyclin A.[292] Cyclins are a family of proteins, highly conserved from yeast to man, that share a stretch of homologous sequence (termed the cyclin box) and play critical roles in cell cycle control in both mitotic and meiotic cells.[171,227,293] Originally described by Joan Ruderman and Tim Hunt as proteins whose levels oscillate sharply during the cell cycles of early clam embryos, cyclin levels also vary dramatically across the cell cycles of higher eukaryotes. Whereas in the clam, cyclin levels are controlled strictly posttranslationally, in cycling higher eukaryotic cells, they are controlled at both the RNA and protein level. The best studied cyclins, termed cyclin A and cyclin B, are abruptly degraded during S (cyclin A) and the G2/S boundary (cyclin B). In addition to these cyclins, a group of G1 cyclins has recently been identified in both yeast and mammalian cells.[203,226,247]

Cyclins appear to function, at least in part, as positive allosteric regulators of the major cell cycle regulated kinase cdc2 (also known as p34 cdc2), and other, cdc2-related kinases. In higher eukaryotes, cyclin B regulates the homolog of the yeast cdc2 gene (see reviews cited above). Although it was initially thought that cyclin A also regulates cdc2,[123] it now appears that it complexes with and regulates a kinase highly related to but distinct from,[372] cdc2. Recent studies in several laboratories[86,292,372] have established the existence of a large family of cdc2-like kinases (cdks). However, the situation may be even more complicated. It now appears that in addition to its role as a kinase regulator, cyclin A binds to a transcription factor, E2F (probably identical to DRTF; see below), which appears to play a key role in controlling the expression of a number of cell cycle-regulated and, presumably, cell cycle-regulating genes.

The binding site for cyclin A on E1A overlaps the binding site for RB; thus the ability to bind cyclin A also appears to be required for E1A-transforming activity.[122] Although cyclin A-binding to E1A does not require RB, it is not clear whether the same E1A molecules that are complexed to RB are also bound to cyclin A-cdc2. The precise stoichiometries of the E1A/cyclin A complex versus E1A/RB complex have not been established.

Similarly, the functional significance of cyclin A-binding by E1A is not yet clear. Harlow's original studies demonstrated that a serine/threonine kinase activity was associated with E1A immunoprecipitates[143]; it has now been established that this kinase activity is comprised mainly of cdk2 associated with cyclin A as well as a small component of cdc2-cyclin A.[121,372] The RB protein is a good substrate for cdc2 kinase in vitro.[219,231] RB is likely to be an in vivo substrate of p34cdc2 or a close relative as well, since most of the sites phosphorylated by cdc2 in vitro are also in vivo phosphorylation sites.[219,231] Since phosphorylation appears to inactivate the growth suppressing activity of RB (see below), the association of cyclin-cdk2 with E1A could be part of the mechanism by which E1A inactivates RB. Alternatively, perhaps cyclin A, when complexed with E1A, is protected from cell cycle-dependent degradation. Since cyclin A is a positive regulator of cdc2-like kinases, which are positive regulators of the cell cycle, this could lead to an unrestrained proliferative signal by means independent of RB.

Studies of the details of complex formation between SV40 large T and RB by Ludlow, DeCaprio, Livingston and their collaborators have also led to a number of important insights into RB function. Unlike E1A, which binds RB promiscuously, these investigators noticed that large T bound only to unphosphorylated RB.[237] Since the consequence of RB-binding by large T is thought to be inactivation of RB's growth inhibitory activity, this finding immediately suggested that both active (unphosphorylated) and inactive (phosphorylated) forms of RB existed in the cell. The notion that phosphorylated RB is "inactive" should be viewed with some caution: an independent, perhaps directly growth stimulatory role for phosphorylated forms of RB has not been excluded. Nevertheless, the implied functional difference between dephospho-and phospho-RB prompted a search by several groups for the mechanism of control of RB phosphorylation.

It was quickly found that RB phosphorylation is regulated in a cell cycle-dependent fashion in all cells tested (Fig. 4).[38,48,65,238,254] In G0 and G1, virtually all RB is in the dephosphorylated form. At the G1/S boundary, RB phosphorylation commences. Phosphorylation appears to precede DNA synthesis; it is obviously attractive to propose that phosphorylation is required for entry into S, although this has not been directly demonstrated. Multiple sites in RB are phosphorylated as cells traverse the cycle from G1/S until M.[219,231] During M, RB is specifically dephosphorylated.[238] Although large T binds only to the dephosphorylated form of RB, it has no effect on this phosphorylation/dephosphorylation cycle. Metabolic labeling experiments by the Livingston group have shown that at G1/S, RB bound to large T becomes phosphorylated and is released from the large T/RB complex. Similarly, when phospho-RB is dephosphorylated at M, it rapidly reassociates with large T.[238]

Several other lines of evidence support a crucial functional role for RB phosphorylation. When hematopoietic cell-lines capable of in vitro differentiation are induced to differentiate, RB phosphorylation ceases within 6 to 10 hours and dephospho-RB accumulates.[48,254] Although dephosphorylated RB accumulates before the full expression of differentiation markers in these lines, it is not clear whether dephospho-RB has any specific role in promoting differentiation. It may simply help promote growth arrest, allowing expression of a default differentiation program. RB phosphorylation also fails to occur when senescent human fibroblasts are stimulated with growth factors.[356] This observation is of some interest because at least some early events following growth factor stimulation (e.g., induction of c-*myc* and several other immediate early genes), although perhaps not all such events (e.g., induction of c-*fos*) appear to occur normally in senescent cells.[335] Four different complementation groups for senescence-inducing genes have been identified[129,287]; it would be interesting to know whether all of these converge on a common event such as control of RB phosphorylation. At least part of the mechanism of action of the well-known negative growth factor, tumor growth factor (TGF-β) may be to prevent RB phosphorylation prevent RB phosphorylation at G1/S.[210] Finally, some naturally occurring RB point mutants have been identified that fail to undergo normal phosphorylation,[184,367] despite the fact that they retain all RB phosphorylation sites. At first glance, these results may appear paradoxical, since dephospho-RB appears to be the growth inhibitory form. The solution to this apparent paradox is likely to be that these mutant forms of RB are unable to assume the correct conformation required for phosphorylation by the RB kinase(s). This same conformation is likely to be the conformation of dephospho-RB which is attained when RB is active for growth inhibition. Notably, such mutants also lose the ability to bind large T.

Obviously, of central importance to understanding the details of cell cycle control of RB is the identification and characterization of the kinase (s) and phosphatases that modify RB. As discussed above, it seems clear that a major kinase contributing to RB phosphorylation at the G1/S boundary is cyclin A/cdk2. However, involvement of other cyclin-dependent kinases, perhaps cdks complexed to G1 cyclins, has not been excluded. Moreover, although RB phosphorylation begins at G1/S, it continues through later stages of the cell cycle, resulting in the phosphorylation of RB at multiple sites. The functional significance of these multiple phosphorylations, as well as the identity of the kinase(s) that catalyze them, are not yet clear. Phosphorylated RB appears to be less tightly bound to the nucleus.[261] Recent data suggest (see below) that RB may interact with a number of different cellular proteins, including some transcription factors. It would indeed be interesting if the relative affinities for these cellular proteins differs with the extent and sites of RB phosphorylation. Changes in RB phosphorylation throughout the cell cycle could then signal cell cycle-dependent release or sequestration of a variety of key cellular control elements. If such a model is correct, then the laborious task of identifying all of the phosphorylation sites of RB (and their respective kinases) as well as understanding the consequences of their mutation, will be crucial to a full understanding of RB function.

The detailed mechanism by which dephospho-RB functions to suppress growth is not yet known. Any model for RB function must take into account several features of the genetics, cell biology, and biochemistry of RB. First, the genetics of retinoblastoma suggest that RB must itself be a pleiotropic cellular regulator. If RB had only a single cellular function, say to negatively regulate protein X, then loss of protein X function should be functionally equivalent to loss of RB. One would then expect that retinoblastoma could arise from homozygous loss of either RB or X, except for the unlikely possibility that the gene for X is somehow not mutable or that mutations in X are lethal. But clinically, retinoblastoma always arises from mutations in Rb. Therefore, whatever pathways RB regulates likely branch at least once immediately distal to RB. Second, RB is located in the nucleus. The importance of this nuclear localization is evinced by the weaker nuclear association of phospho-RB as well as mutant forms of RB. Third, RB has nonspecific DNA-binding activity.

When one considers the possible functions of a nuclear protein that nonspecifically binds DNA resulting in pleiotropic effects, a role in control of transcription and/or DNA synthesis seems most likely. There is no evidence of a direct role for RB in regulating DNA synthesis, but several recent studies strongly suggest that at least one function of RB is to direct transcriptional repression of key cellular regulatory genes. The first indication of a transcription role for RB was provided by Robbins et al.,[313] who demonstrated that Rb expression vectors could block basal and growth factor (serum)-stimulated expression of a CAT reporter gene under the control of the c-*fos* promoter in transient cotransfection assays. Control vectors expressing several mutant RB proteins were unable to block expression of the *fos* promoter. These investigators localized the region in the c-*fos* promoter necessary for Rb-induced repression a region previously found to be important for basal c-*fos* expression (nucleotide [nt] -102 to -71). When appended to a heterologous promoter, this region could confer Rb-repressibility. Notably, this region is distinct from upstream elements of the c-*fos* promoter previously shown to confer growth factor responsiveness.

These early experiments provided tantalizing suggestions of a role for RB in regulating transcription. However, transient transfection experiments cannot distinguish between a direct effect of RB on c-*fos* transcription and an indirect upstream effect on some other event(s), which then leads, potentially through many intervening steps, to inhibition of c-*fos*. Moreover, since transient transfection experiments lead to extremely high levels of expression of transfected genes, one must be wary that potential "pharmacological" effects of high level expression of a gene such as RB on transcription do not reflect true physiological effects.

In view of what is known about c-*fos* and RB regulation, these caveats seem particularly relevant. Induction of c-*fos* transcription occurs at the G0/G1 transition and is followed by repression of c-*fos* transcription to undetectable levels within an hour of stimulation; there is as yet no evidence of a role for c-*fos* elsewhere in the cell cycle. RB, on the other hand, seems to play its major role in controlling the G1/S transition. Moreover, growth factor (serum-) stimulation clearly turns on c-*fos* regardless of the status of the RB gene or protein, so it is uncertain what the physiological role of RB would be in regulating c-*fos*. One way that these apparent discrepancies could be reconciled is if there is a previously unappreciated function for c-*fos* later in the cell cycle, for example in G2 or M; this question has not been studied carefully with appropriately synchronized cells. RB might then serve to turn off basal levels of c-*fos* expression if cells exit M and there are no growth factors in the medium; i.e., to drive cells into G0.

A parallel line of investigation, carried out by Harold Moses' group, has focused on the possible involvement of RB in the regulation of c-*myc* expression by TGF-β[264,289,291]; reviewed in[264]. TGF-β has multiple cell type-dependent functions. In most cell types, however, its most prominent role is to act as a growth inhibitor. The details of the signal-transduction mechanism by which TGF-β causes growth inhibition are largely unknown. However, Moses and his collaborators have demonstrated that, at least in many cell culture systems, addition of TGF-β leads to repression of c-*myc* transcription.[289] This repression is likely to be functionally important for growth inhibition, since (1) c-*myc* expression is a regular feature of actively proliferating cells; (2) c-*myc* expression is downregulated in growth factor depleted cells; and (3) most importantly, treatment of cells with c-*myc* antisense oligonucleotides results in growth inhibition. The TGF-β-induced repression of c-*myc* expression occurs at the transcriptional level. Using deletion constructs of the c-*myc* upstream regulatory region, a *cis*-acting region required for repression of c-*myc* transcription has been identified.[289,290]

A connection between these observations and RB followed from the finding that E1A, large T, and HPV E7 all abrogate TGF-β downregulation of c-*myc*.[290,291] Infection of human keratinocytes with HPV-16 or -18 or with SV40 renders them resistant to TGF-β-induced growth inhibition. Moreover, coexpression of E7, large T, or E1A blocks TGF-β-induced repression of reporter constructs driven by the c-*myc* upstream region in transient cotransfection assays, whereas mutants of these oncoproteins lacking RB-binding capability have no effect. Interestingly, the E1A mutant used in these experiments was able to bind 107K, implicating RB-and not 107K-binding in repression of c-*myc* transcription. Consistent with the presumed locus of RB action in the cell cycle, TGF-β treated cells accumulate at the G1/S boundary.

A caveat must be raised, however, concerning the generality of this model. If TGF-β-induced growth inhibition requires functional RB, one would expect that all cell-lines with functionally inactive RB would be TGF-β nonresponsive. Although recent data on breast carcinoma cell-lines with and without Rb mutations are consistent with this idea (H. Moses, personal communication), there are exceptions in other cell types. For example, bronchial epithelial cells immortalized with large T-antigen (BEAS-2B cells) are induced to stop growing and terminally differentiate in response to TGF-β.[185] Presumably the RB in these cells should be tied up in a nonfunctional complex with large T. Since TGF-β induces squamous differentiation in addition to growth arrest in bronchial epithelial cells, perhaps it acts through a different or additional pathway in these cells. Indeed, there is some evidence that the differentiation-related properties of TGF-β, such as the induction of extracellular matrix protein synthesis, are mediated via an RB-independent pathway.[211] It is also not clear why TGF-β is capable of repressing c-myc transcription in prostate cancer cell-lines lacking functional RB.[408]

As we go to press, several fascinating developments are suggesting that RB's function may be to act as a "squelcher" for a number of important cellular proteins, at least one of which is a key transcription factor. First, the region of RB that binds to large T/E1A/E7 was localized to two noncontiguous streches in the C-terminus.[163] All naturally occurring Rb mutations disrupt these domains, strongly arguing for their functional significance. William Kaelin et al in David Livingston's group constructed a glutathione S-transferase fusion protein to the RB C-terminus and used it as an affinity matrix to identify potential RB-binding proteins.[180] As a key control for specificity of binding, they used a fusion protein to a mutated RB, which was incapable of binding large T. At least seven proteins (Mr 26 kd to 150 kd), all of which appear to be nuclear by crude cell fractionation experiments, bind specifically to the wild type RB fusion protein. A similar approach was taken by Lee's group.[167] They added excess bacterially produced RB to HeLa cell lysates and found that a single, 46 kd cellular protein could now be coimmunoprecipitated with RB. It is not clear why the other proteins identified by Kaelin and Livingston were not detected under these conditions. Perhaps RB complexes with proteins other than the 46 kd protein either could not be recognized by the antiRB antibodies used and/or could not survive the conditions of immunoprecipitation.

One of these proteins has now been identified as the transcription factor E2F/DRTF by several groups, using multiple, complementary approaches.[7,13,46,50] E2F was originally identified as a cellular transcription factor that binds to two sites within the promoter for the adenovirus early gene E2.[271] E1A is required for activation of E2 via a novel mechanism that involves increasing E2F DNA-binding activity, apparently by releasing it from complexes with other cellular proteins. Mutagenesis studies indicate that the same regions of E1A that are required for transformation (and RB-binding) are required to increase E2F DNA-binding activity. Joseph Nevins[46] and Srilata Bagchi[7] and their collaborators found that one of the cellular proteins that bind to E2F is RB itself. E1A, by binding to RB, frees E2F from the RB-E2F complex allowing it to activate E2F-responsive genes. In proliferating cells (but not in G0; see below), E2F DNA-binding activity is constant across the cell cycle, but is associated with different complexes in mobility shift assays in different phases of the cell cycle. RB is bound to E2F in G1, and dissociates around G1/S, consistent with the presumed functional inactivation of RB by phosphorylation at the G1/S boundary. Independently, Kaelin et al[50] showed that a DNA-binding activity elutes from their RB-fusion protein affinity columns. Using a PCR site selection method, they showed that the binding proclivity of this eluted factor resembled that of E2F.

A parallel series of investigations has been carried out by Nicholas La Thangue and his colleague on a transcription factor they call DRTF1, which is probably highly related, if not identical to E2F.[13] DRTF1 was originally identified as a transcription factor whose activity changes upon the in vitro differentiation of the F9 embryonal carcinoma cell-line.[208] DRTF1 binds to the same element as E2F and also forms multiple complexes in mobility shift assays. Interestingly, the relative abundance of these complexes varies among different cell types and changes upon differentiation of F9 cells. Undifferentiated F9 cells have an "E1A-like activity", originally defined as the ability to rescue an E1A-defective adenovirus, which is lacking in differentiated F9 cells.[208,215] LaThangue's group found that at least one of the differences between the DRTF complexes present in undifferentiated and differen-tiated F9 cells is that in differentiated cells RB is in a complex with DRTF. Differentiation leads to a decrease in the endogenous "E1A-like activ-ity," freeing RB to bind to DRTF/E2F, in a manner highly analogous to the actions of authentic E1A in adenovirus-infected cells.

The consequence of RB-binding to DRTF/E2F appears to be the abrogation of transactivation ability. Since DRTF/E2F-binding sites have been identified in a number of key cellular growth promoting genes, the ability of RB to bind and presumably inactivate this factor is presumably essential to its growth inhibitory function. Consistent with this hypothesis, inactive RB mutants fail to bind to DRTF/E2F.

E2F appears to have two additional regulatory roles. First, in a stunning development, the groups of Nevins and LaThangue have also found that E2F complexes with cyclin A (Fig. 4). These complexes are dissociable upon addition of E1A; dissociation requires the same E1A sequence previously shown to be required for E1A-binding of cyclin A. There is one difference between these reports: the Nevins' group has found that E2F forms a complex with cyclin A alone exclusively in S, whereas the E2F/RB complex appears restricted to G1.[266] LaThangue, in collaboration with Tim Hunt et al, reports a tripartite cyclin A/RB/E2F complex in undifferentiated F9 cells.[12]

The precise role of this cyclin A/E2F complex is as yet unclear. Nevertheless, its association with a known transcription factor strongly suggests that cyclin A has some role in modulating transcription. Since it is also clear that cyclin A has a role in control of cell cycle-regulatory kinases, these findings provide the first hint of a connection between cell cycle control events and transcriptional control. The picture that emerges is one of a core group of cell cycle regulatory kinases including cdc2 and the cdks and a parallel group of cell cycle regulatory transcription factors including, but probably not limited to, E2F/DRTF, linked, at least in part, by common allosteric regulators, the first to be identified being cyclin A. Such a scheme provides a framework for understanding how transcriptional and posttranscriptional events might be coordinated throughout the cell cycle.

E2F also appears to function in induction of quiescence. In cycling cells, as discussed above, E2F DNA-binding activity is constant. However, when cells are forced into G0 by growth factor deprivation, E2F-binding activity declines markedly.[46] The mechanism(s) by which this is achieved is not clear, although one obvious possibility, given the nature of other E2F interactions, is that it forms a complex with an as yet unidentified protein that interferes with its ability to bind DNA. Remarkably, the sequences previously identified[290] as critical for TGF-β-mediated repression of c-*myc* (presumably through RB), as well as the sequence required for RB-directed repression of c-*fos* in transient transfection assays,[313] contain reasonably good consensus E2F sites. Thus it seems likely that sequestration of E2F, presumably by RB, contributes to both c-*fos* and c-*myc* regulation.

Although interaction with E2F undoubtedly explains much of RB's growth inhibitory properties, it is not likely to be the whole story. After all, several other proteins interact with RB, at least in vitro. As this review went to press, three of these have been identified. Two partial cDNA clones for putative RB-binding proteins, so far simply known only as RBP-1 and RBP-2 (for retinoblastoma-binding protein), were identified simply by screening a bacteriophage expression library with recombinant RB.[67] The translation products of these clones have appropriate in vitro-binding characteristics, including inability to bind mutant RBs and sensitivity of the binding to competitor viral oncoproteins. The predicted protein sequences of these proteins are unrelated to any other proteins in the current data base. However, since neither is a full-length clone, regions of similarity could have been missed. Both, however, contain regions with significant sequence similarity to the RB-binding sequences of viral oncoproteins, as well as strongly basic stretches that could indicate DNA-binding ability.

The third putative RB-binding protein, the c-*myc* gene product, is the subject of some controversy. Recall that c-*myc* shares the region of sequence homology with large T/E1A/E7 implicated in RB-binding. It was therefore intensively investigated from the outset by several groups as a potential RB-binding protein, but no evidence has yet been presented for any in vivo interaction between RB and *myc*. Recently, however, RB has been shown to be capable of binding to various proteins of the *myc* family members in vitro.[322] The affinity of this interaction appears to be reasonably high. Moreover, RB mutants fail to bind *myc* proteins and the RB/*myc* interaction is blocked by E1A. All of these data are consistent with physiologically significant binding, which has brought the issue of in vivo RB-*myc* interactions back to the forefront.

The reasons for the discrepancy between the in vivo and in vitro results is not clear. Since the in vitro experiments involved either in vitro translated or bacterially produced proteins, it is possible that some cellular modification inhibits RB/*myc*-binding; *myc* proteins are, in fact, heavily phosphorylated in vivo. However if this is the case, then the fraction of total *myc* protein capable of binding RB must be quite small to have avoided detection. A more reasonable explanation is that relatively harsh extraction conditions are required to solubilize *myc*; such conditions could disrupt RB-*myc* complexes. A final possibility is that RB may itself not form an in vivo complex with any *myc* protein. The in vitro results could still be relevant, however, if an RB-related protein, i.e., a protein with binding properties similar to RB, really binds *myc*. An obvious candidate for such a protein, based on its shared binding site with RB on viral oncoproteins, is the 107K/120K protein.

Remarkable progress has been made in understanding the molecular mechanism of the growth inhibitory actions of RB (Fig. 4), as well as the means by which viral oncoproteins such as E1A, large T, and E7 abrogate growth inhibition (Fig. 3). It seems certain that RB functions, at least in large part, to sequester key cellular regulatory proteins, at least some of which are transcription factors. However, we should not jump to the conclusion that all of the RB-binding proteins will turn out to be transcriptional regulators; perhaps RB binds to, and releases in a regulated fashion, proteins important in other key processes such as DNA replication. Since the ability of RB to bind to at least some of these proteins appears to be regulated by phosphorylation, and RB phosphorylation itself is modulated in a complex fashion across the cell cycle, phosphorylation may allow release of different factors at different times. RB is phosphorylated by important cell cycle-regulated serine/threonine kinases including, but not necessarily limited to cdc2 and its close relatives. Conceivably, some or all RB-binding proteins could themselves be targets for phosphorylation, and the ability of a given protein to bind RB might depend on the phosphorylation states of both binding partners.

At least one key target for regulation by RB, the cellular transcription factor E2F, has recognition sequences within a number of important cell cycle regulatory genes; binding to RB appears to

---

Figure 4. *The retinoblastoma protein (RB) and the cell cycle. Shown is a typical mammalian cell cycle diagram with stages G0, G1, S, G2, and M, respectively. Also shown are RB, the transcription factor E2F, and several other important cell cycle regulatory proteins. In G1, RB is unphosphorylated and bound to E2F. The E2F/RB complex is capable of binding to E2F sites, but E2F is in a conformation that does not allow activation of E2F-responsive genes. At G1/S an RB kinase, which is likely to be cdk2, perhaps in association with a G1 cyclin (?G1 CLN/cdk)/and/or cyclin A, phosphorylates RB (-P) leading to release of E2F. During S phase, E2F associates with cyclin A (cycA)-cdk2 (and somewhat with cyclin A cdc-2) to form an active E2F complex, leading to the transcription of E2F-responsive genes (see text). Whether the role of the cyclin A-cdk2 complex is to phosphorylate E2F and/or another component of the transcriptional apparatus to bring about the activation of E2F-responsive genes is not yet known; however, the shape of E2F in the cartoon is shown altered to indicate acquisition of transcriptional activating ability. Throughout S and G2, RB becomes increasingly phosphorylated through the action of cdc-2 and cdc-2-like kinases. The status of E2F in G2 and M has not been well characterized. At G2/M, RB is abruptly dephosphorylated by a serine phosphatase with PP-1 specificity. If the cell is allowed to become quiescent (i.e., to enter G0) via the removal of growth factors, dephospho-RB associates with E2F and perhaps another component (or undergoes a different modification) that prevents RB-E2F-binding to E2F sites. In actively cycling cells, dephospho-RB reassociates with E2F to form a DNA-binding but transcriptionally inactive complex. See text for details.*

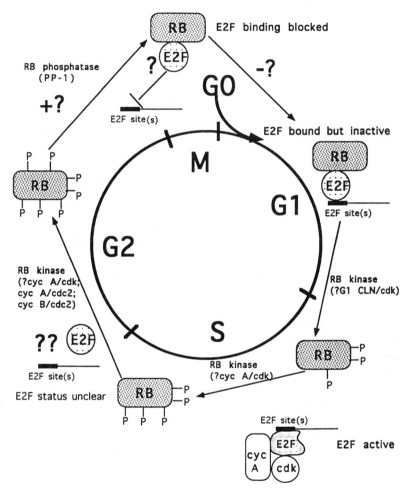

Figure 4. (*see legend on p. 62*)

eliminate transcriptional activation by E2F. At later stages of the cell cycle, E2F complexes with cyclin A, which is itself also a key allosteric regulator of a cell cycle-regulated cdc2-like kinase. We may thus be left with parallel master pathways for cell cycle regulation by, on the one hand, cell cycle-regulated serine/threonine kinases including cdc2 and its relatives, which phosphorylate key substrates at specific times in the cell cycle, and on the other hand, factor repositories such as RB (and perhaps, by inference, the 107/120K protein) that release key factors for action at specific times in the cell cycle. The two pathways "crosstalk" at least at two levels: control of RB's ability to bind certain factors by phosphorylation and interaction of E2F with both RB and cyclin A (Fig. 4). The E1A/large T/E7 family of oncoproteins disrupts this control by mimicking the binding surface of proteins that interact with RB (and presumably 107/120K and cyclin A), thus freeing these proteins at inappropriate times in the cell cycle.

However, many questions remain. What are the identities and functions of the other proteins that interact with RB? Is RB always a negative allosteric regulator of proteins that bind to it, or does it increase the activity of some factors? Recent evidence suggests that RB does, in fact, positively regulate the TGF-β1 gene.[190] Along the same lines, does phosphorylation of RB make it functionally dead, or are there also proteins whose activity is modulated specifically by phospho-RB? Are forms of phospho-RB that differ in their extents of phosphorylation functionally equivalent? What is the identity of the "E1A-like" activity that is present in undifferentiated F9 cells and which disappears upon differentiation; how does this activity relate to factors already known to play a role in F9 differentiation, such as retinoic acid receptors and their target genes? What is the identity of the protein that binds to and inactivates the DNA-binding capacity of E2F in G0 cells? The answers to these questions are likely to come quickly over the next two to three years and to illuminate what has heretofore been a black box between signal transduction and cell cycle control.

The p53 Gene

Origins, Cloning, and Biological Activity

If Rb is the paradigmatic tumor-suppressor gene, the p53 gene certainly holds title as the most confusing.[213,224,225] Indeed, p53 has lived a life of multiple personalities. Originally described independently by Linzer and Levine[232] and Lane and Crawford[214] in 1979, p53 was, for many years, thought to be a dominant cellular proto-oncogene. Within the past few years, this initial impression has been proven incorrect; normal cellular p53 is actually a tumor-suppressor gene. The reason for the discrepancy is that many mutant forms of p53 not only lose their tumor-suppressing activity, but acquire oncogenic activity. Moreover, since loss of p53 function promotes cellular immortalization, many of the immortal cell-lines used as sources for molecular clones of p53 have endogenous p53 mutations. Many of the original studies, which suggested that p53 was a dominant oncogene, actually used mutant forms of p53.

It is easy to see how p53 was miscast. It was originally discovered because it formed a tight complex with SV40 large T-antigen, allowing its coimmunoprecipitation under fairly harsh conditions. Convincing evidence that this interaction was functionally significant came from analysis of complex formation with temperature sensitive large T mutants. At the permissive temperature for transformation, p53 was found in a complex with the mutant T; this complex reversibly dissociated at the nonpermissive temperature.[233] In addition to forming a complex with p53, large T promotes a large increase in the amount of p53 in transformed cells. The increase in p53 levels was shown to be due to posttranslational stabilization of the p53 protein.[279,310] Soon thereafter, it was found that p53 also forms complexes with the product of the adenovirus E1B gene[326] (Fig. 3). When substantially elevated levels of p53 were found in a large number of chemically-transformed and tumor cell-lines, compared with the minute quantitites of p53 present in normal cells,[56,68,72] the correlation between high levels of p53 and cellular transformation seemed well established.

Several groups obtained genomic and cDNA clones for p53 from a variety of sources.[174,278,407] The sequences of these clones predict a protein of approximately 390 amino acids (Fig. 5) which is highly conserved across vertebrate evolution.[175] Comparison of the sequences of p53 proteins from fish to humans indicate five clusters of extensive amino acid similarity; the high degree of sequence conservation in these regions suggest that they are important for p53 function. The p53 protein has three distinct domains (also highly conserved across evolution): a highly acidic N-terminus (approximately the first 75 to 80 aa, human and mouse sequences) followed by a proline-rich hydrophobic region (aa 80 to 150, human and mouse sequences) and a C-terminal basic region (aa 320 to 393, human sequence; aa 275 to 390,

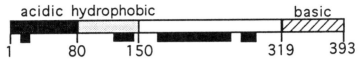

Figure 5. *The p53 tumor suppressor gene product. Shown are structural domains in the human p53 protein. The amino acid positions are as indicated. Solid bars indicate the positions of highly conserved stretches (90% to 100% identity) of sequence in p53 from frogs to mammals. These regions are also frequent targets for mutations in human tumors.[213,224,225] See text for details.*

mouse sequence) which possesses DNA-binding activity and a predicted helix-turn-helix motif. These structural features are similar to those of many transcription factors, which has led to the suggestion that the normal function of p53 is to affect transcription of key cell cycle control genes (see The Normal Function of p53: Perspectives).

Unlike the mammoth Rb, p53 is a relatively small gene, occupying only about 20 kb on chromosome 17 p (chromosome 11 in mice). It consists of 11 exons, including a 5' noncoding exon located significantly upstream from the remaining 10 exons.[224] Little work has been directed towards the control of p53 transcription. There appear to be two separate initiation sites, but both give rise to transcripts differing only in their 5' noncoding exons. The *cis*-acting control sequences for p53 transcription from these two promoters have not yet been well defined. One would expect one or both of these to have features of "housekeeping" promoters, since, like Rb, p53 is ubiquitously expressed. Also like RB, the p53 protein is heavily phosphorylated and located in the nucleus.[277,317] However, the p53 protein is extremely unstable, with a half-life measured in minutes. Many p53 mutants are substantially more stable than wild type, resulting in their accumulating to high levels within the cell (see below).

The cloning and sequencing of both genomic and cDNA clones for p53 from several rodent and human sources allowed a direct test of the biological properties of p53. Several groups demonstrated that expression constructs in which p53 was driven by strong heterologous promoters could cooperate with activated (mutant) dominant *ras* mutations to transform primary rat embryo fibroblasts in a cotransfection assay.[85,173,282] Such p53 constructs also promote immortalization of primary cells.[173] Notably, E1A and the c-*myc* oncogene also cooperate with *ras* in the same type of assay system and have immortalizing capability.[212] This suggests at least some level of functional similarity between the transforming abilities of these genes (see Spectrum and Biological Activity of p53 Mutations). p53 alone was also able to render already established rodent fibroblast lines tumorigenic,[84,186] buttressing its identification as a dominant onco-gene. Further support was provided by a highly influential study in which an Abelson murine leukemia virus-transformed leukemia cell-line lacking p53 expression was identified.[393,394] These cells did not grow as a progressive tumor when inoculated into mice, whereas Abelson virus-transformed cell-lines that did express p53 were highly tumorigenic. More importantly, reintroduction of p53 into the p53-deficient line resulted in highly tumorigenic cells.[393]

In all of these experiments demonstrating oncogenic activity of expression constructs of p53, the transfected cells expressed high levels of p53, consistent with the idea that p53 was a dominant proto-oncogene. The abilities of large T and E1B to contribute to transformation were thought to result, at least in part, from their ability to promote an increase in the level of p53. This notion also conveniently fit the prevailing paradigm of the time, namely, that cancer resulted from dominant oncogenic mutations and that onco-genic retroviruses transformed cells by overexpressing (in some cases mutant) dominant oncogenes.

Other studies also supported a role for p53 in promoting cell growth. p53 mRNA and protein synthesis were found to be regulated across the cell cycle. Quiescent Swiss 3T3 cells have virtually undetect-able levels of p53. Following serum stimulation, p53 RNA and protein synthesis were found to increase in late G1.[309] The observed increase in p53 protein could be explained solely on the basis of increased levels of p53 RNA; there is no apparent cell cycle-dependent alteration in p53 protein stability. Induction of p53 synthesis clearly occurs after early response genes such as c-*fos*, c-*myc*, and actin, but precedes induction of later genes such as histone H3. Similar induction of p53 synthesis occurs when quiescent lymphocytes are mitogenically stim-ulated.[258] Given the transfection results discussed above, these data were reasonably interpreted as indicating that the p53 protein pro-motes cell growth with its time of action probably being late G1 or G1/S. Direct functional support for this hypothesis was provided by microinjection[252] and antisense RNA experiments.[340] These studies indicated that inactivation or elimination of p53 from normal cells rendered them unable to respond to normal mitogenic stimuli.

As the mid-1980s dawned, the case for p53 as an oncogene seemed nearly complete. The first inkling that something was wrong with this idea came from a series of studies by Sam Benchimol's laboratory.[52,265,268,319] These workers were studying the potential involvement of p53 in Friend leukemia virus (FrLV) oncogenesis. What they found presented an intriguing paradox: although many FrLV-induced tumors expressed high levels of p53, a substantial percentage (like the Abelson virus-transformed B cell-line described above) expressed either no p53 or a truncated form. Southern analysis revealed that most of the cases of absent or altered p53 expression arose as a consequence of rearrangements (proviral insertions and/or deletions) in the p53 gene.[52,265,268,319] These rearrangements were homozygous, indicating that loss of the normal, unrearranged homologue had occurred. Such results suggested that loss (or alteration) and overexpression of p53 were somehow functionally equivalent, since both were associated with leukemogenesis in vivo.

A second finding, also from Benchimol's laboratory,[318] cast further doubt on the p53 as oncogene hypothesis. The earlier experiments (discussed above) which tested the biological activity of p53 genomic and cDNA clones had used expression constructs with strong promoters designed to drive high level expression of p53 and thus to mimic the high levels of (at that time, what was presumed to be normal) p53 that had been found in diverse tumor cell-lines. Since such constructs did display oncogenic properties and the resultant transformed cells had high levels of p53 protein, this (in retrospect, circular) argument seemed reasonable. Rovinski and Benchimol,[318] however, found that a purportedly normal genomic clone driven off of its own (weak) endogenous p53 promoter could also complement *ras* in the primary rat embryo fibroblast assay. This cast doubt on the explanation that overexpression was necessary for transformation by (this) genomic clone. But if overexpression was not necessary for transformation, then it was hard to understand the difference between transfected, transformed cells and untransfected, normal cells.

At about the same time, it became clear that not all cDNA clones of p53 were transforming. Levine's group found that a cDNA isolated from F9 teratocarcinoma cells[286] was incapable of complementing *ras*; in the same series of experiments, the original Balb/c mouse-derived genomic clone and several cDNAs derived from other rodent cell-lines displayed transforming activity.[100] These results, along with the availability of sequence information from a number of lower species, focused attention on differences between transforming and nontransforming p53 clones. Remarkably, these differences were, in some cases, minimal. For example, the functional difference between the F9 cDNA clone and the transforming genomic clone was found to be due to a single alanine to valine transition (aa 135) within one of the five blocks of highly conserved sequence (Fig. 5). Comparison of several other cDNAs from frog to man, including cDNAs from normal tissues rather than cell-lines, revealed that, like the F9 clone, they all encoded alanine at position 135. The inescapable conclusion, soon confirmed, was that the Balb/c genomic clone, which had been used for so many experiments focused on the biological activity of p53, was in fact a cloning mutant.[152] Wild type p53, as represented by the F9 cDNA clone, was not able to complement *ras* or to display any other oncogenic biological properties. In fact, subsequent experiments directly demonstrated the opposite: normal p53 has tumor-(transformation) suppressing activity (see below).

At face value, these results alone could still have been interpreted as being consistent with p53 as a dominant proto-oncogene, and this was the initial interpretation of many investigators. After all, several dominant proto-oncogenes (e.g., c-*src*, c-*abl*, etc.) are nontrans-forming in their normal state and require mutations for "activation" of their oncogenic activity. However, much data was still difficult to explain, even with the recognition that mutant and normal p53 clones had been confused. For example, the Friend virus-induced erythroleukemia results suggested that loss and overexpression of p53 were functionally equivalent (see above). Also, how could one explain the finding that multiple independent mutations in p53, distributed across virtually the entire cDNA, resultabed in activation of transforming activity? Typically, one would expect that gain-of-function mutations would only occur within limited regions of a gene; mutations scattered throughout a gene would be expected to result in loss of function. The old paradigm could not fit the emerging data; clearly, a change in thinking was needed.

Normal p53 is a Tumor-Suppressor Gene

That change in thinking was soon provided: normal p53 is not a dominant proto-oncogene but, rather, a tumor-suppressor gene. Mutations in p53 destroy its intrinsic tumor-(growth) suppression ability, which accounted for the fact that mutations in various regions of the p53 gene have similar (although not identical; see below) biological effects. Moreover, p53 mutants may be able to tie up normal p53 in a complex, thus rendering the normal p53 gene product biologically inactive. Mutant p53 may thus act as a "dominant negative."[150]

The first indication that p53 was a human tumor-suppressor gene came from studies by Bert Vogelstein and his colleagues. They had observed that an extremely high percentage (about 80%) of colon cancers show LOH on chromosome 17p.[9,377] Using a series of 17p RFLPs, they were able to narrow the MRO to band 17p13, a region known to contain the p53 gene. Aware of Benchimol's work in FrLV oncogenesis, they looked at the status of p53 in tumors with 17p LOH.[9] Initially, they found no gross abnormalities in the Southern blot pattern of the p53 gene in a sample of over 80 tumors and tumor cell-lines. RNA analysis revealed no gross changes in the size of the p53 transcripts in tumor specimens, although four tumors did show minimal levels of p53 expression (which could have been due to remaining normal cells contaminating a tumor which itself lacked p53 expression). This data certainly gave no firm indication that p53 was the 17p colon cancer gene. However, Southern and Northern analysis could not exclude more subtle defects, such as point mutations or small deletions. Vogelstein and his coworkers then took the extraordinary, one might even say heroic, step of cloning and sequencing p53 cDNAs from colon cancers and matched normal colonic tissue. To their surprise and gratification, they found that both of the first two cDNAs examined had point mutations. Both of these mutations occurred within one of the blocks of highly conserved sequence described above (Fig. 5). Mutations within each of these regions had been found to activate the transforming activity of murine p53, consistent with functional importance of the observed mutations. Most convincingly, these mutant p53 genes were found to display in vitro transforming activity in the *ras* cotransfection assay.[153]

Further studies by the Vogelstein group and others have shown that virtually all colon cancers are homozygous for p53 mutations.[93] In nearly all cases, this homozygosity results in a p53 allele, sometimes reduplicated, bearing a point mutation. Rarely (<10%), there are gross changes in the p53 gene itself in colon cancers; such changes are more common in other types of tumors bearing p53 mutations (see below). Inactivation of p53 in colon cancer is thus subtly different from Rb inactivation in retinoblastoma and other tumors. All Rb mutations thus far examined are true null mutations. Consequently, gross deletions of DNA, and/or absence of RNA, and/or protein are much more common for Rb than for p53. Conversely, most p53 mutations are missense mutations. A colonic neoplasm that acquires a p53 point mutation presumably gains a growth advantage, possibly due to its ability to act as a dominant negative, leading to clonal expansion.[341] The finding of occasional colonic tumors in which one p53 allele is mutated and the other normal is consistent with this model[93,155]; there is no known similar advantage for a cell with one mutant Rb allele. Subsequently, chromosomal mechanisms lead to LOH, leaving the p53 Southern and Northern pattern grossly unaffected. Although a single mutated p53 may provide a selective advantage to cells, the fact that the normal allele is rarely found to remain in colonic tumors suggests that loss of the normal allele results in a further growth advantage. This is reminiscent of the findings (discussed above) of both Wolf et al. in the Abelson system and Benchimol's group in the Friend system, where the addition of (now recognized to be mutant) p53 expression constructs to leukemic cells completely lacking p53 renders them more tumorigenic.

Mutations of p53 are by no means limited to colon cancers.[272] Allele loss on 17p is commonly observed in a wide variety of human tumors.[155] In most of these tumors, the gene on 17p targeted for deletion is p53. Vogelstein's group, as well as a number of other laboratories, have found p53 mutations in virtually all types of malignancy studied, including common carcinomas such as breast, lung (small cell and nonsmall-cell), bladder, glioblastomas, sarcomas, and leukemias. For some of these malignancies, such as lung cancer, p53 mutation occurs in virtually all cases. In others, the true frequency of p53 mutation in clinical specimens has not been clearly established. Overall, however, mutation of p53 is clearly the single most common known cancer-associated genetic event.

Whether p53 mutation is a necessary event in the genesis of other cancers—indeed, most cancers—or instead, contributes to tumor progression, remains to be determined. In chronic myelogenous leukemia (CML), p53 mutation is clearly associated with progression to blast crisis, rather than initiation of the malignancy.[2] The degree to which p53 mutation is responsible for this conversion remains to be rigorously determined. Since the chronic phase of CML is relatively well tolerated clinically, understanding (and ultimately preventing) progression to blast crisis is potentially of great importance. Clonal expansion of cells with mutations in p53 also occurs during brain tumor progression.[341]

Most of the mutations identified map within four of the five highly conserved regions of the p53 gene (aa 117 to 142, 171 to 181, 234 to 258, and 270 to 286). As is also the case for mutations in the *ras* oncogene,[14,96] the frequency distribution of mutations within the p53 gene varies among different tumor types.[155] It is not clear whether this is because different mutagens lead to different types of mutation or whether it reflects selection for mutations with different biological properties in different cell types, or some combination of both. Regardless of whether or not there is selection for different types of p53 mutations in different tumor types, it seems likely from many in vitro studies that different p53 mutations will have different biological effects (see below). Such differences may ultimately prove to be clinically important.

Mutations in p53 are not limited to sporadic human tumors. Stephen Friend's laboratory, in collaboration with Frederick Li et al, has found that the rare autosomal dominant Li-Fraumeni syndrome is associated with, and presumably caused by germ-line mutations in p53.[243] Li-Fraumeni syndrome is characterized by increased suscepti-bility to a variety of tumors, including breast carcinomas, brain tumors, leukemias, osteosarcomas, and soft tissue sarcomas.[228] The types of tumors that arise in patients with this syndrome also have p53 mutations when they arise sporadically in nonaffected individuals. A similar spectrum of tumors is also observed in mice carrying a mutant p53 transgene; such animals are effectively the murine equivalent of Li-Fraumeni patients. The somatic tissues of individuals are heterozy-gous for p53 mutations. A small number of tumors arising from Li-Fraumeni patients were also analyzed; these tumors had lost the remaining normal copy of p53 and were now homozygous for the initial germ-line mutation. This provides further support for the general paradigm that familial and sporadic cancers arise from the same set of genetic events, familial tumors occurring earlier and with higher frequency because one of the events has already occurred in the germ line.

Different point mutations were found in different families with the syndrome. However, the mutations in the six families studied all clustered within a single region of the p53 gene (conserved region IV). Li-Fraumeni patients, although they have a high cancer incidence, show no developmental abnormalities.[109] It is perhaps surprising that patients carrying a mutation in all of their cells for a gene such as p53, which appears to be universally important in growth control, would develop normally. It may be that only certain p53 mutations will allow normal development to occur; hence the clustering of mutations within a limited region of the gene. For example, any p53 mutation that could function in vivo as a dominant negative (and thus functionally inactivate the remaining normal p53 allele) might not be tolerated during development. Indeed, the p53 protein in fibroblasts from several Li-Fraumeni patients did not display the prolonged half-life associated with most p53 mutations. Friend and his coworkers noted that since the Li-Fraumeni p53 mutant protein did not accumulate to high levels in these cells, it presumably could not interfere with the remaining normal protein as a dominant negative. Such mutations might be phenotypically silent until the remaining normal allele was lost, thus allowing normal growth and development to occur.

Another reason for the apparent clustering of mutations in a specific region of the p53 gene in Li-Fraumeni patients may be selection imposed by identifying a patient as having Li-Fraumeni syndrome. Only some p53 mutations might be compatible with the development of tumors in a wide variety of tissues. It is conceivable that other familial cancer syndromes might also have p53 mutations, perhaps localized to other regions of the p53 gene. Such mutations could predispose to a more limited spectrum of tumors than the Li-Fraumeni syndrome, depending on the particular biological properties of the mutation. The finding that different spectra of p53 mutations are found in different types of tumors (analogous to the relative frequency of *ras* mutations in different types of tumors) is consistent with this possibility. Indeed, somatic p53 mutations have recently been found in some pediatric cancer patients lacking other features of the Li-Fraumeni syndrome.[242,369]

Direct tests of the biological activity of normal p53 have been provided by a number of groups using several systems. In experiments using cotransfection assays, Levine's[99] and Moshe Oren's[83] groups showed that wild type p53 cDNA could block the ability of mutant p53 to complement *ras* in the transformation of primary rat embryo fibroblasts (REFs). The rare foci that grew out of these triple transfections contained no normal p53 protein. Mutations in the wt p53 gene completely abrogated its ability to suppress transformation. The ability of wild type p53 to inhibit mutant p53 plus *ras* transformation did not appear to be due to a nonspecific toxic effect of wild type p53, since wild type p53 did not affect the plating efficiency of normal fibroblasts. Interestingly, wild type p53 also appeared to inhibit E1A's (and *myc*'s) ability to complement *ras* in the same cotransfection assay, although the potency of p53 towards blocking E1A-(*myc*) transforming ability was somewhat less than towards interfering with mutant p53.

Oren's group subsequently provided additional, particularly graphic confirmation of these results.[83] They discovered that the Val 135 mutant of p53 behaved as a temperature sensitive conditional mutant. At the nonpermissive temperature, cells transfected with *ras* and the mutant p53 are growth arrested, whereas at the permissive temperature, they are transformed. Levine's group has obtained similar evidence with inducible mutant p53 constructs (A. Levine, personal communication).

Levine's and Oren's experiments showed that normal p53 could block transformation by mutant p53 and dominant nuclear onco-genes. A complementary series of experiments, performed in a number of laboratories, indicated that restoration of normal p53 to tumor cell-lines that have p53 mutations causes growth arrest.[8,42,47,71,253] Tumor cells reconstituted with wild type p53 arrest in late G1,[71] suggesting that normal p53 functions, at least in part, at this stage of the cell cycle. This idea is consistent (although for exactly opposite reasons) with the earlier studies showing increased p53 mRNA and protein in late G1. An important feature of these reconstitution studies is that introduction of additional copies of normal p53 into cells that have not undergone p53 mutations, e.g., certain colonic adenoma cell-lines, has no deleterious effects; the growth inhibitory effect of normal p53 appears to be restricted to cells that have undergone p53 mutations.

Most studies have suggested that restoration of normal p53 to tumor cells results in growth arrest. Wen-Hwa Lee and his collaborators have introduced normal p53 into the same retroviral vector they had used earlier to restore Rb to Rb-cells.[47] This construct can restore normal p53 expression to Saos 2 cells, which completely lack p53. Although these p53-reconstituted cells grew much more slowly and displayed morphological alterations compared to uninfected or parental virus-infected cells, they were able to be maintained stably as a cell-line. However, the p53-reconstituted cells had completely lost the ability to grow in soft agar or as tumors in nude mice. Lee and his colleagues also introduced mutant p53 genes into the same cell-line with the same vector system. Interestingly, the mutant p53 gene, in a background of no endogenous p53, increased the saturation density of the Saos 2 line in vitro. Although under the conditions of their nude mouse assay, the mutant p53-expressing cell clones displayed comparable tumorigenicity to the parental line, the higher saturation density achieved by these cells suggests at least some selective advantage to expression of a mutant p53 compared with no p53 expression—at least in this cell-line. This observation is, of course, consistent with the situation in most tumors, in which p53 missense mutations are usually retained.

Although Lee's studies suggested selective advantage for mutant p53 against a background of no p53, they also called into question the notion of a selective advantage of mutant p53 against a background of normal p53. Using retroviral vectors marked with two different drug resistance markers, they introduced one copy of normal p53 and one copy of mutant p53 into Saos 2 cells. Cells expressing both genes showed no difference in growth behavior from those expressing just the normal p53 gene; in other words, one copy of normal p53 was dominant to one copy of mutant p53. This dominance of normal p53 to mutant p53 was found despite the accumulation of the mutant p53 protein to tenfold higher levels than the normal protein, owing to the prolonged half-life of the mutant. These findings certainly challenge the idea that p53 can function as a dominant negative during normal tumorigenesis. They are also at variance with the in vitro studies in tissue culture cells described earlier where, at least under some conditons, p53 mutants do appear capable of acting as dominant negatives. Moreover, in a small number of tumors, heterozygous p53 mutations have been found. Although it has been argued that these tumors may have been removed at a time in their development wherein only one p53 mutation had occurred, it is difficult to understand why they would be clonal for the p53 mutation if that mutation was not providing some selective advantage. Perhaps only extremely high ratios of mutant to normal p53 protein—greater than tenfold—can result in dominant negative effects. How often such levels are obtained during oncogenesis in vivo is unclear. It does seem clear, however, that only some mutant p53 proteins in some cell types would be able to accumulate to such high levels. It also seems clear that normal p53 functions biologically as a growth suppressor gene in tumor cells, with relatively little effect on normal cells. This apparently selective toxicity imbues the notion of a molecular pharmacological approach to p53 replacement with a measure of optimism.

However, the overall interpretation of this phenomenology is still somewhat confusing. Normal p53 appears to be selectively growth inhibitory for transformed cells or cells that are partly along the pathway to full malignant transformation. This likely explains the extremely high frequency of p53 mutations in virtually all types of naturally occurring tumors: cells that have progressed a certain extent towards tumorigenicity can no longer tolerate normal p53 expression.

Mutant p53 behaves like E1A or *myc* in the two gene transfection system. At first glance, this would seem to imply that inhibition of mutant p53 plus *ras* transformation by normal p53 is due to normal p53's ability to interfere with an E1A-like function. However, the ability of normal p53 to block E1A plus *ras* transformation (or *myc* plus *ras* transformation) need not and probably should not be interpreted as indicating a direct effect of normal p53 on the pathway of E1A-induced oncogenesis. Instead, it may reflect the ability of normal p53 to inhibit the growth of transformed cells in general. In fact, normal p53 may be antagonizing the function provided by *ras* in the two gene transfection assay, rather than directly antagonizing the effect of E1A, *myc*, or mutant p53. This idea is consistent with the independent requirement of E1A and E1B for transformation by adenoviruses, since E1B's function presumably is to inactivate endogenous p53: if E1A's function is "*myc*-like," then E1B (and hence p53 inactivation) must be "*ras*-like."

If this explanation is correct, then why does mutant p53 substitute for E1A (or *myc*)? The solution to this apparent paradox may be that normal p53 is bifunctional (see also, The Normal Function of p53: Perspectives). During the normal cell cycle, p53 clearly serves a growth inhibitory role, since its loss or inactivation promotes cell growth. Nevertheless, the microinjection and antisense experiments described above imply a growth stimulatory role for p53 in normal cells. During the normal cycle, p53 could oscillate between a form that inhibits growth and a form that stimulates growth. The transition between these two forms could be controlled by posttranslational modification; an obvious candidate, given that p53 is a phosphoprotein, is phosphorylation. There is evidence for phosphorylation of p53 in vivo and in vitro by at least two cell cycle-regulated serine/threonine kinases, casein kinase II[250,251] and cdc 2.[22] These kinases appear to phosphorylate p53 at different sites, suggesting that they may direct p53 phosphorylations with different functional consequences.

A bifunctional model for p53 also predicts the existence of p53 mutants with different biological properties. Some mutant p53s (those which effectively complement *ras* in the REF assay) could have lost growth inhibitory function but retained growth stimulatory ability. One might further infer that the growth inhibitory activity would be mediated along the pathway by which *ras* stimulates growth, whereas the growth stimulatory activity would be mediated along a pathway similar to that by which *myc* (and E1A) stimulates growth. An additional prediction of this model is that mutant p53s might exist which have lost both their growth inhibitory and their growth stimulatory function. For example, in the REF cotransfection assay, such mutants would be both unable to suppress mutant p53 (or E1A or *myc*) plus *ras* transformation (suppression function) and themselves be unable to complement *ras* (stimulation function); indeed such mutations have been found (see below).

The Spectrum and Biological Properties of p53 Mutations

The biochemical and biological properties of different p53 mutations, both naturally occurring (in tumors) and genetically engineered, display both important similarities and differences. All mutant p53 proteins have markedly diminished ability to bind to SV40 large T-antigen.[225] Since, obviously, no selection for inability to bind SV40 large T was applied during the generation of these mutants, this finding has been taken to indicate that some vital function of normal p53 involves interaction with a protein(s) (or other macromolecule) containing a domain(s) mimicked by large T. Moreover, since all p53 mutants that have lost tumor-suppressor activity also lose the ability to bind large T, the tumor-suppressor activity of p53 may well be mediated through these presumptive interactions with as yet unidentified cellular proteins.

p53 also has been shown to bind to DNA both nonspecifically and, more recently, specifically (see below). Although detailed tests of only a relatively small number of mutations have been reported, thus far there is an absolute correlation between p53 mutation (i.e., inactivation of p53 suppression function) and loss of both nonspecific and specific DNA-binding ability.[225] Interestingly, mutants that differ in several other properties, including their ability to bind conformation-specific antibodies and to collaborate with *ras* in transforming REF cells (see below), all have markedly decreased ability to bind DNA. Moreover, large T interferes with the ability of p53 to bind to DNA in a sequence-specific fashion and, as indicated above, there is apparently an absolute correlation between p53 mutation and inability to bind large T. Whether large T is "seeing" the same surface of p53 that binds DNA is not clear. If it is, there may not have to be protein targets for p53; the p53-binding surface on large T may be mimicking the DNA target(s) of p53. Alternatively, large T may be "seeing" a conformation that is only attained (and attainable) by p53 molecules that are competent to bind DNA. In this case, there are likely to be cellular proteins whose normal function is to recognize this surface, interacting with, and perhaps transmitting a signal for, DNA-bound p53.

Most mutant p53 proteins have prolonged half-lives and therefore accumulate to substantially higher levels than normal p53.[100] This has led to the suggestion that the ability to detect p53 by immunostaining of tissue sections is indicative of mutation. Although this may be a relatively specific test, it is certainly not sufficiently sensitive to be clinically useful. For example, a study of colon cancers revealed that only about 50% had immunostainable p53, yet virtually all such tumors have p53 mutations.[314] Some p53 mutations clearly do not increase the stability of the p53 protein, at least in some cell types; the p53 mutations associated with the Li-Fraumeni syndrome are a prime example (see above). Moreover, the stability of a given p53 mutation may vary in different cells. To the extent the accumulation of high levels of mutant protein helps contribute to transformation, these differences may help explain the preponderance of specific p53 mutations in certain tumors.

Most but, again, not all, p53 mutations that have increased half-lives also bind to a heat shock protein, hsc 70, as well as to normal p53, to form large oligomeric complexes.[53,100,358,359] Again, however, there are exceptions. Oren's group has described a mutant at position 270 which occurs naturally in human tumors.[136] This mutant accumulates substantially in tumor cell-lines carrying it, as well as when it is introduced into REFs via expression constructs. Nevertheless, it fails to form detectable complexes with hsc 70 or endogeneous p53. Although, as expected, this mutant cannot suppress transformation, it also does not cooperate with *ras* to transform REFs. It is therefore an example of the type of mutation described above, in which both activities of p53 appear to have been lost.

Most mutations that are "activated" for transforming ability share the feature of failing to be recognized by the conformation-specific monoclonal antibody PAb 246.[403] These mutants instead are recognized by monoclonal antibody PAb 240, which does not react with normal p53.[114] The properties of these monoclonal antibodies support the idea that activating mutants of p53 are "locked" in a particular conformation; this is consistent with a (bifunctional) normal p53 that oscillates between conformational (and possibly different functional) states. In support of this hypothesis, Milner and coworker have reported[259] that during the normal cell cycle, p53 oscillates between PAb 246-reactive and nonreactive conformations. However, it is not clear whether the conformation attained by mutant p53 proteins that allows recognition by PAb 240 is ever achieved under physiological conditions by wild type p53.

Finally p53 mutations differ in their ability to transactivate. Recent studies using fusions of p53 to the yeast transcriptional activator GAL4 deleted for its trans-activation function have shown that either the entire p53 protein[306] or its N-terminus[97] can transactivate a reporter gene under the control of a GAL4 DNA-binding site. Interestingly, some p53 mutants, but not all,[305,306] have lost their ability to transactivate in such assays. It is intriguing that a mutation at position 175, which has lost the ability to transactivate, has substantially greater ability to complement *ras* in the REF assay than a mutant at position 273, which retains transactivation ability. These two mutants also differ in their gross conformations, as indicated by their relative abilities to be immunoprecipitated by the ("normal") conformation-specific PAb246. These studies raise the tantalizing possibility of a correlation between inability of a p53 mutant to transactivate and its acquisition of transforming ability.

Interactions Between p53 and DNA Tumor Virus Oncogene Products

The significance of the p53/large T interaction was not fully appreciated until after the discovery of the RB/E1A and RB/large T complexes, despite the fact that p53 was the first normal gene product demonstrated to form complexes with a DNA tumor virus oncoprotein.[214,232] Among such proteins, the ability to bind p53 is not restricted to large T (Fig. 3). Shortly after the discovery of the large T/p53 interaction, p53 was shown to complex with adenovirus E1B[326] and, more recently, the E6 protein of human papillomaviruses (HPVs) 16 and 18 has been found to bind p53.[386] Initially, large T was believed to activate p53-transforming ability, perhaps by preventing p53 proteolysis and thus promoting its accumulation to high levels. Now, by analogy to the RB complexes with viral oncoproteins and given our revised view of p53 as a tumor-suppressor gene, it is believed that the function of the p53 complexes is to inactivate the growth suppressing function of p53.

Perhaps the most convincing evidence of inactivation of p53 function by a viral oncoprotein comes from the HPV system. E6 forms a complex with p53 in vitro and in vivo. The affinity of the E6/p53 interaction is directly related to the relative oncogenicity of the HPV strain; highly oncogenic strains such as HPV 16 and 18 bind p53 with substantially higher affinity than nononcogenic strains.[386] Unlike E1B and large T, which stabilize normal p53 and thus cause it to accumulate to high levels in infected cells, HPV-infected cells have low levels of p53. In vitro studies using p53 translated in reticulocyte lysates suggest that this is probably because E6 targets normal p53 for proteolytic degradation by the ubiquitin system.[332] If confirmed in vivo, this would be the first unambiguous demonstration of functional inactivation of a tumor-suppressor gene product by a viral oncogene product.

Further evidence for the functional importance of E6-mediated inactivation of p53 in HPV oncogenesis comes from analysis of cervical carcinomas. As discussed above, HPV is increasingly recognized as a major human pathogen. A high percentage of cervical carcinomas are associated with HPV[161]; these all invariably express E6 (as well as E7). If E6 is functionally important in transformation by HPV, and if this function includes inactivation of p53, then cervical carcinomas not associated with HPV infection would be expected to inactivate p53 by other means. Indeed, it appears that such tumors have p53 mutations. Conversely, p53 mutations would be superfluous in cervical carcinomas associated with oncogenic HPV. As predicted, such tumors have wild type p53.[57,58,331,396]

The potential clinical implications of these findings should not be underemphasized. Although developing an agent that would effectively mimic the function of a tumor-suppressor gene such as Rb or p53 is a formidable task, it may be considerably easier to develop a drug that antagonizes the E6 and/or E7 gene products. Such a drug would restore normal p53 and/or RB function to cervical cancer cells, since the actual p53 and Rb gene products would be expected to be normal in these tumors. The in vitro Rb and p53 reconstitution experiments described above (see The Retinoblastoma Gene and Normal p53 is a Tumor-Suppressor Gene) suggest that such pharmacological interventions might reasonably be expected to suppress the tumorigenicity of cervical carcinoma cells.

The finding that both Rb and p53 are complexed by the gene products of three distinct classes of DNA tumor viruses, the polyomaviruses, the adenoviruses, and the papillomaviruses, emphasizes the central importance of Rb and p53 in growth control of a wide variety of cell types. Since these viruses target both tumor-suppressor genes, it seems likely that Rb and p53 serve parallel functions in the cell, both of which must go awry before uncontrolled growth ensues. This dual requirement for Rb and p53 inactivation in vivo is remarkably similar to the requirement for both "*myc*-like" (E1A, mutant p53, other nuclear oncogenes) and *ras*-like (E1B) functions to transform primary REFs. Although it is probably unwise to push this analogy too far, these groupings of genes may provide a rough idea of the members of these parallel cellular pathways. Furthermore, it suggests that other viruses that have been implicated as carcinogens, for example hepatitis B virus and, perhaps, the Herpesvirus, may target other tumor-suppressor genes. Even if they do not, it seems likely that determining the mechanism(s) by which they do contribute to cancer may lead to important new insights into oncogenesis.

The Normal Function of p53: Perspectives

Normal p53 has been implicated in two separate cellular functions: control of DNA replication and transcription. These two roles need not be mutually exclusive; indeed, as discussed in detail above, a bifunctional role for p53 could help account for some apparently conflicting data.

The notion that p53 might be involved in DNA replication arose out of attempts to understand the large T/p53 interaction. In addition to its ability to bind tumor-suppressor gene products, large T also functions directly to promote SV40 viral replication. It binds to the SV40 origin and serves both as a helicase and to bind DNA polymerase α,[115] which is required for replication of SV40 viral DNA. Wild type, but not mutant, p53 blocks the ability of large T to bind DNA polymerase α,[115] blocks its helicase function,[381] and prevents its ability to stimulate SV40 DNA replication.[35,381] This is a general feature of p53 molecules from all species, including those which are permissive for SV40 replication. Together with the aforementioned absolute correlation between mutations of p53 and loss of its ability to bind large T-antigen, these findings suggested that the (a) function of normal p53 was to bind to cellular proteins with similar structural features to the p53-binding surface of large T, and with cognate functions in cellular DNA replication. An implication of such a model, given the growth suppressive actions of p53, was that p53's function in such a complex was to inhibit cellular DNA replication. Furthermore, since T-antigen binds DNA, it was inferred that the putative cellular protein(s) that bind p53 would bind DNA.

Recent findings suggest that the converse may actually be true. The laboratories of Carol Prives and Bert Vogelstein collaboratively were studying the ability of p53 to modulate T-antigen-binding to the SV40 origin of replication. To the surprise of these investigators, control experiments indicated that wild type (but not mutant) p53 was able to bind specifically to the GC boxes of the SV40 origin.[15,110] T-antigen interfered with p53's ability to bind to these sequences.[15] These data suggested that sequence-specific p53-binding to cellular DNA sequences might directly interfere with DNA replication. T-antigen might then serve to strip p53 away from sequences that inhibit viral DNA replication, which would help explain why p53-binding was selected for during the evolution of a lytic virus such as SV40.

Using a site-selection PCR approach, Vogelstein's laboratory independently demonstrated that p53 could bind to the specific DNA sequence TGCCT.[189] Intriguingly, this motif is not found within the GC boxes of the SV40 origin where p53 also binds.[15] All of the cellular sites thus far shown to bind p53 appear to be near replication origins, further supporting a role for p53 in DNA replication.

However, based on the presence of several stuctural features commonly found in transcription factors (acidic region, proline-rich region, potential amphipathic helix; see Fig. 5), and its ability to transactivate a reporter gene when fused to GAL4 (as discussed above), a role for p53 in transcriptional control has also been suggested. The p53 transactivation results must be interpreted with some caution, because the N-terminal acidic domain alone was found to be a strong trans-activator. Classic work by Mark Ptashne and his collaborators has shown that highly acidic surfaces ("acid blobs") alone can confer trans-activation ability to DNA-binding proteins.[241] It has been argued that a "nonspecific" effect of the acidic domain is not responsible for the transactivation activity of p53 because some p53 point mutations, which have no net change in charge, have completely lost transactivation ability, whereas others, also with no net change in charge, retain it.[97,306] However, this argument is not quite convincing, since these same point mutations are known to result in conformational changes global enough to affect ability to be recognized by various monoclonal antibodies; thus the acidic domain could simply be rendered inaccessible to the transcriptional apparatus in these mutants.

Nevertheless, the strength of the transactivation effect of p53—it is approximately as strong as the Herpesvirus VP16 protein, one of the most potent known transactivators—along with the demonstration of sequence-specific DNA-binding activity—mandates that a role for p53 in transcription be investigated seriously. If p53 does have a role in transcription, it probably helps stimulate expression of growth inhibitory genes and/or inhibits transcription of growth stimulatory genes. It remains to be seen whether p53-binding sites will also be found in the regulatory regions of growth regulatory genes, consistent with its postulated role as a transcription factor. In addition, it is not clear whether p53 acts by itself or in combination with another factor(s) to modulate transcription.

It will not be too surprising if p53 has roles in control of both replication and transcription. These roles may be exerted at slightly different stages of the cell cycle and/or by p53 molecules differing in extent and/or sites of phosphorylation. In this way, both kinases (casein kinase II and cdc2) that are thought to phosphorylate p53 may fine-tune p53 function. The possible roles of such fine-tuning in cell cycle control are obviously analogous to those discussed earlier for RB. In addition, the possible implications of mutants that distinguish between the two functions are intriguing. Since all mutants that lose suppressor activity lose DNA-[188] and large T-(see above) binding activity, it seems likely that these functions are linked. It certainly will be important to determine whether the apparent correlation between loss of transactivation ability and activation of transforming activity holds. Such studies are likely to be important not just for understanding the molecular details of p53 action, but may also affect prognosis in cancer patients bearing different p53 mutations in different cell types. Although p53 has been an enigma for quite some time—and in many ways still is—the next few years should bring rapid progress in unraveling its mysteries.

The Wilms' Tumor Gene

WT, also known as pediatric nephroblastoma, is a rare childhood embyonal kidney tumor, with an incidence of approximately 1:10,000 live births.[246] WT usually occurs in children <two years old and almost always before 10. Like retinoblastoma and other embryonal tumors, WT occurs in familial and sporadic forms. Familial WT displays autosomal dominant inheritance and is characterized by earlier onset (including presence of tumors at birth) and multiple, often bilateral tumors. The sporadic form, which is more common (>90%), presents as single tumors.

However, unlike retinoblastoma, which arises as a consequence of mutations at a single locus, the molecular genetics of WT are more complex. A small subset of WTs (<5%) occurs together with a variable number of associated developmental abnormalities,[246,255] including aniridia (absence of the iris of the eye), genitourinary abnormalities, and mental retardation; this constellation of abnormalities has been termed the WAGR syndrome (for Wilms' tumor, Aniridia, Genitourinary abnormalites, and mental Retardation). Aniridia itself occurs in familial and sporadic forms.[269] In addition to the association of familial aniridia with WT (usually as part of the WAGR syndrome), sporadic aniridia is associated with a high risk of developing WT, suggesting linkage between these two disorders.[269] However, it should be emphasized that familial and sporadic forms of WT can occur without any associated developmental defects.

Early cytogenetic studies by Francke and coworkers[106,311] revealed an association between aniridia and deletions of chromosomal region 11p13. These studies, which followed relatively soon after the association of retinoblastoma with deletion of 13q14, prompted a search for LOH on 11p. Several groups subsequently demonstrated that 11p LOH was, in fact, quite frequent in WT.[92,205,280,307] Studies using finer RFLP probes confirmed that 11p13 was a common region of allele loss in such tumors.[124,299,375] Taken in the context of the Rb model, these data suggested that a WT tumor-suppressor gene probably resided in 11p13, near a gene(s) required for normal development of the iris, the genitourinary tract, and the nervous system. The presence or absence of associated developmental abnormalities in patients with WT was thought to be dependent on the size of the lesion affecting the presumptive WT locus: large deletions would be more likely to involve nearby genes than small ones.

This simple model was called into question by later studies. In some WTs, LOH was demonstrated at 11p15,[148,204,308] whereas 11p13 markers remained heterozygous. This work suggested that the relevant tumor-suppressor gene in these tumors was at 11p15, not 11p13. Interestingly, 11p15 allele loss has also been found in a number of other malignancies, including breast[4] and bladder cancer[90] (Table 2). In addition, Beckwith-Wiedeman syndrome, a rare disorder associated with a number of embryonal malignancies including WT, adrenocortical carcinoma, hepatoblastoma, and embryonal rhabdosarcoma, has been mapped to 11p15.[204,206,294] Thus, there may be a tumor-suppressor gene at 11p15 whose inactivation can contribute to a wide variety of tumors besides WT. Other studies suggest the existence of a third WT locus: two groups have found that familial WTs that are not associated with WAGR display negative evidence for linkage (i.e., evidence that there is no linkage) to either 11p13 or 11p15 markers.[133,169]

The resolution of these conflicting data is not yet completely clear. It may be that loss of more than one tumor-suppressor gene locus is required for the development of WT. Perhaps, for example, loss of a gene at both 11p13 and 11p15, or 11p13 and the as yet unlocated familial WT locus, is required. The finding of a point mutation in the recently cloned 11p13 gene and LOH at 11p15 in the same tumor supports such a multiple gene model.[135] It does not seem likely that all three genes must be inactivated in all WTs. WT is not uncommonly present at birth; the occurrence of six genetic events (mutation plus LOH at three loci) in utero is hard to envision. Of course, such an occurrence could be imagined if the function of one of the three presumptive WT genes is to maintain chromosomal stability. In addition, it may be that one or more of these genes could function as dominant negatives; interestingly, in the aforementioned tumor with 11p15 LOH and WT-1 mutation, the 11p13 gene remained heterozygous. Alternatively, it may be that there are molecular genetic subtypes of WT, some of which arise from 11p13 mutation, some from 11p15, and some from a gene or genes unlinked to 11p. It will be interesting to see if these genes are all on a common growth or differentiation regulatory pathway; if they are, then mutation of any of them might be functionally equivalent. Finally, the "WT" produced by these different genetic alterations may, in fact, not be exactly the same disease, since it has been suggested[18,164] that tumors associated with 11p13 deletions (heterogeneous histology) can be distinguished histopathologically from those with 11p15 deletions (homogeneous histology).

With its recent molecular cloning and characterization, it is clear, however, that the 11p13 gene associated with WAGR is inactivated in at least a subset of WT. The cloning of this gene, termed WT-1, independently by two groups headed by D. Hausman[40,315] and G. Bruns,[120] respectively, was a true triumph of modern gene mapping techniques. The location and finally the cloning of WT-1 involved a long, laborious grind of RFLP mapping and chromosome walking. A key strategy employed was to use pulse field gel electrophoresis of irradiation-induced somatic cell hybrids[315] containing the WAGR region as its only human DNA against a hamster background to obtain a complete genetic map of the WAGR locus. This map allowed the WT gene to be delimited to a 350 kb region. Search of this region for evolutionarily conserved and transcribed regions led to the identification of the WT-1 gene. In addition, these mapping studies delineated the regions within which the genes for the associated developmental abnormalities of the WAGR syndrome reside. Although it was initially believed that the loci responsible for these various developmental abnormalities were separable from the WT-1 gene,[40,315] more recent evidence clearly indicates that WT-1 itself plays a role in normal genitourinary development.[283–285,300,374] The cloning of WT-1 has also led to the demonstration that another rare inherited disorder, Denys-Drash syndrome, which is characterized by severe developmental abnormalities of the urogenital system and increased risk of WT (but no aniridia or mental retardation), is also due to mutations in the WT-1 gene.[283]

WT-1 encodes an approximately 3.5 kb mRNA. The WT-1 gene itself is spread out over more than 50 kb. Recent studies have identified another transcriptional unit (confusingly termed WIT-1) closely linked to WT-1 and transcribed in the opposite direction to generate a 2.5 kb RNA.[164] It appears that these two genes are within a kilobase of each other, but they appear to be nonoverlapping. In normal tissues and nearly all WTs, they appear to be coordinately controlled. Sequence analysis of WIT-1 indicates only a small potential open reading frame. Whether WIT-1 actually encodes a protein or is a pseudogene remains to be determined. However, it has been suggested that its transcription may affect the level of WT-1 expression.[164]

Although it was considerably more difficult to identify WT-1 than other tumor-suppressor genes, pain and diligence were rewarded when analysis of WT-1 cDNAs immediately suggested its likely function. Unlike Rb and p53, which are ubiquitously expressed, WT-1 expression is strikingly restricted to a limited number of tissues. The highest level of WT-1 expression is found in embryonic kidney.[40] In mouse and baboon, but apparently not in humans, WT-1 RNA is found in adult kidney as well. Using in situ hybridization, WT-1 expression has been detected in the developing genitourinary system, including fetal testis and ovary, and the metanephric and mesonephric kidney.[285,300] The restricted tissue distribution of WT-1 suggests that its normal function may be to induce or control some aspect of normal genitourinary differentiation. It also suggests that mutations in WT-1, unlike those in Rb or p53, are unlikely to play a role in other malignancies.

The predicted protein sequence of WT-1 strongly suggested that it was a transcription factor.[40,120] There are four consecutive zinc fingers[198] at its C-terminus. WT-1 also has an upstream proline/glutamine-rich domain; in other transcription factors, such domains function in transcriptional activation or repression.[260] Intriguingly, the WT-1 zinc fingers share over 50% sequence identity with the EGR-1[361] and EGR-2[178] proteins, two transcription factors whose expression is highly induced when quiescent fibroblasts are stimulated by growth factors to enter the cell cycle. This homology is likely to be functionally significant, since recent experiments indicate that WT-1 and EGR-1 and -2 bind to the same recognition sequences.[304] This suggests a model in which WT-1 and EGR-1 and -2 affect transcription of a common set of genes. Since EGR-1 and -2 are early growth response genes,[178,361] whose function is presumably to help stimulate proliferation-associated genes, it is tempting to speculate that WT-1 antagonizes transcription of this same set of genes.

Strong evidence that WT-1 is, indeed, the gene involved in at least a subset of WTs has come from analysis of DNA and RNA of WT patients.[135,170,283,284,320,370] In patients with WT and known homozygous deletions, including submicroscopic deletions, of 11p13, there is complete absence of WT-1 expression. Some WTs without gross deletion of 11p13 markers also show absent or greatly decreased WT-1 expression. One such tumor was found to have a deletion of <11 kb completely contained within WT-1.[170] Although the majority of WT show normal levels of expression of WT-1 compared with age-matched, normal kidney, reverse transcription PCR analysis has indicated that at least some of these contain small deletions in WT-1 undetectable by Southern or Northern blotting. In one such tumor, one of the predicted zinc fingers was deleted.[135] Similarly, several independent point mutations have been found in WTs from patients with Denys-Drash syndrome.[283] Clearly, these mutations are functionally significant because the mutant proteins cannot bind to the WT/EGR recognition sequence.[283,304]

It seems clear that all WT associated with WAGR, as well as at least some other WTs, have mutations in WT-1. However, the overall frequency of WT-1 mutations in WT remains to be established. Moreover, conclusive proof of the biological significance of WT-1 mutations awaits its reintroduction into WT cells. Nevertheless, the vast and ever-emerging literature on the mechanism of action of transcription factors should promote rapid progress into the detailed mechanism of action of normal WT-1 and its perturbation in cancer.

The DCC Gene

Among the several consistent genetic abnormalities found in colorectal carcinomas are allelic deletions of 18q, which are found in more than 70% of cases.[377,378] This led to the suggestion that this region harbored a tumor-suppressor gene. Vogelstein and his colleagues identified a new gene that has several characteristics of such a gene,[94] which they termed DCC (for Deleted in Colon Carcinoma).

A panel of RFLP probes was used to localize the presumptive gene to 18q21-qter. No DNA rearrangements were noted in several known genes that map to this region. However, an anonymous probe detected a homozygous deletion in a colon cancer DNA. This same probe also detected an unusual event in another patient: the patient's normal DNA was homozygous with the RFLP probe; however, tumor DNA was heterozygous. In other words, the tumor displayed a "gain of heterozygosity mutation." When this region was cloned and sequenced, it was noticed that a possible consequence of the lost Msp 1 site was the creation of new potential splice donor site. This same probe detected allelic deletions in about 70% of colon carcinomas. The detection of independent somatic mutations, especially a potential point mutation, by a probe that also detected such a high frequency of allele loss strongly suggested that this probe was within the proposed DCC gene.

Proof that this was, in fact, the case required a herculean effort, involving a bidirectional chromosome walk spanning nearly 400 kbp, the cloning and sequencing of numerous genomic fragments that were highly conserved in other higher vertebrate species to detect potential exons, and, finally, a novel "exon-connection" strategy to obtain pieces of the DCC cDNA.[94] Ultimately, overlapping cDNA clones representing approximately 2.9 kb of contiguous sequence were obtained. These clones defined a large locus, perhaps a megabase in size. A 10 to 12 kb transcript was detectable only in brain poly(A) RNA. Using RNA based PCR, low levels of DCC transcripts were found in virtually all tissues examined, with highest levels in brain. The majority of colon cancers showed no detectable transcript even with the highly sensitive PCR assay. More importantly, Southern analysis revealed that about 10% of primary tumors and tumor xenografts in nude mice contained gross abnormalities in the DCC gene, including one example of a homozygous deletion involving the 5' end of the gene defined by the existing cDNA. The other novel fragments apparently all arose from insertions within a single intron, characterized by two unusual streches of long repeats of T-A. The functional significance of this region, and why it appears to be such a frequent target for mutation, are unclear. None of the insertions in this region could be cloned either in bacteriophage or plasmid or successfully amplified by PCR, suggesting some unusual DNA structure.

The high frequency of somatic mutation and its lack of expression in colon cancer are consistent with the identification of DCC as the 18q gene. Interestingly, as yet, no point mutations within the coding sequence of DCC have been found. It is not clear why DCC inactivation is accomplished most often by mutations that completely eliminate DCC RNA. It is also not clear whether DCC mutations occur in other types of malignancy, especially in other malignancies of gastrointestinal epithelia. Since DCC appears to be expressed in a variety of different tissues, it is possible that abnormalities in DCC may occur in other cancers.

Its predicted protein sequence suggests that DCC is a transmembrane protein, presumably on the plasma membrane. More importantly, its presumptive extracellular domain has strong similarity to sequence features of the cell-adhesion molecule (CAM) family, including four Ig repeats and a fibronectin type III domain. Overall, DCC has greatest sequence similarity to NCAM. Given the large body of evidence that intercellular interactions are perturbed in cancer, e.g., loss of contact inhibition, invasion, and metastasis, the discovery of a putative tumor-suppressor gene with sequence features of a CAM is of great interest.

The functional significance of this similarity has not yet been demonstrated, but it seems likely that DCC is somehow involved in cell surface interactions. If this is the case and if the level of DCC protein in cells reflects its extremely low mRNA level (detectable only by PCR), it seems very unlikely that DCC functions as a traditional CAM like NCAM. Such CAMs physically bind cells together by homotypic or heterotypic interactions. In order for these interactions to be physically significant, they must occur in reasonably large numbers; if DCC is present at the dimishingly low levels suggested by the level of its transcript, it is hard to see how it could meaningfully participate in adhesion per se. Instead, it seems most likely that DCC has co-opted the extracellular structural features of CAMs to serve as a signal-transducer (receptor) for some type of adhesion signal, either cell-cell or cell-extracellular matrix. Such a model would predict that DCC interacts with an intracellular catalytic subunit. Elucidating the molecular details of DCC action awaits the generation of appropriate immunological reagents capable of recognizing DCC and its potential partners in normal and neoplastic cells.

The Neurofibromatosis (NF-1) Gene

In 1882, von Recklinghausen described an autosomal recessive syndrome inherited at high frequency (1:3,000), characterized by a variety of abnormalities. These mainly affect tissues of neuro-ectodermal origin but also include widespread general effects such as dwarfism. The pathognomonic findings include multiple "cafe-au-lait" spots and variable numbers of neurofibromas.[6] Although neurofibromas are benign, affected patients have a high incidence of central nervous system tumors, including some malignancies. The cause of these symptoms remained undetermined for over a century. Recently, the combined contributions of cytogenetics, population genetics, and molecular biology have resulted in the isolation of a single large gene, NF-1, responsible for these abnormalities.[45,379] Very recent biochemical and genetic analysis of the protein encoded by this gene has helped establish a direct correlation between the NF-1 gene and the multiple disease phenotypes.[245,397]

As was earlier the case for the Rb and WT genes, initial determination of the approximate chromosomal localization of NF-1 on the long arm of chromosome 17 resulted from a combination of careful clinical and cytogenetic observations. Finer mapping placed the gene within a 600 kb segment on 17q11.[16] The serendipitous discovery that a putative murine c-*onc* gene *evi*-2 (initially discovered as a gene located at retroviral integration sites in murine lymphomas) mapped to this region[376] raised the possibility that NF-1 might be the human counterpart of *evi*-2. However, analysis of DNA from multiple NF-1 patients eliminated this possibility. Nevertheless, *evi*-2 served as a useful starting point to clone four additional genes in the region. Three of these were also eliminated as candidates for the elusive gene, since they were not consistently mutated in NF-1 patients.[45,379]

The fourth gene displayed several interesting properties. First, it was found to be deleted in many cases of NF-1. Some of these deletions were internal, consistent with it being the target of the larger deletions in other patients. Second, it encoded a very long transcript (13 kb). A cDNA of the transcript of this gene was cloned from both normal and affected individuals. Analysis by PCR and sequencing and/or by SSCP indicated that a significant percentage (about 10%) of NF-1 patients without gross structural rearrangement of NF-1 had subtle mutations within the small region of the gene subjected to initial analysis.[45,379] This high frequency of mutation made it highly likely that this was the gene for NF-1.

Remarkably, sequence analysis of the cDNA revealed that NF-1 encoded a protein highly similar to the mammalian and yeast *ras*-GTPase activating proteins (*ras*-GAP). GAPs, as their name implies, enhance the weak intrinsic GTPase activity of *ras* and other small G-proteins (see also Chapter 10).[137,392] Subsequent work demonstrated that NF-1 has GTPase activating protein activity for *ras* proteins.[11,245,397] Indeed, the in vitro GTPase activating protein activity of NF-1 for *ras* proteins is significantly higher than that of *ras*-GAP.[245] Moreover, expression of NF-1 (or *ras*-GAP) in S. *cerevesiae* can functionally complement mutations in the yeast genes IRA-1 and -2,[11,397] which themselves display GAP activity.

The reason for multiple GAPs for *ras* gene products is not yet clear. Both NF-1 and *ras*-GAP clearly coexist within all mammalian cells.[25,66,134] The majority of cellular ras-GAP is cytosolic, whereas NF-1 is predominantly membrane-bound.[66] It is not yet clear whether GAPs function solely to discharge activated ras proteins to their inactive state or, instead, themselves serve to transmit downstream signals; some evidence clearly supports a role for ras-GAP as a signal-transducer.[401] An intriguing possible model is that ras-GAP has a bifunctional role, both deactivating ras and sending a downstream signal, whereas NF-1 is just a ras-deactivator. Such a model would account for the demonstrable signaling activity of ras-GAP, the failure of ras-GAP to also be a gene for NF-1, and for the fact that loss of (a single copy of) NF-1 (with ras-GAP intact) results in neurofibroma generation. Of course, other explanations are also possible. Moreover, a simple model in which NF-1 serves as the primary ras deactivator would predict that patients with NF-1 type I should also have an increased risk of tumors that have been associated with activating *ras* gene mutations, such as pancreatic carcinoma, lung adenocarcinoma, and colon carcinoma (since NF-1 loss should be equivalent to ras activation). Although von Recklinghausen's disease is associated with increased risk of central nervous system (CNS) tumors, it is not known to be associated with the aforementioned epithelial tumors.

Regardless of the precise role of NF-1 in normal and neoplastic cell signaling, its identification and the characterization of its encoded protein has great potential value in the diagnosis and treatment of patients with NF-1. In addition, the similarity between the IRA gene products and NF-1 has suggested approaches to rapid enzymatic assays and screening methods for potential therapeutic agents.

Retinoic Acid Receptors as Tumor-Suppressor Genes: Acute Promyelocytic Leukemia and Other Malignancies

Nearly all cases of acute promyelocytic leukemia (APML) display a characteristic translocation between chromosomes 15 and 17. Among the leukemias, this disease is also remarkable because it shows a dramatic clinical response to retinoic acid (RA), the active form of Vitamin A.[166] APML patients treated with retinoic acid usually go into complete remission. More importantly, as opposed to conventional chemotherapeutic agents which work by selectively killing dividing cells, retinoic acid appears to induce remission in APML by inducing terminal differentiation of the malignant promyeloblasts.[382] Those APML patients that do not have 15;17 translocations fail to respond to retinoic acid.[256,382]

Recently, the connection between the 15;17 translocation and the retinoic acid responsiveness of APML has begun to be understood. The cloning and characterization of the translocation breakpoints and the genes that reside there, initially by deThe and Dejean,[51,70] and independently by several other groups[29,236,257] indicates that the chromosome 17 breakpoint is located within the retinoic acid receptor (RAR) α gene.

Retinoids (including vitamin A and its active derivative retinoic acid) exert profound effects on the growth and differentiation of nearly all cell types. Signaling by retinoic acid is, at least in large part, accomplished through the action of nuclear RARs, which are members of the steroid-thyroid hormone superfamily of ligand-specific transcription factors.[131] Ligand-binding to members of this gene family results in transcriptional activation of a variety of target genes; some of them also serve as specific repressors in the absence of ligand. There are three human RAR genes, termed RAR-α , RAR-β, and RAR-γ, each located on different chromosomes (17, 3, and 12, respectively). Each of these genes gives rise to multiple transcripts, due to alternative promoter usage and alternative splicing.[69] These transcripts encode several proteins from each gene, which differ at their N-termini. The alternative splice products are likely to have functionally distinct roles because the N-terminus in other members of the steroid-thyroid superfamily often functions to direct cell type and promoter-specific transcriptional activation.[69,131] Support for this notion comes from the high degree of evolutionary conservation of these alternative spliced forms.

Previous work had suggested that RAR-α gene played an important role in myeloid differentiation. Initial studies indicated that RAR-α was the only member of the RAR family expressed at detectable levels in myeloid cells.[118] The HL60 cell-line normally differentiates in response to retinoic acid in cell culture. HL60 mutants that failed to respond to retinoic acid had been isolated. When one of these mutants was examined in detail, it displayed defective nuclear-binding of retinoic acid.[54] Although the detailed status of the RAR-α gene and its protein product in this line was not reported, a retroviral construct directing the expression of RAR-α was able to restore retinoid responsiveness.[54] These data support the notion that the differentiation response to retinoic acid in myeloid cells is mediated by RAR-α.

The 15;17 translocation in APML results in the disruption of both RAR-α and a gene on chromosome 15, originally termed *myl*, but recently renamed PML. Two novel fusion proteins result.[62,182] The RAR-α N-terminus is replaced with sequences from the PML N-terminus. This results in a PML-RAR-α fusion protein. The reciprocal event generates an RAR-α-N-terminus-PML C-terminus fusion protein. It is not clear which of these fusion proteins, if not both, are required for leukemogenesis. Normal PML is expressed constitutively in myeloid cells and itself has interesting structural features, including three cysteine/histidine-rich regions resembling, but distinct from zinc fingers.[62,182] Similar domains have recently been recognized in several transcription factors. Thus the normal PML gene product may itself bind DNA and participate in modulating transcription. Alternatively, PML may normally participate in another process involving DNA-binding, since one of its cysteine/histidine-rich domains is most similar to the recombination gene RAG-1.[62,182]

The status of the unrearranged RAR-α and PML alleles, although grossly normal by Southern and Northern analysis, has not been established at the sequence level. It is therefore not clear whether RAR-α (or PML) should be viewed as a tumor-suppressor gene or a dominant oncogene. Indeed, these results pose something of a paradox. The ability of retinoids to induce differentiation appears to be restricted to APML, and within APMLs to those cases that have 15;17 translocations. It therefore appears as if *acquistion* of retinoid responsiveness correlates with disruption of RAR-α. This apparent gain-of-function suggests that the PML-RAR-α fusion protein may function as a dominant negative repressor at physiological levels of RA, interfering with the transcription of key retinoid-responsive genes required for normal myeloid differentiation. At higher, pharmacological levels of RA, this repression may be relieved, resulting in induction of differentiation. Recently, evidence consistent with such a model has been published by two groups.[62,182] This model is in many ways analogous to the actions of the v-*erb*A oncogene, which is essentially a dominant negative mutant of the thyroid hormone receptor-α.[60] For this reason, we have chosen to discuss RAR-α as a tumor-suppressor gene, even though its disruption in APML does not fit the classic two-hit Knudson model.

If RAR-α is a tumor-suppressor gene, then what of the other RARs? Although the jury is still out, it seems likely, based on the profound physiological effects of retinoids on both normal and neoplastic cells, that other RARs may be the target for mutations in other neoplasms. The possible involvement of the RAR beta (RAR-β) gene in human lung cancer has been examined in the author's laboratory,[119] and in the laboratories of Anton Jetten[270] and Ted Bradley.[159] Several features of the physiology of bronchial epithelial cells (the target cells in lung cancer) as well as the molecular biology of lung cancer suggest such involvement[119]: (1) Retinoic acid deficiency leads to squamous metaplasia, in which the normal mucociliary cells of the airway are replaced by squamous cells resembling those found in skin; (2) Bronchial squamous metaplasia is considered to be a preneoplastic lesion; (3) Most lung cancers and lung cancer cell-lines are resistant to the differentiating actions of retinoic acid; (4) A particularly important role for RAR-β in normal bronchial epithelial differentiation is suggested by a number of observations: (a) RAR-β is first expressed in developing lung concurrent with commencement of bronchial epithelial differentiation; (b) In adults, RAR-β is expressed at highest levels in bronchial epithelium, along with genitourinary and intestinal epithelium; and (c) RAR-β expression is induced by retinoic acid, with a time course consistent with its requirement for preventing squamous metaplasia and/or inducing mucociliary differentiation; and (5) Nearly all lung cancers have, as one of their many consistent genetic abnormalities, deletions of the short arm of chromosome 3 (Table 2). Although the precise boundaries of these deletions are somewhat controversial, and there may be more than one tumor-suppressor locus on 3p, several studies have suggested that the region 3p21–24 is involved. RAR-β has been mapped by in situ hybridization to 3p23–24.[248] Interestingly, 3p deletions in the same general region have also been found in several other epithelial malignancies, although it is by no means clear that these deletions all target the same loci.

In a study of a large number of tumor cell-lines and a smaller sample of primary tumors, frequent RAR-β expression abnormalities were observed.[119] Normally, RAR-β is expressed as two transcripts of 3.1 and 2.8 kb. These two transcripts probably represent at least two N-terminal isoforms of RAR-β.[36] The levels of both transcripts are markedly increased by treatment with retinoic acid.[119] Expression abnormalities in lung cancer include complete absence of RAR-β expression, even in the presence of pharmacological levels of retinoic acid in about one-third of cases, selective absence of the 2.8 kb transcript in 15% to 20%, and two examples of what is either selective loss of the 3.1 kb transcript or expression of a novel, truncated transcript. The remaining 40% of the cell-lines express widely varying levels of both RAR-β transcripts; the significance of these quantitative variations is uncertain. Quantitative differences in the expression of RAR-α and RAR-γ were also noted in these samples, although at much lower frequency. No cases of absent RAR-α or RAR-γ expression were observed.

Although it is clear that RAR-β expression abnormalities are frequent in lung cancer, and it seems likely that these abnormalities, perhaps in combination with abnormal expression of the other RARs, are responsible, at least in part, for the abnormal growth and differentiation found in lung cancer cells, the molecular basis of abnormal RAR expression is not yet understood. Southern analysis has revealed heterozygous rearrangements of RAR-β in a few cases.[119] In addition, abnormally high expression of RAR-α in one cell-line appears to correlate with (and presumably is due to) significant amplification of the RAR-α gene.[119] However, the majority of samples analyzed have no grossly detectable abnormality in their RAR genes. If RAR-β is the 3p tumor-suppressor gene in lung cancer (and there is a single 3p gene involved in all lung tumors), then one would expect that tumors that retain RAR-β expression would have mutations too small to be seen at the Southern or Northern blot level. However, analysis of four such tumors by RNA based PCR and sequencing the complete RAR-β coding region corresponding to the 3.1 kb transcript failed to reveal any such mutations.[119] It remains possible that these tumors contained mutations in the region of the 2.8 kb transcript(s) that differ from the 3.1 kb transcript (the N-terminus of the predicted protein), since the 2.8 kb transcript could not be analyzed with the available human reagents. Although this may seem unlikely, it bears repeating that it is this region of RAR-α that is disrupted in APML and which functions in cell type and promoter-specific transcriptional activation in other members of the steroid-thyroid hormone superfamily (see above).

Further studies are required to resolve the issue of whether RAR-β is itself a tumor-suppressor gene in lung cancer or whether its expression is deranged in *trans* as a consequence of mutations in other tumor-suppressor genes and/or dominant oncogenes. Since RAR-β is itself a retinoic acid-responsive gene, it is possible that mutations in other RARs are responsible for the abnormalities in RAR-β expression. These mutations would, in most cases, have to be small (point mutations, small deletions), since no gross abnormalities in other RAR genes were observed in Southern blots. Conceivably, some lung tumors have mutations in RAR-β, whereas others have mutations in other RARs. Such combinatorial abnormalities could account for the different histopathological subtypes observed.

Although no firm data is yet available, RARs are also good candidates for tumor-suppressor genes in other malignancies. A small study of RAR expression in cell-lines of squamous cell carcinomas of the head and neck compared with matched normal cells revealed absent (and uninducible) RAR-β expression in a significant proportion.[162] As in the lung cancer studies, the mechanism of altered expression is not clear: no gross rearrangements of the RAR-β gene were observed. The possibility that RAR-α may be involved in other malignancies is suggested by at least two findings. First, several malignancies, notably breast cancer and ovarian cancer, show LOH for 17q loci.[59,328] Second, recent studies have shown strong genetic linkage between familial breast cancer and 17q21 markers; these studies strongly suggest that a breast cancer tumor-suppressor gene is located at 17q21 which, coincidentally, is the location of RAR-α.[138] Since breast epithelium is known to be retinoid-responsive in vivo and in vitro,[337] detailed examination of the RAR-α gene in familial and sporadic breast cancer seems warranted. Interestingly, breast cancers also show frequent LOH for 3p alleles,[3] involving the same general region implicated in the development of lung cancer and other epithelial malignancies (3p14–24). Whether RAR-β is the gene targeted by these deletions also bears investigation.

Familial Adenomatous Polyposis and Other 5q Tumor-Suppressor Genes

Familial adenomatous polyposis (FAP), also known as familial polyposis *coli*, is a relatively common inherited cancer syndrome accounting for approximately 5% of all colon cancer. In addition, hereditary colon cancer without polyposis has been described; together these inherited syndromes account for up to 8% of colonic malignancies. Even more common than FAP are unlinked familial cancer syndromes not associated with polyposis, the so-called hereditary nonpolyposis colon cancer (HNPCC) syndromes.[240] Since colon cancer is the second most common malignancy in the United States, inherited colon cancer syndromes are the most common familial cancer syndromes, and thus a significant clinical problem.[249]

FAP and its allelic relative Gardner's syndrome, in which colonic polyps are associated with other tumors and systemic manifestations, are inherited as highly penetrant autosomal dominant traits. They are characterized by the development in the second to third decade of life of hundreds to thousands of adenomatous polyps throughout the colon. Each polyp is itself monoclonal,[91,377] presumably representing the outgrowth of different colonic epithelial stem cells. Adenomatous polyps are preneoplastic growths. The sheer number of premalignant polyps in FAP patients virtually ensures that the requisite secondary events necessary for progression to carcinoma will occur in one or more polyps. Accordingly, unrecognized or untreated patients almost inevitably develop colon cancer by their third to fifth decade.

The FAP gene was localized to 5q (5q21–22), initially by fortuitous cytogenetic observations,[149] followed by linkage analysis with 5q markers.[23,223] The FAP gene, and/or a closely linked locus is also involved in sporadic colon carcinomas. LOH of 5q alleles in the region of the FAP gene has been detected in 30% to 50% of sporadic colonic adenomas and carcinomas.[5,93,327,347,377,378] LOH is *not* observed in FAP adenomas.[93,327,347,377,378] This suggests that heterozygous FAP mutation is sufficient to contribute to the genesis of colonic adenomas. In this context, it is not clear whether the FAP mutation acts as a dominant negative, by analogous mechanisms to those suggested for p53, or whether gene dosage at the FAP locus is critically important. Since sporadic adenomas show LOH at the FAP locus,[93,377] the latter mechanism is more likely. This conclusion has received support from molecular analyses of the mutations present in the recently cloned gene for FAP, which suggest loss of function (see below). Nevertheless, loss of both FAP alleles does appear to provide a selective advantage over a single FAP mutation, since colon carcinomas arising in FAP patients often display 5q LOH.[24,94,276,327,377,378]

Two 5q genes that may play a role in colon carcinogenesis have recently been cloned. The first of these, termed MCC (for Mutated in Colon Carcinoma), was identified by searching for transcribed sequences mapping to the 5q21 region with a cosmid that detected a rearranged restriction fragment in a colonic tumor.[193] Cloning of overlapping cDNAs, representing 4.1 kb of contiguous nucleotide sequence, revealed an open reading frame capable of encoding an 829 amino acid protein that has a small region of sequence similarity to the G-protein-coupled muscarinic receptor. This sequence similarity, though weak, is interesting because it occurs in a region of the muscarinic receptor conserved in evolution and demonstrated by mutagenesis studies to be functionally important. The coding region of the MCC gene was found to be disrupted in the tumor with the large rearrangement. More importantly, somatically acquired point mutations were found in two other tumors out of a screen of 100 tumors analyzed by PCR and RNase protection of four exons. Because only a few exons were screened, this could represent a substantial underestimate of the true frequency of mutation in MCC in colon cancer.

However, at present, the significance of this gene in colon carcinogenesis is unclear. All of the detected mutations, including the large rearrangement, were apparently heterozygous, and one of the two point mutations predicts a highly conservative substitution. Since these are heterozygous mutations, MCC conceivably could function as an oncogene, rather than a tumor-suppressor gene. MCC was originally believed to be a candidate FAP gene, but with the recent cloning of adenomatous polyposis coli (APC) (see below), it now seems clear that if MCC is involved in colon carcinogenesis, it represents a second 5q locus that is targeted mainly in sporadic colon cancer. No germ-line mutations have been found in MCC,[273] arguing against it being a second FAP gene, although the entire MCC gene has not been analyzed in all FAP patients. Nevertheless, the high frequency of somatic mutation in MCC in colon cancer argues for its involvement in at least a subset of colon cancers.

Two groups, one headed by Bert Vogelstein and Yusuke Nakamura[192,273] and the other by Ray White[132,179] have recently reported the cloning and identification of the gene for FAP. The

Vogelstein group used MCC as a starting point and screened approximately four megabases of contiguous sequence for candidate transcribed sequences. The White group used pulse field gel analysis of the APC region to define a common region of deletion in two independent FAP patients with large (100 kb and 260 kb, respectively) deletions in the APC locus, and searched for mutations within the three candidate genes that map to this common region of deletion. Both groups identified the same gene, termed APC, and found that it is mutated in the somatic tissue of a number of patients with either FAP or Gardner's syndrome. Analysis of multiple exon-intron boundaries by PCR-RNase protection[273] or SSCP (single strand conformational polymorphism) analysis,[132] followed by DNA sequencing, revealed that these mutations included nonsense and missense mutations, small deletions, and splice site mutations. These mutations were not found in a large screen of unaffected individuals. More importantly, the mutations exactly cosegregated with the disease phenotype in APC families, arguing against their being mere sequence variants. Further proof was provided by the study of a patient who apparently developed FAP de novo. The patient's parents had no detectable abnoramality of the APC gene, nor did the patient's wife. On the other hand, the patient had a 2 bp deletion in one APC allele, which was then transmitted to two of his children.[132] The obvious prediction is that these children, but not the patient's third child who inherited the wild type allele, will develop FAP.

Interestingly, a patient with Gardner's syndrome and an FAP patient without extracolonic manifestations were found to have identical point mutations in APC.[273] This suggests that the extracolonic features unique to Gardner's syndrome are either epigenetically determined or determined genetically by a locus other than APC (epistasis). A caveat to this interpretation must be raised, however. Since the entire APC gene was not sequenced in these two patients, it remains theoretically possible that another (second site) mutation exists in the Gardner's syndrome patient elsewhere in APC.

Both nonsense and missense APC mutations were also detected in several sporadic colon cancers.[273] Comparison of the APC sequence in the normal tissue of these individuals indicated that the mutations were somatically acquired. Taken together, this constitutes strong evidence that APC is the gene for FAP and its relative, Gardner's syndrome. Moreover, it suggests that the same gene is also targeted in at least some sporadic tumors. It will be interesting to see if mildly defective alleles of APC are associated with some HNPCC syndromes.

It is even possible that some apparently "sporadic" colon cancers will also occur in patients with mild constitutional APC mutations. This would be interesting in view of epidemiologic data that suggest that all colon cancer is inherited.[39,41] Even if this is true, however, it seems clear that constitutional APC mutations do not occur in all cases of sporadic colon cancer, since the data of Vogelstein and White clearly establish that at least some APC mutations are somatically acquired.

Overlapping cDNA clones allowed the construction of a near full-length clone for the large (9.5 kb) transcript corresponding to the APC gene.[179,192] The White group noted that alternative splicing occurs within exon 9, resulting in a protein's differing by 101 amino acids.[132] Interestingly, both splice isoforms of APC appear to be expressed in all tissues tested, although the reverse transcription-PCR analysis used would not be expected to provide accurate quantitation of relative expression. Expression in extracolonic tissues would be expected given that Gardner's syndrome and FAP can result from the same mutation. It will be interesting to see if APC expression patterns are the same in these two classes of patients.

Sequence analysis of APC revealed a long open reading frame predicting a protein of approximately 300 kd. The predicted APC protein shows no strong similarity to any protein in the data base. Interestingly, it is mildly similar to MCC. APC also shows some degree of relatedness to intermediate filament proteins and myosins, but the functional significance of this similarity is unclear. The absence of any apparent signal sequence or transmembrane domain suggests that APC is a cytoplasmic or nuclear protein. Both APC and MCC have sequence features suggesting the ability to form coiled-coils; hence the possibility of oligomerization exists. Such a possibility is of course intriguing, in view of the prediction, discussed above, that heterozygous mutation in the gene for FAP should be sufficient to promote polyp formation. The ability of a mutant APC protein to oligomerize with its normal counterpart, or potentially with MCC, conceivably could lead to inactivation of normal APC function via a dominant negative mechanism. However, it is difficult to understand how nonsense and/or frameshift mutants, some of which map to the domains likely to mediate oligomerization, could be effective dominant negatives. Overall, molecular analyses of APC mutations are more consistent with loss of function. A final, tantalizing possibility, based solely on the predicted molecular weight of APC and its presumed ability to mediate protein-protein interactions, is that APC could be the 300 kd E1A-associated protein.

The cloning of the APC gene is exciting not just because its analysis promises new insights into basic mechanisms of colon carcinogenesis. For the first time, the gene for a major familial cancer syndrome has been cloned. Reagents derived from APC should be available soon for prenatal and antenatal diagnosis. This should spare many patients the discomfort associated with colonoscopic screening. More importantly, since 5q mutations, presumably in either APC or MCC, are among the earliest events in colon carcinogenesis (see below), the design of drugs that antagonize the effects of these mutations could provide valuable chemopreventative agents.

Suppression of Angiogenesis and Metastasis

An alternative approach to identifying genes that suppress malignancy is to "work backwards" from the functional consequences of malignancy to the responsible genetic alterations. The most fruitful of these studies have focused on two characteristic features of most malignancies: their ability to promote their own vascularization (angiogenesis) and their ability to invade and metastasize to distant sites. Although deranged growth control may be the sine qua non of cancer, acquisition of angiogenic capacity is required for the growth of tumors to any significant size, and nearly all cancers kill because of their ability to metastasize to other organs. Two different lines of investigation have identified novel gene products whose absence promotes either angiogenesis or metastasis. This subject has recently been extensively reviewed[235] and will be considered only briefly here.

There is controversy over whether genes of this type should be viewed as tumor-suppressor genes. Instead, they have been alternatively termed "angiogenesis suppressors" or "metastasis suppressors." The normal function of "metastasis suppressor" genes certainly is not to prevent metastasis, since under normal physiological conditions, metastasis, a pathological disorder, should not have to be prevented. Moreover, it is clear that mutations in dominant oncogenes and/or tumor-suppressor genes can lead to altered angiogenic and/or metastatic capabilities.

Noel Bouck and her colleagues have devoted considerable effort towards understanding chemically induced transformation of BHK cells. Coordinate suppression of several parameters of transformation occurs when these cells are fused to either normal BHK cells or to normal human fibroblasts.[32–34] Cytogenetic studies of transformed segregants of the the human x BHK hybrids have established that the suppressing activity resides on human chromosome 1.[34,357]

In attempting to understand the mechanism by which normal cells suppress tumorigenicity of the transformed cells, these workers discovered that normal cells and suppressed hybrids secreted a potent angiogenesis inhibitor.[303] They purified this inhibitor and, in subsequent work, identified it as the hamster homologue of thrombospondin, a platelet and extracellular matrix protein of previously unknown function.[130] Thrombospondin itself is not the tumor-suppressor gene resident on chromosome 1, since it maps to human chromosome 15.[130] However, since there is an absolute correlation between tumor suppression and expression of thrombospondin, it seems likely that thrombospondin gene expression is under the control (directly or indirectly) of the chromosome 1 tumor-suppressor gene. This strong correlation between suppression of tumorigenicity and thrombospondin synthesis also indicates, at least in this system, that some tumor-suppressor genes may function to prevent neovascularization. Other genes may be controlled by the chromosome 1 tumor-suppressor gene in a manner identical to thrombospondin, so it should not be inferred from these studies that suppression of angiogenic capability is the only important function of this tumor-suppressor gene. Nevertheless, these studies suggest that defining the mechanism of differential control of thrombospondin expression in normal and transformed cells could lead to the identification of the chromosome 1 tumor-suppressor. Since several regions of chromosome 1 have been proposed to harbor tumor-suppressor genes (see Tables 1 and 2), such studies may have applications beyond the BHK cell system.

Patricia Steeg, Lance Liotta, and their colleagues have identified a novel gene that appears to functionally suppress metastasis. Using differential hybridization of cDNA libraries, they looked for genes that were expressed in derivatives of a murine melanoma cell-line with low metastatic potential but not expressed, or expressed at substantially lower levels, in clonal relatives with high metastatic potential.[355] A key feature of their approach was the availability of several clonal derivatives of the same original melanoma line that differed in metastatic potential. The common origin of these lines reduced the likelihood that differences in gene expression would be due to cell-line differences. The gene they isolated, termed *nm23*, was not only found to be expressed at markedly lower levels in the melanoma lines with high metastatic potential,[355] but decreased or absent *nm23* expression subsequently was shown to correlate well with increased likelihood of metastasis in several other experimental systems,[316] as well as in some human tumors.[20,147] When *nm23* is reexpressed in cell-lines with high metastatic capability, metastatic ability is markedly depressed, supporting a direct role for *nm23* involvement in metastasis suppression.[221]

The sequence of *nm23* revealed strong resemblance to the *Drosophila* gene, *awd*.[316] The degree of sequence similarity is so great that it is virtually certain that *nm23* is the mammalian homologue of *awd*. Mutations in *nm23/awd* lead to pleiotropic abnormalities in the postembryonic fly, including abnormalities of wing, leg, brain, eye, and gonadal function.[63] The disordered development observed is not inconsistent with the disruption of intercellular boundaries seen in metastasis.

More recently, information on the mechanism of *nm23/awd* action has come from another direction. Several groups have obtained cDNA clones from various species for nucleoside diphosphate (NDP) kinases, enzymes whose function is to catalyze the phosphorylation of nucleoside diphosphates to nucleotide triphosphates. Sequence analysis of these cDNA clones demonstrated strong similarity to *nm23/awd*[191,380]; indeed direct demonstration of *awd* NDP kinase enzymatic activity has been obtained.[21] Proposed cellular roles for such enzymes include involvement in control of microtubule polymerization and modulation of G protein activity.[234] How mutations in or absence of an NDP kinase might lead to the multiple abnormalities seen in *awd* flies or the deranged cell-cell interactions found in metastasis is unclear and obviously will be the focus of future work. In addition, since NDP kinases constitute a heterogeneous family of enzymes,[234,235] it will be interesting to study the effects of other members of the family on metastasis.

The *nm23/awd* gene has been mapped by both somatic cell hybrid analysis and in situ hybridization to 17q22. Significant LOH encompassing this locus has been found in several human tumors.[222] One metastatic tumor had homozygous deletion of *nm23/awd*. However, rigorous demonstration that *nm23/awd* is the target for these chromosomal abnormalities (e.g., by finding point mutations or small deletions affecting only *nm23/awd*) has not yet been reported. Moreover, decreased *nm23/awd* expression is not universally associated with more agressive human tumors; in colon cancer, for example, there is no correlation between *nm23/awd* expression and metastatic potential.[146] Thus, it is not yet completely clear whether *nm23/awd* should be viewed as the metastasis analogue of a tumor-suppressor gene or is better characterized as an "effector" gene. Nevertheless, the isolation of *nm23/awd* and the identification of its biochemical activity have provided new insights into the molecular biology of metastasis.

Putting It All Together: Oncogenes and Tumor-Suppressor Genes in Human Cancer

Over the past six years, Bert Vogelstein and his colleague have carried out an extraordinary series of studies aimed at elucidating the detailed molecular basis of colon carcinogenesis.[93] These studies have identified multiple genetic events, including activation of a dominant oncogene (*ras*), and inactivation of multiple tumor-suppressor genes, including p53, DCC, and one or more genes on 5q (FAP, MCC). Together, these studies approach a complete molecular description of a major carcinoma. Moreover, they have provided a general theoretical framework for the analysis of other common solid tumors.

The main experimental advantage of analyzing colonic carcinogenesis, so presciently realized by Vogelstein, is that it proceeds through a macroscopically recognizable series of well-defined intermediate events. This, plus the accessibility of the colonic epithelium via endoscopy provided adequate material from each of the steps in colon carcinogenesis from small adenomatous polyp to larger polyp to carcinoma in situ to frank invasive carcinoma. Since solid tumors are often heavily contaminated with stromal and/or inflammatory cells, complicating the analysis of genetic changes specific for the tumor cells, a key innovation was the use of cryostat sectioning to select regions of tumors enriched for neoplastic cells.

A number of general principles have been established. First, all of the events from adenoma onward occur in clonal populations of cells. Studies of foci of carcinoma arising within adenomas revealed that the carcinomas contained all of the genetic changes present in the adenomas. In addition, carcinomas had sustained further mutations. This established unambiguously that carcinomas arise directly from adenomas, a point of previous dispute. Second, cancer appears to result from the *accumulation* of mutational events in both dominant oncogenes and tumor-suppressor genes; there may also be contributory epigenetic events.

Polyp generation usually involves mutations at the APC locus, and possibly the MCC locus. In FAP patients, mutation at APC is inherited, accounting for their high rate of polyp generation. However, since FAP patients have intervening nonpolypoid epithelium there may be another requisite event, as yet unidentified, for polyp generation. As discussed above, the unaffected APC allele does not appear to be lost in FAP adenomas (although it *is* lost in *carcinomas* arising in FAP patients—see above). In sporadic colon cancer, LOH for the 5q region harboring APC (and MCC) presumably is functionally equivalent to inherited APC mutation.

Mutation of 5q gene(s) is followed by hypomethylation of approximately one third of the genome.[95,128] Whether hypomethylation is induced by the FAP mutation itself, by an as yet undefined mutation(s), perhaps in some component of the methylation apparatus, or is epigenetic is not known. However, the consequences of global hypomethylation are likely to be substantial. Demethylation is correlated with a change from transcriptionally inactive to active chromatin. Thus the transcriptional program of hypomethylated adenoma cells is likely to be dramatically different from that of normal colonic epithelium. In addition, demethylation is clastogenic and thus might predispose adenomas to further genetic changes.[333] In particular, events such as nondisjunction, which could then induce LOH, might be promoted.

The conversion between small adenomas and larger adenomas is accompanied by, and presumably caused by, mutations in a *ras* oncogene (nearly always Ki-*ras*), in about 50% of cases.[30,103,377] The mechanism by which large adenomas develop in the remaining 50% of cases is not known. An obvious possibility is that other proteins that help mediate *ras* signal-transduction, e.g., GTPase activating protein, NF-1, or perhaps upstream mediators of *ras* action, such as GTP-GDP exhange proteins, are the targets for mutation in these tumors. Presumably *ras* mutation gives a proliferative advantage to adenoma cells, allowing clonal expansion.

Conversion to malignancy is associated with the loss of at least two tumor-suppressor genes, the aforementioned p53 and DCC genes, located on 17p and 18q, respectively. Loss of 18q tends to occur in earlier stages of tumor progression than 17p LOH. However, the four genetic changes, 5q mutation, *ras* mutation, loss of 17p, and loss of 18q, are probably not sufficient for development of carcinoma, since large but nonmalignant adenomas that have all of these changes have been found.[377,378] In addition to these consistent changes, colonic carcinomas average two to three additional allelic losses (for an average of four to five allelic losses per tumor). Unlike the 17p and 18q allelic losses, which occur in 75% or more of tumors, the other allelic losses are spread throughout the genome, although certain regions (1q, 4p, 6p and q, 8p, 9q, and 22q) are targeted more frequently.[378] Although these additional losses could be epiphenomena due to the increased genomic instability of tumors, it is interesting that several of these same regions have been implicated as potential tumor-suppressor loci in other malignancies (Tables 1 and 2). It seems reasonable that genes within some of these regions are, in fact, tumor-suppressor genes, and their loss leads to progression to colon carcinoma. If this is the case, then at least some of the biological variability observed between different colonic tumors may be due to these later genetic events. For example, the invasive and metastatic capabilities of a tumor may vary depending on which additional (progression) events occur after the central four. The total number of genetic events predicted by the Vogelstein model to be necessary for carcinoma development is remarkably consistent with predictions based on the age-related increased incidence of colon cancer.[73,93,288]

Although statistically, the events associated with and presumably leading to colon carcinogenesis tend to occur in the order 5q (APC, MCC) mutation → hypomethylation → *ras* mutation → DCC mutation → p53 mutation → other mutation(s), this order is by no means fixed. Some adenomas have 17p allelic losses, but no *ras* mutations, and in others 18q deletions have preceded *ras* mutations. It appears that the combination of genetic events, rather than the order, is critical to the development of cancer. This is consistent with the existence of redundant growth control pathways in the cell, most or all of which must be perturbed before decontrolled growth results. It is also strikingly reminiscent of the requirement for DNA tumor viral oncoproteins to inactivate multiple suppressor gene products to promote malignant transformation.

The reason why the events tend to occur in a certain order may be due to the relative mutability of the different genes, which may in turn depend on the type of carcinogen. The order of subsequent events may depend in part on the initial events. For example, hypomethylation may be more likely to lead to nondisjunction events in some chromosomes rather than others (see also Perspectives and a Look to the Future).

Although the model discussed above accounts for most colon cancers, there are a few exceptions that do not appear to fit the general scheme. For example, a small number of carcinomas have been found to contain one or fewer mutations of the analyzed loci.[93,377] It could be that these cancers are not the same disease as the vast majority of those tumors which do fit the model, in much the same way in which chronic myelogenous leukemia without Philadelphia chromosome behaves differently clinically than Philadelphia chromosome-positive CML, and APML with and without the 15;17 translocation behave differently. However, since each of the proposed target genes in colon cancer has not been analyzed down to the nucleotide level in each tumor, it may be that the apparent "exceptions" just represent unusual mutations (for example, *ras* mutations at sites other than positions 12, 13, or 61, or p53 mutations outside the four conserved regions).

The power of the Vogelstein model is enhanced by its ability to predict prognosis and its implications for diagnosis and therapy. Clinical course correlates with the number of genetic events found in the tumors; those patients with more than four changes have a worse prognosis than those with fewer.[187] The elucidation of the key events in colon carcinogenesis offers the hope of developing a molecular exfoliative cytology approach to colon cancer screening. The feasibility of such an approach for detecting p53 mutations in bladder cancer by PCR of urine samples[343] suggested that similar methods could be applied to stool samples. Screening for Ki-*ras* mutations, which usually occur early in the carcinogenic process and can be detected easily by oligonucleotide hybridization panels, may be a particularly useful application of such technology. Indeed, *ras* mutations have recently been detected in the stool of patients with potentially curable colon tumors.[342] If all colon cancer has a genetic component, it is likely that different germ-line mutations in the genes key to colon cancer development will be responsible, suggesting that antemorbid molecular screening is a realistic possibility. Since colon cancer is curable if surgically excised early in its course, and has a dismal prognosis regardless of therapy if discovered late, the successful development of such techniques may have a dramatic impact on the natural history of this major human cancer.

Obviously, the long-range hope and promise of discovering the key cellular targets for mutation in colon cancer is the development of specific pharmacological agents designed to reverse the effects of these mutations. Although this goal is likely to take longer than successful diagnostic applications, Vogelstein has recently pointed out how the structure of the MCC and APC genes may be help explain the mechanism by which Sulindac, an antiinflammatory drug which inhibits cyclooxygenase, antagonizes the growth of polyps in patients with FAP.[192]

As important as these discoveries are in explaining colon carcinogenesis, of even greater importance is their implication for carcinogenesis in general. The general scheme, that cancer is the result of the progressive accumulation of mutations in a small number (4 to 6) of dominant oncogenes and tumor-suppressor genes, appears to hold for a number of other solid tumors. For example, studies of small-cell carcinoma of the lung have revealed that p53 and Rb mutations are nearly always present, along with deletions on chromosome 3p. Moreover, amplification of various members of the *myc* family of oncogenes is found in a subset of such tumors, although the occurrence of *myc* mutations may, at least in part, be due to chemotherapy.[96] Nonsmall-cell lung cancer also has consistent p53 mutations, as well as a significant, albeit lower, percentage of Rb mutations, and nearly universal 3p deletions. In addition, adenocarcinomas of the lung (a type of nonsmall lung cell cancer), as well as all pancreatic carcinomas, are associated with a high frequency of Ki-*ras* mutations.[96] Similarly, multiple, progressive changes in tumor-suppressor genes and oncogenes have been demonstrated in common malignancies such as breast cancer and brain tumors.

Proposed and Candidate Tumor-Suppressor Genes

A few groups have attempted to identify "tumor-suppressor" genes by directly screening for genes with the ability to suppress transformation by viral oncogenes. Such genes, if obtained, may be "pharmacological" suppressors; e.g., genes that normally play no direct role in negative growth control or even in regulation of the cellular counterpart of the oncogene being tested, but which, expresssed at inappropriately high levels, can antagonize oncogene actions. These genes, while interesting in their own right, clearly do not fall into the same category as genes such as p53, Rb, etc.

M. Noda and his colleagues have taken such an approach to isolate a gene that has weak "suppressing" activity for v-Ki-*ras*.[194,274] They prepared an expression cDNA library from normal human fibroblasts and introduced this library en masse into DT cells, which are transformed NIH3T3 cells bearing two copies of the Kirsten sarcoma virus provirus. Multiple independent revertant clones, derived from distinct transfected cDNAs, were obtained[274]; one of these, named K-*rev*-1, was recovered as a full-length cDNA and characterized in detail.[194] Sequence analysis revealed that K-*rev*-1 is a relative of the *ras* family of small G proteins and is identical to the *rap*-1 gene independently cloned by other investigators on the basis of its *ras* homology.

The biological activity of K-*rev*-1 as a "suppressor" of *ras* transformation is weak. Fewer than 5% of DT cells receiving K-*rev*-1 expression plasmids actually revert, although Noda and his colleagues report "partial reversion" in up to 30%. The authors have argued that reversion correlates with, and presumably requires, a very high level of K-*rev*-1 expression. Close examination of the K-*rev*-1 expression levels indicates that if this idea is correct, there must be a marked threshold effect, since the difference in K-*rev*-1 expression levels between some "partial revertants" and "revertants" is minimal. In general, there seems to be a rough correlation between reversion and high levels of K-*rev*-1 expression, but other genetic or epigenetic changes in addition to K-*rev*-1 overexpression may be required to fully revert DT cells.

The resemblance of K-*rev*-1 to *ras* genes suggested a model in which K-*rev*-1 competes with *ras* for key effector molecules. Consistent with this notion, K-*rev*-1 can bind ras-GAP. Interestingly, the affinity of K-*rev*-1 for ras-GAP is substantially higher (about $10\times$) than the affinity of *ras* for ras-GAP.[109] There are two potential problems with this model. First, it requires that ras-GAP be a downstream effector of *ras*; whether ras-GAP has any downstream effector function is a subject of some controversy.[137,392] Second, if the affinity of K-*rev*-1 for ras-GAP is so much higher than *ras* for ras-GAP, then why is overexpression of K-*rev*-1 required to induce reversion? One possible resolution to this problem would be if K-*rev*-1 is not normally located in the proper place in the cell to interact with ras-GAP. In that case, it is possible that overexpression would lead to "spillover" of K-*rev*-1 into a compartment in which it could compete for ras-GAP-binding.

Regardless of the mechanism by which K-*rev*-1 antagonizes *ras* transformation in vitro, the requirement for such high levels of expression to see this effect makes it unlikely that K-*rev*-1 is a physiological antagonist of *ras*. It remains possible that K-*rev*-1 may itself play a role in normal growth control, but the emerging literature on the protean functions of small G-proteins makes it equally likely that it plays some other role in cellular physiology. As yet, there is no evidence for K-*rev*-1 mutation in any human tumor, and based on the analysis above, it seems unlikely that such a role will be found.

A similar approach to identifying genes with *ras* suppressor activity was taken by Schaefer and colleagues.[330] These workers transfected total human DNA into a ras-transformed rat cell-line and screened for flat revertants. Using successive rounds of transfection and cloning of human DNA by probing with human highly repetitive DNA (Alu repeats), they obtained a piece of genomic DNA with apparently high reversion-inducing activity. Although the apparent potency of this clone makes it potentially of great interest, there has been no subsequent report from this group identifying a gene(s) associated with the initial cloned DNA, so its significance remains unclear.

The existence of dominant revertants of ras-transformed cells has suggested a different, but complementary approach. These revertants presumably have undergone a mutation in a gene or genes that can antagonize ras action. Moreover, since they are dominant revertants, inactivation of the gene(s) responsible for reversion should lead to a return to the transformed state (retransformation). If inactivation could be attained by insertion of a molecular tag into the putative suppressor gene, then it should be possible to recover the gene of interest using the molecular tag. In prokaryotes and lower eukaryotes, such an approach, termed insertional mutagenesis, has been employed with great success using transposable elements (transposon tagging), including retrotransposons.

Retroviruses provide a potential mutagen for application of this approach to higher eukaryotes. An attempt has been made to use this approach to identify gene(s) that suppress Ki-ras in dominant revertants (F2 cells) of the DT line described above. F2 cells retain the two copies of the KiSV provirus, which are biologically active in transfection assays and express apparently normal levels of v-Ki-ras RNA and protein. Nevertheless, these cells display flat morphology and fail to grow in soft agar or to form tumors in nude mice.[275] Using retroviral insertional mutagenesis, our laboratory has identified a number of retransformants bearing integrated retroviral genomes. One of these retransformants has been characterized in some detail (D. Simmons and B. Neel, unpublished observations). The integration site in this clone identifies a novel locus that has several properties consistent with its involvement in reversion. Sequence analysis of this gene, which has been named skr-1, predicts a 130 kd protein with a domain at the N-terminus that is very likely to form a leucine zipper and a markedly hydrophilic C-terminus, but no other obvious structural features or similarities to other proteins in the data base. Multiple attempts to stably express this gene in higher cells have been unsuccessful, suggesting that it may be growth inhibitory. However, recent experiments suggest that transient overexpression of skr-1 may inhibit the ability of ras to activate the c-fos gene (U. Lorenz and B. Neel, unpublished observations). If confirmed, it will be interesting to determine how this inhibition is mediated and whether skr-1 is a target for mutational inactivation in tumor cells.

A related approach to the identification of genes that negatively affect cell growth involves the study of senescence.[129] When normal human fibroblasts are serially passaged in culture, they reproducibly lose proliferative capability at approximately the same passage number. Somatic cell hybrid studies have indicated that senescence most often behaves as a dominant trait, and at least four complementation groups for senescence have been identified.[287] Recently, microtransfer of a single chromosome (human chromosome 1) has been shown to confer senescence, suggesting that at least one of these "senescence" genes resides on chromosome 1.[360] Moreover, microinjection of poly(A) RNA from senescent cells has been reported to induce growth arrest in normal fibroblasts.[239] Despite dilution experiments, which argue that the senescence-inducing RNA should be relatively abundant, this RNA has not yet been molecularly cloned.

Although many tumor cells appear to be immortal (i.e., to have lost their capacity for senescence) in vivo, it is not at all clear that immortalization is necessary for oncogenesis. Many tumors cannot be easily established either as immortal cell-lines in culture or as successful xenografts in immunodeficient mice. Although it is difficult to be sure that these failures are not simply technical, it seems equally likely that at least some tumor cells are not immortalized. There is clear evidence for this in some experimental systems. For example, primary cells transformed by Rous sarcoma virus (RSV) and other oncogenic retroviruses are fully capable of forming a large tumor that kills its host, but the cells derived from these tumors will exhibit senescence in tissue culture at around the same passage as normal, uninfected cells (T. Martins and B. Neel, unpublished observations). Thus, immortalization may be part of the pathway to some malignancies, but it does not seem to be necessary for all. Clarification of the relationship between senescence and oncogenesis will have to await molecular definition of the genes associated with senescence and examination of their status in malignancy.

Another popular avenue of inquiry concerns the biological roles of tyrosine phosphatases (PTPs). This stems from the straightforward deduction that since many dominant oncogenes are tyrosine kinases, at least some PTPs, which would presumably function in opposition to tyrosine kinases, are tumor-suppressor genes. PTPs form a large multigene family which, like the tyrosine kinases, can be subdivided into transmembrane and nontransmembrane classes.[101] The presumed function of the transmembrane PTPs is to serve as receptors for as yet largely unidentified ligands. The extracellular domains of several of these PTPs display strong sequence similarity to CAMs, suggesting that they may transduce similar signals. In particular, it has been suggested that some of these putative receptor-PTPs may mediate such phenomena as contact inhibition of cell growth and invasion, which are deranged in many cancer cells. Thus it seems possible that mutations in transmembrane PTPs might contribute to oncogenesis. The functions and mechanism of regulation of the nontransmembrane PTPs are completely unknown. However, a reasonable possibility is that at least some of them function to counteract the phosphorylation events induced by receptor and nonreceptor tyrosine kinases. Thus, mutations in nontransmembrane PTPs might also be oncogenic.

However, there is, as yet, no strong evidence for involvement of PTPs in any human malignancy. The chromosomal locations of several of these genes have been determined. Two map within regions that are frequent targets for deletion in human tumors. A transmembrane PTP termed rPTP-γ, maps to 3p21.1,[209] which is within the region of 3p that is commonly deleted in lung cancer, renal cancer, and several malignancies (Table 2). RFLP studies demonstrated LOH for rPTP-γ in about 30% to 40% of a small sample of lung tumors.[209] In addition, some tumors show LOH for rPTP-γ with retained heterozygosity for other 3p loci. However, no rearrangements or homozygous deletions of rPTP-γ were found in this sample of tumors, nor was there any other evidence of mutation within the gene itself. In addition, although the RFLP data certainly indicate significant LOH, the percentage of LOH observed is not particularly high, certainly less than that observed for RFLPs mapping close to or within Rb or p53 in retinoblastomas or colon cancers, respectively. The chromosomal localization of this rPTP to 3p21.1 is interesting, but it far from establishes involvement of this gene in carcinogenesis.

Recently, several groups[295,336,404] have independently identified a novel nontransmembrane PTP containing src-homology-2 (SH2) domains. SH2 domains are stretches of approximately 100 amino acids that are present in a number of key secondary signaling molecules such as ras-GAP, PLC-γ, the regulatory subunit of phosphatidylinositol-3 kinase, and, as the name implies, members of the *src* family of nontransmembrane tyrosine kinases. Several recent studies have demonstrated that SH2 domains direct interactions with specific phosphotyrosyl proteins.[202] The newly identified SH2-containing PTP, termed PTP1C,[336] SH-PTP1,[295] or HCP,[404] respectively, is expressed predominantly in hematopoietic cells of all lineages.[295,404] Chromosomal localization studies have positioned this gene at 12p12–13, a region involved in deletions or translocations in a high percentage of pediatric precursor B-cell acute lymphoblastic leukemias.[296,404] These varied cytogenetic abnormalities suggest that a 12p12–13 locus harbors a tumor-suppressor gene, rather than a dominant oncogene. Studies in progress should resolve whether this PTP is the target gene.

Overexpression of nontransmembrane PTPs can block transformation of fibroblasts transformed by tyrosine kinase oncogenes, such as *neu*[37] and v-*src*.[395] It is difficult to assess the implications of such results. A large body of evidence indicates that tyrosine kinase oncogenes transform cells by virtue of their ability to induce aberrant tyrosine phosphorylation, so it hardly seems surprising that inappropriate expression of a PTP could pharmacologically antagonize the actions of these oncogenes. The physiological significance of these results is even more questionable in view of the fact that, in some cases, only truncated versions of the PTPs were effective in causing reversion. These truncations remove the PTP C-terminus, which is essential for association of these proteins with their appropriate cellular compartment,[108,395] and appears to have negative regulatory effects[55] (J. Frangioni and B. Neel, unpublished observations). Thus, as for the transmembrane PTPs, the jury is still out on the potential role of nontransmembrane PTPs as human tumor-suppressor genes.

Perspective and a Look to the Future

Although only five years have elapsed since the field of tumor-suppressor genes entered the molecular era with the cloning of Rb, progress has been extremely rapid. It is already possible to arrive at some general conclusions regarding the functions of these genes. One class (growth inhibitory genes), consisting of genes such as Rb, p53, and, most likely, NF-1, largely appear to inhibit cell growth. Whether they have any direct effect on cytodifferentiation is unclear. Damage to growth inhibitory genes may help promote malignancy in a wide variety of cell types. Consistent with a general role in growth control, one would expect that such genes would be expressed ubiquitously; indeed, this is observed. One would also expect to see mutations in such genes in a number of different malignancies; this is certainly the case for Rb and p53, although involvement of NF-1 in diseases other than NF-1 has not yet been reported. Furthermore, one would expect that newly identified genes with growth inhibitory properties, including genes identified from lower species, would be candidate tumor-suppressor genes of this type. At the very least, initial attempts to characterize the human counterparts of such genes should include chromosomal localization studies to look for possible coincident localization with regions implicated in tumor suppression by linkage or LOH studies.

Other genes, such as WT-1, may have a more direct effect on differentiation of a particular tissue, rather than a direct effect on cell growth. The restricted expression of WT-1 to certain tissues and to limited times during development argues for such a role. Accordingly, one would not expect genes such as WT-1 to be involved in other cancers. Although no other examples of such genes have yet been found for human tumors, *Drosophila* genetics may provide fertile ground for identifying them. Elisabeth Gateff and her colleagues, notably Bernard Mechler, have identified over 20 *Drosophila* "tumor-suppressor" genes.[117] Homozygous inactivation of these genes lead to abnormal cellular proliferations that resemble tumors at various stages of *Drosophila* development. When these abnormal masses are injected into adult flies, progressive tumors that kill the fly result, further implicating them as malignant growths. Where analyzed in detail, these mutations appear to cause altered differentiation. Many of these genes are likely to have mammalian homologues, and it would not be at all surprising if several of these homologues are tumor-suppressor genes of the WT type.

It is not yet clear how the other identified tumor-suppressor genes should be classified, because little is known of their function. The widespread expression of APC (and, for that matter, MCC) as well as the extracolonic manifestations in Gardner's syndrome suggest that these genes may have general growth inhibitory functions. Similarly, DCC's widespread expression, and its adhesion molecule-like structure suggests that it may fall into this class. It is more difficult to categorize a gene like RAR-α. It is ubiquitously expressed, and thus by our simple scheme, might be expected to have a growth inhibitory role. Nevertheless, in APML, differentiation is blocked, presumably because of the 15;17 translocation disrupting RAR-α. More importantly, a direct role for RAR-α in promoting differentiation is suggested by the finding that treatment of APML patients with retinoic acid, the ligand for RAR-α, induces remission by promoting terminal differentiation of myeloid cells. Perhaps RAR-α plays a more general role in induction of differentiation in a wide variety of tissues. For example, liganded RAR-α may be a signal for the cell to switch to the differentiation state for which that cell type is preprogrammed. If so, mutations in RAR-α should probably be sought actively in many tumors, particularly those in which a role for a 17q gene is suspected by LOH or linkage studies. As mentioned above, a particularly good candidate for such a tumor is breast cancer, since linkage studies have implicated 17q21, the location of RAR-α in familial breast cancer, and LOH studies have implicated 17q in sporadic tumors (see above).

Although distinguishing between "growth inhibitory" (Rb, p53, NF-1) and "differentiation-inducing" (WT-1) tumor-suppressor genes is useful conceptually, it should not be rigidly interpreted as implying a specific mechanism of action. For example, although Rb and p53 may play no direct role in differentiation, they may promote differentiation indirectly. By promoting growth arrest in a cell faced with a decision to divide or differentiate, such genes may induce differentiation by default. Similarly, a gene such as WT-1 may promote differentiation in a tissue-restricted fashion by interfering with a generalized growth promoting stimulus. The shared DNA-binding site between EGR-1 and -2 and WT-1 would be consistent with such a mechanism.

Perhaps tumor-suppressor gene products are best viewed as components of (growth inhibitory and/or differentiation-inducing) signal-transduction pathways (Fig. 6). Such pathways would be expected to contain receptors, perhaps exemplified by DCC, transducers/second messengers such as NF-1 (and perhaps APC and/or MCC), and nuclear proteins, some (e.g., RAR-α, WT-1, Rb) or all (?p53) of which may serve to directly modulate transcription. It would not be at all surprising if the genes for negative growth factors (e.g., TGF-β and other members of the activin/inhibin family) are also found to be mutated in some cancers. Clearly, filling in the gaps (no pun intended) between the members of these pathways will be one of the main challenges of the next 5 to 10 years. Many of these missing components are themselves likely to be tumor-suppressor genes. The remainder should include the key regulators and effectors of tumor-suppressor gene action.

If tumor-suppressor gene products comprise a signal-

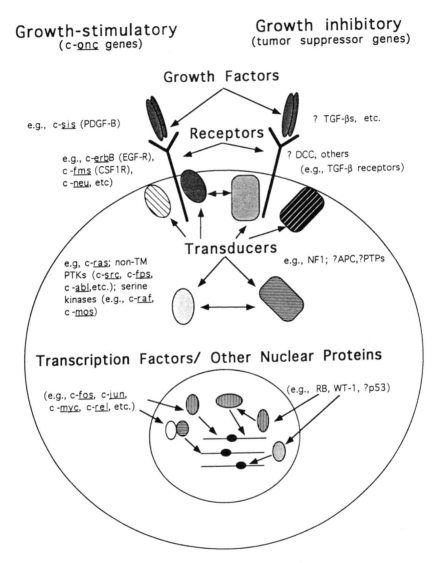

Figure 6. *(see legend on p. 117)*

transduction pathway, then what signals do they transduce? Here, the tumor-suppressor gene field is likely to benefit greatly from analogies with better studied signal-transduction pathways for stimulating growth (Fig. 6). All cells receive at least two different types of signal from their environment. Soluble signals, in the form of growth factors (and negative growth factors), cytokines, and hormones, give up-to-the-minute information about environmental conditions. Such signals, however, can only be interpreted in the context of a cell's starting environment, i.e., its cell-cell interactions and cell-matrix interactions. Growth factors such as epidermal growth factor (EGF), platelet-derived growth factor (PDGF), fibroblast growth factor (FGF), and others, transmit their signals through tyrosine kinase receptors, many of which, when mutationally deranged, are oncogenic. Similarly, mutation and/or overexpression of many of the downstream targets of these growth factors also can contribute to oncogenesis. These signals alone, however, are not sufficient to promote growth. Saturating levels of such factors will not stimulate DNA synthesis or cell division if the cells are not residing on an appropriate matrix.[172] The nature and transmission of cell-matrix and cell-cell signals is less well understood.

It is likely that a parallel set of pathways for both soluble and solid-state signals exists for growth inhibition/induction of differentiation. There is already evidence that a soluble negative growth factor, TGF-β, can modulate the activity of a tumor-suppressor gene product, Rb. Conversely, the structure of DCC suggests that it may transmit a solid state signal.

These growth promoting and growth inhibiting signal-

Figure 6. *Oncogenes and tumor-suppressor genes as members of growth stimulatory and growth inhibitory signal-transduction pathways. On the left half of the figure growth stimulatory pathways are schematized. Oncogenes have been found to arise as a consequence of mutation and/or altered regulation of proteins at every level of these pathways. Representative examples of such genes are indicated. In some cases, for example, the transcription factors c-jun and c-fos, c-onc genes physically interact. At the right of the figure, the known tumor-suppressor gene products are arranged along a putative growth inhibitory pathway. Possible positions of as yet incompletely characterized gene products (e.g., DCC, APC) are denoted with "?." Examples of potential, but as yet undemonstrated, tumor-suppressor genes (e.g., PTPs, TGF-βs and their receptors) are also denoted with "?." In some cases (e.g., ras proteins and NF-1), there are likely to be direct interactions between c-onc and tumor-suppressor gene products (indicated by double arrows).*

transduction pathways are likely to crosstalk at all levels, from receptor to transcription factor. For example, the TGF-β pathway appears to involve crosstalk between the growth inhibitory Rb gene and the growth stimulatory c-*myc* gene. There is also likely to be crosstalk between WT-1 and the EGRs. Members of the *ras* gene family crosstalk at the level of *ras*-GAP and NF-1. Our knowledge of the number and complexity of these interactions is likely to increase dramatically in the next few years. Ultimately, it should be possible to determine how (or whether) mutation in a particular tumor-suppressor gene leads to altered response(s) to signaling by soluble and solid-state mediators. Such studies may identify subtle differences in cellular physiology between normal, preneoplastic, and malignant cells— differences that may prove to be novel targets for chemoprevention and/or chemotherapy.

The existence of parallel signal-transduction pathways for growth stimulation and inhibition, and for different types of signals, soluble and solid state, fits nicely with the notion that multiple genetic events are needed for full malignant transformation. Presumably, a single "hit" can perturb one or more of these pathways, but the remaining normal components can react in a homeostatic fashion to prevent uncontrolled cellular growth. In some conditions, a single mutation, or very few mutations, may be sufficient to drive a benign proliferation, for example a colonic polyp or a neurofibroma. But for frank malignancy, multiple hits must occur in order to inactivate the remaining restraining pathways. This is true even for viral carcinogenesis, as we have seen from the emerging data on interactions of DNA tumor viral oncoproteins with multiple tumor-suppressor gene products.

Theoretically, one would expect that this could be accomplished either by activating oncogenes or by inactivating tumor-suppressor genes, or by some combination of both. In practice, in human malignancies, tumor-suppressor gene mutations appear to be more common than oncogene activation mutations. The reason(s) for this are not clear. It could be that negative regulation of cell growth is physiologically more important (or more refractory to disruption) than positive regulation. Alternatively, it may indicate more about the relative sensitivity of different genes to mutagenesis than the importance of their gene products in regulation. Perhaps some combination of these two explanations approaches the true answer.

It is also not yet clear why mutations in some tumor-suppressor genes occur only in some tumors. Mutations in p53, which appears to be a key cell cycle regulatory gene, have been found in nearly all malignancies examined. But Rb mutations, although found in malignancies other than retinoblastoma, are not nearly so common. There are two general classes of explanation for this apparent specificity. First, it is frequently argued that redundant pathways exist for negative growth control, and the Rb pathway is "more important" in some cell types than in others; in such cells, Rb inactivation is more likely to contribute to oncogenesis. Although redundant pathways undoubtedly exist, there is no evidence as yet to support the notion that Rb is more important or less important in different tissues. Alternatively, it may be that what is different between different tissues is the sensitivity of Rb to mutagenesis.

For example, Rb may be more or less likely to undergo certain chromosomal events (such as deletion, translocation, or mitotic recombination) in different cell types. Recent experiments using a tissue culture model system support this general notion.[74] Transfection of several different dominant oncogenes into NIH3T3 cells carrying an enhancerless retrovirus encoding neomycin phosphotransferase led to the induction of secondary chromosomal events which were detected by conversion of the cells to neomycin resistance. These studies imply that initial, random oncogenic events in tumorigenesis might predispose to secondary chromosomal events involving specific tumor-suppressor genes. A colonic epithelial cell having undergone a *ras* mutation, for example, might be predisposed to chromosomal events involving 17p (p53) and/or 18q (DCC), but not 13q (Rb).

At the organismic level, the relative accessibility and susceptibility of certain tissues to carcinogenic agents could also contribute to apparent specificity. Previous work has demonstrated that different carcinogens induce distinct subsets of *ras* mutations.[14,96] Recently, similar data have been obtained for mutations in p53.[154,301] Specific subsets of *ras* and p53 mutations are also found in different human tumors, arguing for the clinical relevance of these experimental models.[155,177] Obviously, lining epithelia of the gastrointestinal tract are likely to be exposed to different types of carcinogens than mammary epithelia or central nervous system neurons. Certain candidate tumor-suppressor genes, such as the as yet unidentified 3p gene(s) associated with lung cancer and other epithelial malignancies (Table 2), are located in chromosomal regions containing fragile sites. Such genes might be particularly susceptible to chromosomal events induced by potent clastogenic agents such as cigarette smoke or radiation. Most likely, the association of mutations in Rb (and probably other tumor-suppressor genes) with subsets of tumors reflects both the relative importance of Rb in growth control in that cell type and the relative susceptibility of the Rb gene to mutation in that cell type.

In any event, it seems clear that when the roster of tumor-suppressor genes is filled and combined with that of the dominant oncogenes, nearly all of the key players in control of normal cell growth will stand identified. Together, these genes are likely to constitute the vast majority of the genes whose structure and function are deranged in neoplasia, although there will probably be a few others. We have already mentioned the existence of genes that appear to modulate tumor angiogenesis and metastasis. Alterations in at least one different class of genes, which we have not discussed, are also likely to be involved in cancer. These include genes whose function is to maintain genomic integrity, including those responsible for DNA repair and chromosome stability. Although beyond the scope of this review, mutations in such genes clearly occur in the germ line (e.g., xeroderma pigmentosum, ataxia telangiectasia, and the chromosome breakage syndromes such as Bloom's syndrome) and are likely to occur in sporadic cancer as well. It is even conceivable, based on its sequence similarity to RAG-1, that PML belongs to this gene class. It is arguable whether such genes should be called "tumor-suppressor" genes, but it seems clear that in the most general sense, they do suppress tumors; their absence leads to increased genomic instability and thus favors mutation of tumor-suppressor genes and oncogenes. It should also be mentioned in passing that, as opposed to classic tumor-suppressor genes, germ-line mutations in these genes lead to inherited cancer predisposition with autosomal recessive inheritance.

In summary, we truly stand on the threshold of a full molecular description of normal and neoplastic growth. It would not at all be surprising if 10 years from now all of the fundamental circuits in growth control have been deciphered. In fact, what would probably be more surprising is if this revolution in molecular oncology does not transform the way we understand, diagnose, prognosticate, and treat the heretofore mysterious diseases we call cancer.

Acknowledgments: The author thanks Ms. Maureen Magane and Mr. John Frangioni for their valuable help in preparing the manuscript, as well as members of his laboratory for their tolerance of the many hours he spent working on this review. Work from the author's laboratory described in this chapter was supported by grants from the NIH (RO1 CA49152) and the Harvard Medical School/Hoffman-Laroche Institute for Chemistry and Medicine.

References

1. Abramson D, Ellsworth R, Kitchin F, et al. Second monocular tumors in retinoblastoma survivors. Ophthalmology 1984; 91:1351–1355.
2. Ahuja H, Bar-Eli M, Advani S, et al. Alterations of the p53 gene and the clonal evolution of the blast crisis of chronic myelocytic leukemia. Proc Natl Acad Sci USA 1989; 86:6783–6787.
3. Ali I, Lidereau R, Callahan R. Presence of two members of the c-*erb*A receptor gene family (c-*erb*A beta and c-*erb*A2) in smallest region of somatic homozygosity on chromosome 3p21–25 in human breast carcinoma. J Natl Cancer Inst 1989; 81:1815–1820.
4. Ali I, Lidereau R, Theillet C, et al. Reduction to homozygosity of genes on chromosome 11 in human breast neoplasia. Science 1987; 238:185–188.
5. Ashton-Rickardt PG, Dunlop MG, Nakamura Y, et al. High frequency of APC loss in sporadic colorectal carcinoma due to breaks clustered in 5q21–22. Oncogene 1989; 4:1169–1174.
6. Bader J, Miller R. Neurofibromatosis and childhood leukemia. J Pediatr 1978; 92:925–929.
7. Bagchi S, Weinmann R, Raychaudhuri P. The retinoblastoma protein copurifies with E2F-1, an E1A-regulated inhibitor of the transcription factor E2F. Cell 1991; 65:1063–1072.
8. Baker S, Markowitz S, Fearon E, et al. Suppression of human colorectal carcinoma cell growth by wild type p53. Science 1990; 249:912–915.
9. Baker SJ, Fearon ER, Nigro JM, et al. Chromosome 17 deletions and p53 gene mutations in colorectal carcinomas. Science 1989; 244:217–221.
10. Balaban G, Gilbert F, Nichols W, et al. Abnormalities of chromosome #13 in retinoblastomas from individuals with normal constitutional karyotypes. Canc Genet Cytogenet 1982; 6:213-221.
11. Ballester R, Marchuk D, Boguski M, et al. The NF1 locus encodes a protein functionally related to mammalian GAP. Cell 1990; 63:851–859.
12. Bandara LR, Adamczewski JP, Hunt T, et al. Cyclin A and the retinoblastoma gene product complex with a common transcription factor. Nature 1991; 352:249–251.
13. Bandara LR, La Thangue NB. Adenovirus E1A prevents the retinoblastoma gene product from complexing with a cellular transcription factor. Nature 1991; 351:494–497.
14. Barbacid M. *ras* genes. Annu Rev Biochem 1987; 56:779-827.
15. Bargonetti J, Friedman P, Kern S, et al. Wild-type, but not mutant p53 immunopurified proteins bind to sequences adjacent to the SV40 origin of replication. Cell 1991; 65:1083–1091.
16. Barker D, Wright E, Nguyen K, et al. Gene for von Recklinghausen neurofibromatosis is in the pericentromeric region of chromosome 17. Science 1987; 236:1100–1102.

17. Barski G, Cornefert F. Characteristics of "hybrid"-type clonal cell lines obtained from mixed cultures in vitro. J Natl Canc Inst 1962; 28:801.

17a. Fougere C, Ruiz C, Ephrussi B. Gene dosage dependence of pigment synthesis in melanoma X fibroblast hybrid. Proc Natl Acad Sci USA 1972; 69:330–334.

18. Beckwith J, Kiviat N, Bonadio J. Nephrogenic rests, nephroblastomatosis, and the pathogenesis of Wilms' tumor. Pediatr Pathol 1990; 10:1–36.

19. Benedict WF, Xu H-J, Hu S-X, et al. Role of the retinoblastoma gene in the initiation and progression of human cancer. J Clin Invest 1990; 85:988–993.

20. Bevilaqua G, Sobel M, Liotta L, et al. Association of low *nm23* levels in human primary infiltrating ductal breast carcinomas with lymph node involvement and other histopathological indicators of high metastatic potential. Cancer Res 1989; 49:5185–5190.

21. Biggs J, Hersperger E, Steeg PS, et al. A *Drosophila* gene that is homologous to mammalian gene associated with tumor metastasis codes for a nucleoside diphosphate kinase. Cell 1990; 63:933–940.

22. Bischoff JR, Friedman PN, Marshak DR, et al. Human p53 is phosphorylated by p60-cdc2 and cyclin B-cdc2. Proc Natl Acad Sci USA 1990; 87:4766–4770.

23. Bodmer WF, Bailey CJ, Bodmer J, et al. Localization of the gene for familial adenomatous polyposis on chromosome 5. Nature 1987; 328:614–616.

24. Bodmer WF, Cottrell S, Frischauf A-M, et al. Genetic analysis of colorectal cancer. Toyko 1991; 20:49–52.

25. Bollag G, McCormick F. Differential regulation of *ras*GAP and neurofibromatosis gene product activities. Nature 1991; 351:576–579.

26. Bookstein R, Lee E-H, Peccei A, et al. Human retinoblastoma gene: Long-range mapping and analysis of its deletion in a breast cancer cell line. Mol Cell Biol 1989; 9:1628–1634.

27. Bookstein R, Rio P, Madreperla SA, et al. Promoter deletion and loss of retinoblastoma gene expression in human prostate carcinoma. Proc Natl Acad Sci USA 1990; 87:7762–7766.

28. Bookstein R, Shew J-Y, Chen P-L, et al. Suppression of tumorigenicity of human prostate carcinoma cells by replacing a mutated RB gene. Science 1990; 247:712–715.

29. Borrow J, Goddard A, Sheer D, et al. Molecular analysis of acute promyelocytic leukemia breakpoint cluster region on chromosome 17. Science 1990; 249:1577–1580.

30. Bos J, Fearon E, Hamilton S, et al. Prevalence of *ras* gene mutations in human colorectal cancers. Nature 1987; 327:293-297.

31. Botstein D, White R, Skolnick M, et al. Construction of a genetic linkage map in man using restriction fragment polymorphisms. Am J Hum Genet 1980; 32:314.

32. Bouck N, diMayorca G. Chemical carcinogens transform BHK cells by inducing a recessive mutation. Mol Cell Biol 1982; 2:97-105.

33. Bouck N, Head M. The majority of independently transformed BHK cell clones share a single functional lesion which determines anchorage independence and influences tumorigenicity. In Vitro Cell Dev Biol 1985; 21:463–469.

34. Bouck N, Stoler A, Polverini P. Coordinate control of anchorage independence, actin cytoskeleton, and angiogenesis by human chromosome 1 in
hamster-human hybrids. Cancer Res 1986; 46:5101–5105.
35. Braithwaite AW, Sturzbecher H-W, Addison C, et al. Mouse p53 inhibits
SV40 origin-dependent DNA replication. Nature 1987; 329:458–460.
36. Brand N, Petkovich M, Krust A, et al. Identification of a second human
retinoic acid receptor. Nature 1988; 332:850–853.
37. Brown-Shimer S, Johnson K, Hill D, et al. Effect of protein tyrosine
phosphatase 1B expression on transformation by the human *neu* oncogene. Cancer Res 1992; 52:478–482.
38. Buchkovich K, Duffy LA, Harlow E. The retinoblastoma protein is
phosphorylated during specific phases of the cell cycle. Cell 1989;
58:1097–1105.
39. Burt R, Bishop D, Cannon L, et al. Dominant inheritance of adenomatous
colonic polyps and colorectal cancer. N Engl J Med 1985; 312:1540–1544.
40. Call KM, Glaser T, Ito CY, et al. Isolation and characterization of a zinc
finger polypeptide gene at the human chromosome 11 Wilm's tumor
locus. Cell 1990; 60:509–520.
41. Cannon-Albright L, Skolnick M, Bishop D, et al. Common inheritance of
susceptibility to colonic adenomatous polyps and associated colorectal
cancers. N Engl J Med 1988; 319:533–537.
42. Casey G, Lo-Hsueh M, Lopez M, et al. Growth suppression of human
breast cancer cells by the introduction of a wild-type p53 gene. Oncogene
1991; 10:1791–1797.
43. Cavenee WK, Dryja TP, Phillips RA, et al. Expression of recessive alleles
by chromosomal mechanisms in retinoblastoma. Nature 1983; 305:779–
784.
44. Cavenee WK, Hansen MF, Nordenskjold M, et al. Genetic origin of
mutations predisposing to retinoblastoma. Science 1985; 228:501–503.
45. Cawthon RM, Weiss R, Xu G, et al. A major segment of the neurofibromatosis type 1 gene: cDNA sequence, genomic structure, and point mutations. Cell 1990; 62:193–201.
46. Chellappan SP, Hiebert S, Mudryj M, et al. The E2F transcription factor is
a cellular target for the RB protein. Cell 1991; 65:1053–1061.
47. Chen P, Chen Y, Bookstein R, et al. Genetic mechanisms of tumor
suppression by the human p53 gene. Science 1990; 250:1576-1580.
48. Chen PL, Scully P, Shew JY, et al. Phosphorylation of the retinoblastoma
gene product is modulated during the cell cycle and cellular differentiation. Cell 1989; 58:1193–1198.
49. Cherington V, Brown M, Paucha E, et al. Separation of simian virus 40
large-T-antigen-transforming and origin-binding functions from the ability to block differentiation. Mol Cell Biol 1988; 8:1380–1384.
50. Chittenden T, Livingston DM, Kaelin WGJ. The T/E1A-binding domain of
the retinoblastoma product can interact selectively with a sequence-
specific DNA-binding protein. Cell 1991; 65:1073-1082.
51. Chomienne C, Ballerini P, Balitrand N, et al. The retinoic acid receptor α
gene is rearranged in retinoic acid-sensitive promyelocytic leukemias.
Leukemia 1990; 4:802–807.
52. Chow V, Ben-David Y, Bernstein A, et al. Multistage Friend erythroleuke-

mia: Independent origin of tumor clones with noraml or rearranged p53 cellular oncogenes. J Virol 1987; 61:2777-2781.

53. Clarke C, Cheng K, Frey A, et al. Purification of complexes of nuclear oncogene p53 with rat and *Escherichia coli* heat shock proteins: In vitro dissociation of hsc70 and dnaK from murine p53 by atp. Mol Cell Biol 1988; 8:1206–1215.

54. Collins SJ, Robertson KA, Mueller L. Retinoic acid-induced granulocytic differentiation of HL-60 myeloid leukemia cells is mediated directly through the retinoic acid receptor (RAR-alpha). Mol Cell Biol 1990; 10:2154–2163.

55. Cool D, Tonks N, Charbonneau H, et al. Expression of a human T-cell protein-tyrosine-phosphatase in baby hamster kidney cells. Proc Natl Acad Sci USA 1990; 87:7280–7284.

56. Crawford LV, Pim DC, Gurney EG, et al. Detection of a common feature in several human tumor cell lines-a 53,000 dalton protein. Proc Natl Acad Sci USA 1981; 78:41–45.

57. Crook T, Wrede D, Tidy J, et al. Clonal p53 mutation in human cervical cancer: Association with human papillomavirus-negative tumors. Lancet 1992; 339:1070–1073.

58. Crook T, Wrede D, Vousden K. p53 point mutation in HPV negative human cervical carcinoma cell lines. Oncogene 1991; 6:873–875.

59. Cropp C, Lidereau R, Campbell G, et al. Loss of heterozygosity on chromosomes 17 and 18 in breast carcinoma: Two additional regions identified. Proc Natl Acad Sci USA 1990; 87:7737–7741.

60. Damm K, Thompson C, Evans R. Protein encoded by v-*erb*A function as a thyroid-hormone receptor antagonist. Nature (London) 1989; 339:593–597.

61. De Mars R. 23rd Annual Symposium, Fundamental Cancer Research 1969. Baltimore, Williams and Wilkins 1970; pp. 105–106.

62. de The H, Lavau C, Marchio A, et al. The PML-RAR-α fusion mRNA generated by the t(15;17) translocation in acute promyelocytic leukemia encodes a functionally altered RAR. Cell 1991; 66:675–684.

63. Dearolf C, Hersperger E, Shearn A. Developmental consequences of *awd*^b3, a cell-autonomous lethal mutation of *Drosophila* induced by hybrid dysgenesis. Dev Biol 1988; 129:159–168.

64. DeCaprio JA, Ludlow JW, Figge J, et al. SV40 large tumor antigen forms a specific complex with the product of the retinoblastoma susceptibility gene. Cell 1988; 54:275–283.

65. DeCaprio JA, Ludlow JW, Lynch D, et al. The product of the retinoblastoma susceptibility gene has properties of a cell cycle regulatory element. Cell 1989; 58:1085–1095.

66. DeClue J, Cohen B, Lowy D. Identification and characterization of the neurofibromatosis type 1 protein product. Proc Natl Acad Sci USA 1991; 88:9914–9918.

67. Defeo-Jones D, Huang PS, Jones RE, et al. Cloning of cDNAs for cellular proteins that bind to the retinoblastoma gene product. Nature 1991; 352:251–254.

68. DeLeo AB, Jay G, Apella E, et al. Detection of a transformation-related

antigen in chemically induced sarcomas and other transformed cells of the mouse. Proc Natl Acad Sci USA 1979; 76:2420–2424.

69. DeLuca L. Retinoids and their receptors in differentiation, embryogenesis, and neoplasia. FASEB J 1991; 5:2924–2933.

70. deThe H, Chomienne C, Lanotte M, et al. The t(15;17) translocation of acute promyelocytic leukaemia fuses the retinoic acid receptor α gene to a novel transcribed locus. Nature 1990; 347:558–561.

71. Diller L, Kassel J, Nelson CE, et al. p53 functions as a cell cycle control protein in osteosarcomas. Mol Cell Biol 1990; 10:5772–5781.

72. Dippold WG, Jay G, DeLeo AB, et al. p53 transformation-related protein: Detection by monoclonal antibody in human and mouse cells. Proc Natl Acad Sci USA 1981; 78:1695–1699.

73. Dix D. The role of aging in cancer incidence: An epidemiologic study. J Gerontol 1989; 44:10–18.

74. Drews R, Chan V-W, Schnipper L. Oncogenes result in genomic alterations that activate a transcriptionally silent, dominantly selectable reporter gene. Mol Cell Biol 1992; 12:198–206.

75. Dryja T, Rapaport J, Epstein J, et al. Chromosome 13 homozygosity in osteosarcoma without retinoblastoma. Am J Hum Genet 1986; 38:59–66.

76. Dryja T, Rapaport J, Joyce J, et al. Molecular detection of deletions involving band q14 of chromosome 13 in retinoblastomas. Proc Natl Acad Sci USA 1986; 83:7391–7394.

77. Dryja TP, Mukai S, Petersen R, et al. Parental origin of mutations of the retinoblastoma gene. Nature 1989; 339:556-558.

78. Dunn J, Phillips R, Becker A, et al. Identification of germline and somatic mutations affecting the retinoblastoma gene. Science 1988; 241:1797–1800.

79. Dunn J, Phillips R, Zhu X, et al. Mutations in the RB1 gene and their effects on transcription. Mol Cell Biol 1989; 9:4596-4604.

80. Dyson N, Buchkovich K, Whyte P, et al. The cellular 107K protein that binds to the adenovirus E1A also associates with the large T antigens of SV40 and JC virus. Cell 1989; 58:249–255.

81. Dyson N, Howley P, Munger K, et al. The human papilloma virus-16 E7 oncoprotein is able to bind to the retinoblastoma gene product. Science 1989; 243:934–936.

82. Ejima Y, Sasaki MS, Kaneko A, et al. Types, rates, origin and expressivity of chromosome mutations involving 13q14 in retinoblastoma patients. Hum Genet 1988; 79:118–123.

83. Eliyahu D, Michalovitz D, Eliyahu S, et al. Wild type p53 can inhibit oncogene-mediated focus formation. Proc Natl Acad Sci USA 1989; 86:8763–8767.

84. Eliyahu D, Michalovitz D, Oren M. Overproduction of p53 antigen makes established cells highly tumorigenic. Nature 1985; 316:158–160.

85. Eliyahu D, Raz A, Gruss P, et al. Participation of p53 cellular tumour antigen in transformation of normal embryonic cells. Nature 1984; 312:646–649.

86. Elledge SJ, Spottswood MR. The new human p34 protein kinase, CDK2, identified by complementation of a CDC28 mutation in *Saccharomyces cerevesiae*, is a homolog of *Xenopus* Eg1. EMBO J 1991; 10:2653–2659.

87. Evans EP, Burtenshaw M, Brown BB, et al. The analysis of malignancy by cell fusion. IX. Reexamination and clarification of the cytogenic problem. J Cell Sci 1982; 56:113–130.

88. Ewen M, Ludlow J, Marsilio E, et al. An N-terminal transformation-governing sequence of SV40 large T antigen contributes to the binding of both p110^{Rb} and a second cellular protein, p120. Cell 1989; 58:257–267.

89. Ewen ME, Xing YG, Lawrence JB, et al. Molecular cloning, chromosomal mapping, and expression of the cDNA for p107, a retinoblastoma gene product-related protein. Cell 1991; 66:1155-1164.

90. Fearon E, Feinberg A, Hamilton S, et al. Loss of genes on the short arm of chromosome 11 in bladder cancer. Nature 1985; 318:377–380.

91. Fearon E, Hamilton S, Vogelstein B. Clonal analysis of human colorectal tumors. Science 1987; 238:193.

92. Fearon E, Vogelstein B, Feinberg A. Somatic deletion and duplication of genes on chromosome 11 in Wilms' tumor. Nature 1984; 309:176–178.

93. Fearon ER, Vogelstein B. A genetic model for colorectal tumorigenesis. Cell 1990; 61:759–767.

94. Fearon ER, Cho KR, Nigro JM, et al. Identification of a chromosome 18q gene that is altered in colorectal cancers. Science 1990; 247:1046–1049.

95. Feinberg A, Gehrke C, Kuo K, et al. Reduced genomic 5-methylcytosine content in human colonic neoplasia. Cancer Res 1988; 48:1159–1161.

96. Field JK, Spandidos DA. The role of *ras* and *myc* oncogenes in human solid tumours and their relevance in diagnosis and prognosis. Anti-cancer Res 1990; 10:1–22.

97. Fields S, Jang SK. Presence of a potent transcription activating sequence in the p53 protein. Science 1990; 249:1046-1049.

98. Figge J, Webster T, Smith T, et al. Prediction of similar transforming regions in simian virus 40 large T, adenovirus E1A, and *myc* oncoproteins. J Virol 1988; 61:1814–1818.

99. Finlay CA, Hinds PW, Levine AJ. The p53 protooncogene can act as a suppressor of tranformation. Cell 1989; 57:1083–1093.

100. Finlay CA, Hinds PW, Tan T-H, et al. Activating mutations for transformation by p53 produce a gene product that forms an hsc70-p53 complex with an altered half-life. Mol Cell Biol 1988; 8:531–539.

101. Fischer E, Charbonneau H, Tonks N. Protein tyrosine phosphatases: A diverse family of intracellular and transmembrane enzymes. Science 1991; 253:401–406.

102. Ford G, Gallie B, Phillips R, et al. A physical map around the retinoblastoma gene. Genomics 1990; 6:284–292.

103. Forrester K, Almoguera C, Han K, et al. Detection of high incidence of K-*ras* oncogenes during human colon tumorigenesis. Nature 1987; 327:298–303.

104. Francke U. Retinoblastoma and chromosome 13. Birth Defects 1978; 12:131–137.

105. Francke U, Holmes LB, Atkins L, et al. Anirdia-Wilm's tumor association: evidence for specific deletion of 11p13. Cytogenet Cell Genet 1979; 24:185–192.

107. Francke U, Kung F. Sporadic bilateral retinoblastoma and 13q-chromosomal deletion. Med Pediatr Oncol 1976; 2:379–385.

108. Frangioni J, Beahm P, Shifrin V, et al. The nontransmembrane tyrosine phosphatase PTP1B localizes to the endoplasmic reticulum via its 35 amino acid C-terminal sequence. Cell 1992; 68:545-560.

109. Frech M, John J, Pizon V, et al. Inhibition of GTPase activating protein stimulation of RAS-p21 GTPase by the Krev-1 gene product. Science 1990; 249:169–171.

110. Friedman P, Kern S, Vogelstein B, et al. Wild-type, but not mutant, human p53 proteins inhibit the replication activities of simian virus 40 large tumor antigen. Proc Natl Acad Sci USA 1990; 87:9275–9279.

111. Friend SH, Bernards R, Rogelj S, et al. A human DNA segment with properties of the gene that predisposes to retinoblastoma and osteosarcoma. Nature 1986; 323:643–646.

112. Fung YK, Murphee AL, Tang A, et al. Structural evidence for the authenticity of the human retinoblastoma gene. Science 1987; 236:1657–1659.

113. Gallie BL, Squire JA, Goddard A, et al. Biology of disease: Mechanism of oncogenesis in retinoblastoma. Lab Invest 1990; 62:394–408.

114. Gannon JV, Graves R, Iggo R, et al. Activating mutations in p53 produce a common conformational effect: A monoclonal antibody specific for the mutant form. EMBO J 1990; 9:1595–1602.

115. Gannon JV, Lane DP. p53 and DNA polymerase α compete for binding to SV40 T antigen. Nature 1987; 329:456–458.

116. Gardner H, Gallie B, Knight L, et al. Multiple karyotypic changes in retinoblastoma tumor cells: Presence of normal chromosome 13 in most tumors. J Canc Genet Cytogenet 1982; 6:201.

117. Gateff E, Mechler BM. Tumor-suppressor genes of Drosophila melanogaster. Oncogenesis 1989; 1:221–245.

118. Gaub M, Lutz Y, Ruberte E, et al. Antibodies specific to the retinoic acid nuclear receptors alpha and beta. Proc Natl Acad Sci USA 1989; 86:3089–3093.

119. Gebert J, Moghal N, Frangioni J, et al. High frequency of retinoic acid receptor β abnormalities in human lung cancer. Oncogene 1991; 6:1859–1868.

120. Gessler M, Poustka A, Cavenee W, et al. Homozygous deletion in Wilms' tumours of a zinc-finger gene identified by chromosome jumping. Nature 1990; 343:774–778.

121. Giordano A, Lee JH, Scheppler JA, et al. Cell cycle regulation of histone H1 kinase activity associated with the adenoviral protein E1A. Science 1991; 13:1271–1275.

122. Giordano A, McCall C, Whyte P, et al. Human cyclin A and the retinoblastoma protein interact with similar but distinguishable sequences in the adenovirus E1A gene product. Oncogene 1991; 6:481–485.

123. Giordano A, Whyte P, Harlow E, et al. A 60 kd cdc2-associated polypeptide complexes with the E1A proteins in adenovirus-infected cells. Cell 1989; 58:981–990.

124. Glaser T, Lewis W, Bruns G, et al. The β-subunit of follicle-stimulating hormone is deleted in patients with aniridia and Wilms' tumour, allowing a further definition of the WAGR locus. Nature 1986; 321:882–887.

125. Godbout R, Dryja T, Squire J, et al. Somatic inactivation of genes on chromosome 13 is a common event in retinoblastoma. Nature 1983; 304:451–453.
126. Goddard A, Balakier H, Canton M, et al. Infrequent genomic rearrangement and normal expression of the putative RB1 gene in retinoblastoma tumors. Mol Cell Biol 1988; 8:2082.
127. Goddard A, Phillips R, Greger V, et al. Use of the RB1 cDNA as a diagnostic probe in retinoblastoma families. Clin Genet 1990; 37:117–126.
128. Goelz S, Vogelstein B, Hamilton S, et al. Hypomethylation of DNA from benign and malignant human colon neoplasms. Science 1985; 228:187–190.
129. Goldstein S. Replicative senescence: The human fibroblast comes of age. Science 1990; 249:263–266.
130. Good D, Polverini P, Rastinejad F, et al. A tumor suppressor-dependent inhibitor of angiogenesis is immunologically and functionally indistinguishable from a fragment of thrombospondin. Proc Natl Acad Sci USA 1990; 87:6624–6628.
131. Green S, Chambon P. Nuclear receptors enhance our understanding of transcription regulation. Trends Genet 1988; 4:309–314.
132. Groden J, Thilveris A, Samowitz W, et al. Identification and characterization of the familial adenomatous polyposis coli gene. Cell 1991; 66:589–601.
133. Grundy P, Koufos A, Morgan K, et al. Familial predisposition to Wilms' tumour does not map to the short arm of chomosome 11. Nature 1988; 336:374.
134. Gutmann D, Wood D, Collins F. Identification of the neurofibromatosis type 1 gene product. Proc Natl Acad Sci USA 1991; 88:9658–9662.
135. Haber DA, Buckler AJ, Glaser T, et al. An internal deletion within an 11p13 zinc finger gene contributes to the development of Wilms' tumor. Cell 1990; 61:1257–1269.
136. Halevy O, Michalovitz D, Oren M. Different tumor-derived p53 mutants exhibit distinct biological activities. Science 1990; 250:113–116.
137. Hall A. *ras* and GAP—who's controlling whom. Cell 1990; 61:921–923.
138. Hall J, Lee M, Newman B, et al. Linkage of early-onset familial breast cancer to chromosome 17q21. Science 1990; 250:1684–1689.
139. Hansen M, Cavenee W. Genetics of cancer disposition. Cancer Res 1987; 47:5518–5527.
140. Hansen M, Koufos A, Gallie B, et al. Osteosarcoma and retinoblastoma: A shared chromosomal mechanism revealing recessive predisposition. Proc Natl Acad Sci USA 1985; 82:6216-6220.
141. Harbour JW, Lai S-L, Whang-Peng J, et al. Abnormalities in structure and expression of the human retinoblastoma gene in SCLC. Science 1988; 241:353–357.
142. Harlow E, Franza BJ, Schley C. Monoclonal antibodies specific for adenovirus early region 1A proteins: Extensive heterogeneity in early region 1A products. J Virol 1985; 55:533-546.
143. Harlow E, Whyte P, Franza B Jr, et al. Association of adenovirus early-region 1A proteins with cellular polypeptides. Mol Cell Biol 1986; 6:1579–1589.

144. Harris H. The analysis of malignancy by cell infusion: The position in 1988. Cancer Res 1988; 48:3302–3306.
145. Harris H, Miller OJ. Suppression of malignancy by cell fusion. Nature 1969; 223:363–368.
146. Haut M, Steeg P, Willson J, et al. Induction of *nm23* gene expression in human colonic neoplasms and equal expression in colon tumors of high and low metastatic potential. J Natl Cancer Inst 1991; 83:712–716.
147. Hennessy C, Henry J, May F, et al. Expression of the anti-metastatic gene *nm23* in human breast cancer: An association with good prognosis. J Natl Cancer Inst 1991; 83:281–285.
148. Henry I, Grandjouan S, Couillin P, et al. Tumor-specific loss of 11p15.5 alleles in *del* 11p13 Wilm's tumor and in familial adrenocortical carcinoma. Proc Natl Acad Sci USA 1989; 86:3247–3251.
149. Herrera L, Kakati S, Gibas L, et al. Gardner syndrome in a man with an interstitial deletion of 5q. Am J Med Genet 1986; 25:473–476.
150. Herskowitz I. Functional inactivation of genes by dominant negative mutations. Nature 1987; 329:219–222.
151. Hibi K, Takahashi T, Yamakawa K, et al. Three distinct regions involved in 3p deletion in human lung cancer. Oncogene 1992; 7:445–449.
152. Hinds P, Finlay C, Levine A. Mutation is required to activate the p53 gene for cooperation with the *ras* oncogene and transformation. J Virol 1989; 63:739–746.
153. Hinds P, Finlay C, Quartin R, et al. Mutant p53 DNA clones from human colon carcinomas cooperate with *ras* in transforming primary rat cells: A comparison of the "hot spot" mutant phenotypes. Cell Growth Differ 1990; 1:571–580.
154. Hollstein M, Peri L, Mandard A, et al. Genetic analysis of human esophageal tumors from two high incidence geographic areas: Frequent p53 base substitutions and absence of *ras* mutations. Cancer Res 1991; 51:4102–4106.
155. Hollstein M, Sidransky D, Vogelstein B, et al. p53 mutations in human cancers. Science 1991; 253:49–53.
156. Hong F, Huang H-J, To H, et al. Structure of the human retinoblastoma gene. Proc Natl Acad Sci USA 1989; 86:5502-5506.
157. Horowitz JM, Park S-H, Begenmann E, et al. Frequent inactivation of the retinoblastoma anti-oncogene is restricted to a subset of human tumor cells. Proc Natl Acad Sci USA 1990; 87:2775–2779.
158. Horowitz JM, Yandell DW, Park SH, Canning S, et al. Point mutational inactivation of the retinoblastoma antioncogene. Science 1989; 243:937–940.
159. Houle B, Leduc F, Bradley W. Implication of RAR-β in epidermoid (squamous) lung cancer. Genes, Chromosomes & Cancer 1991; 3:358–366.
160. Houweling A, van den Elsen PJ, van der Eb AJ. Partial transformation of primary rat cells by the leftmost 4.5% fragment of adenovirus 5 DNA. Virology 1980; 105:537–550.
161. Howley P. Role of the human papillomaviruses in human cancer. Cancer Res 1991; 51:5019s-5022s.
162. Hu L, Crowe D, Rheinwald J, et al. Abnormal expression of retinoic acid

receptors and keratin 19 by human oral and epidermal squamous cell carcinoma cell lines. Cancer Res 1991; 51:3972–3981.

163. Hu Q, Dyson N, Harlow E. The regions of the retinoblastoma protein needed for binding to adenovirus E1A or SV40 large T antigen are common sites for mutations. EMBO J 1990; 9:1147-1155.

164. Huang A, Campbell C, Bonetta L, et al. Tissue, developmental, and tumor-specific expression of divergent transcripts in Wilms' tumor. Science 1990; 250:991–994.

165. Huang H-JS, Yee J-K, Shew J-Y, et al. Suppression of the neoplastic phenotype by replacement of the RB gene in human cancer cells. Science 1988; 242:1563–1566.

166. Huang M, Ye Y, Chen S, et al. Use of all-*trans* retinoic acid in the treatment of acute promyelocytic leukemia. Blood 1988; 72:567–572.

167. Huang S, Lee W-H, Lee EY-H. A cellular protein that competes with SV40 T antigen for binding to the retinoblastoma gene product. Nature 1991; 350:160–162.

168. Huang S, Wang N, Tseng BY, et al. Two distinct and frequently mutated regions of the retinoblastoma protein are required for binding to SV40 T antigen. EMBO J 1990; 9:1815-1822.

169. Huff V, Compton DA, Chao LY, et al. Lack of linkage of familial Wilms' tumour to chromosomal band 11p13. Nature 1988; 336:377–378.

170. Huff V, Miwa H, Haber D, et al. Evidence for WT1 as a Wilms' tumor gene: Intragenic germinal deletion in bilateral WT. Am J Hum Genet 1991; 48:997–1003.

171. Hunter T, Pines J. Cyclins and cancer. Cell 1991; 66:1071-1074.

172. Ingber D, Folkman J. Mechanochemical switching between growth and differentiation during fibroblast growth factor-stimulated angiogenesis in vitro: Role of extracellular matrix. J Cell Biol 1989; 109:317–330.

173. Jenkins JR, Rudge K, Currie GA. Cellular immortalisation by a cDNA clone encoding the transformation-association phosphoprotein p53. Nature 1984; 312:651–654.

174. Jenkins JR, Rudge K, Redmond S, et al. Cloning and expression analysis of full length mouse cDNA sequnces encoding the transformation associated protein p53. Nucleic Acids Res 1984; 12:5609–5626.

175. Jenkins JR, Sturzbecher H-W. The p53 Oncogene. Amsterdam, Elsevier Science Publications 1988; pp. 403–423.

176. Jonasson J, Povey S, Harris H. The analysis of malignancy by cell fusion. VII. Cytogenic analysis of hybrids between malignant and diploid cells and of tumours derived from them. J Cell Sci 1977; 24:217–254.

177. Jones P, Buckley J, Henderson B, et al. From gene to carcinogen: A rapidly evolving field in molecular epidemiology. Cancer Res 1991; 51:3617–3620.

178. Joseph L, LeBeau M, Jamieson G, et al. Molecular cloning, sequencing and mapping of EGR2, a human early growth response gene encoding a protein with "zinc-binding finger" structure. Proc Natl Acad Sci USA 1988; 85:7164–7168.

179. Joslyn G, Carlson M, Thliveris A, et al. Identification of deletion mutations and three new genes at the familial polyposis locus. Cell 1991; 66:601–613.

180. Kaelin W Jr, Pallas D, DeCaprio J, et al. Identification of cellular proteins that can interact specifically with the T/E1A-binding region of the retinoblastoma gene product. Cell 1991; 64:521–532.
181. Kaelin WGJ, Ewen ME, Livingston DM. Definition of the minimal simian virus 40 large T antigen-and adenovirus E1A-binding domain in the retinoblastoma gene product. Mol Cell Biol 1990; 10:3761–3769.
182. Kakizuka A, Miller WHJ, Umesono K, et al. Chromosomal translocation (t(15;17) in human acute promyleocytic leukemia fuses RARα with a novel putative transcription factor, PML. Cell 1991; 66:663–674.
183. Kalderon D, Smith AE. In vitro mutagenesis of a putative DNA binding domain of SV40 large T. Virology 1984; 139:109–137.
184. Kaye FJ, Kratke RA, Gerster JL, et al. A single amino acid substitution results in a retinoblastoma protein defective in phosphorylation and oncoprotein binding. Proc Natl Acad Sci USA 1990; 87:6922–6926.
185. Ke Y, Reddel RR, Gerwin BI, et al. Human bronchial epithelial cells with integrated SV40 virus T antigen genes retain the ability to undergo squamous differentiation. Differentiation 1988; 38:60–66.
186. Kelekar A, Cole M. Tumorigenicity of fibroblast lines expressing the adenovirus E1a, cellular p53, or normal c-myc genes. Mol Cell Biol 1986; 6:7–14.
187. Kern S, Fearon E, Tersmette K, et al. Clinical and pathological associations with allelic loss in colorectal carcinomas. JAMA 1989; 261:3099–3103.
188. Kern S, Kinzler K, Baker S, et al. Mutant p53 proteins bind DNA abnormally in vitro. Oncogene 1991; 6:131–136.
189. Kern S, Markowitz S, Fearon E, et al. Identification of p53 as a sequence-specific DNA-binding protein. Science 1991; 252:1708–1711.
190. Kim SJ, Lee HD, Robbins PD, et al. Regulation of transforming growth factor beta 1 gene expression by the product of the retinoblastoma-susceptibility gene. Proc Natl Acad Sci USA 1991; 88:3052–3056.
191. Kimura N, Shimada N, Nomura K, et al. Isolation and characterization of a cDNA clone encoding rat nucleoside diphosphate kinase. J Biol Chem 1990; 265:15744–15749.
192. Kinzler K, Nilbert M, Su L-K, et al. Identification of FAP locus genes from chromosome 5q21. Science 1991; 662:661–665.
193. Kinzler K, Nilbert M, Vogelstein B, et al. Identification of a chromosome 5q21 gene that is mutated in colorectal carcinomas. Science 1991; 251:1366–1370.
194. Kitayama H, Sugimoto Y, Matsuzaki T, et al. A ras-related gene with transformation suppressor activity. Cell 1989; 56:77–84.
195. Klein G. The approaching era of the tumor suppressor genes. Science 1987; 238:1539–1545.
196. Klinger HP. Suppression of tumorigenicity in somatic cell hybrids. I. Suppression and reexpression of tumorigenicity in diploid human X D98AH2 hybrids and dependent segration of tumorigenicity from other cell phenotypes. Cytogenet Cell Genet 1980; 27:254–266.
197. Klinger HP. Suppression of tumorigenicity. Cytogenet Cell Genet 1982; 32:68–84.
198. Klug A, Rhodes D. 'Zinc fingers': A novel protein motif for nucleic acid recognition. Trends Biochem Sci 1987; 12:464–467.

199. Knudson A. Hereditary cancers: Clues to mechanisms of carcinogenesis. Brit J Canc 1989; 59:661–666.
200. Knudson AG. Mutation and cancer: statistical study of retinoblastoma. Proc Natl Acad Sci USA 1971; 68:820–823.
201. Knudson AJ. Genetics of human cancer. Ann Rev Genet 1986; 20:231–251.
202. Koch C, Anderson D, Moran M, et al. SH2 and SH3 domains: Elements that control interactions of cytoplasmic signaling proteins. Science 1991; 252:668–672.
203. Koff A, Cross F, Fisher A, et al. Human cyclin E, a new cyclin that interacts with two members of the CDC2 gene family. Cell 1991; 66:1217–1228.
204. Koufos A, Grundy P, Morgan K, et al. Familial Weidemann-Beckwith syndrome and a second Wilms' tumor locus both map to 11p15. Am J Genet 1989; 44:711–719.
205. Koufos A, Hansen M, Lampkin B, et al. Loss of alleles at loci on human chromosome 11 during genesis of Wilms' tumor. Nature (London) 1984; 309:170–172.
206. Koufos A, Hansen MF, Copeland NG, et al. Loss of heterozygosity in three embryonal tumours suggests a common pathogenetic mechanism. Nature 1985; 316:330–334.
207. Kuhn T. The Structure of Scientific Revolutions, Chicago, University of Chicago Press; p. 210, 1970.
208. La Thangue NB, Thimmappaya B, Rigby PW. The embryonal stem cell E1A-like activity involves a differentiation-regulated transcription factor. Nucleic Acids Res 1990; 18:2929–2938.
209. LaForgia S, Morse B, Levy J, et al. Receptor protein-tyrosine phosphatase γ is a candidate tumor suppressor gene at human chromosome region 3p21. Proc Natl Acad Sci USA 1991; 88:5036–5040.
210. Laiho M, DeCamprio JA, Ludlow JW, et al. Growth inhibition by TGF-β linked to suppression of retinoblastoma protein phosphorylation. Cell 1990; 62:175–185.
211. Laiho M, Ronnstrand L, Heino J, et al. Control of *jun*B and extracellular matrix protein expression by transforming growth factor-beta 1 is independent of simian virus 40 T antigen-sensitive growth-sensitive growth-inhibitory events. Mol Cell Biol 1991; 11:972–978.
212. Land HF, Parada LF, Weinberg RA. Cellular oncogenes and multistep carcinogenesis. Science 1983; 222:771–778.
213. Lane D, Benchimol S. p53: Oncogene or anti-oncogene? Genes & Dev 1990; 4:1–8.
214. Lane D, Crawford LV. T-antigen is bound to host protein in SV40-transformed cells. Nature 1979; 278:261–263.
215. La Thangue NB, Rigby PW. An adenovirus E1A-like transcription factor is regulated during the differentiation of murine embryonal stem cells. Cell 1987; 22:507–513.
216. Lee EY-HP, To H, Shew Y-H, et al. Inactivation of the retinoblastoma susceptibility gene in human breast cancers. Science 1988; 241:218–221.
217. Lee W-H, Shew J-Y, Hong FD, et al. The retinoblastoma susceptibility gene encodes a nuclear phosphoprotein associated with DNA binding activity. Nature 1987; 329:642–645.

218. Lee W-H, Bookstein R, Hong F, et al. Human retinoblastoma susceptibility gene: Cloning, identification, and sequence. Science 1987; 235:1394–1399.
219. Lees J, Buchkovich K, Marshak D, et al. The retinoblastoma protein is phosphorylated on multiple sites by human cdc2. EMBO J 1991; 10:4279–4290.
220. Lele K, Penrose L, Stallard H. Chromosome deletion in a case of retinoblastoma. Ann Hum Genet 1963; 27:171–174.
221. Leone A, Flatow U, King C, et al. Reduced tumor incidence, metastatic potential, and cytokine responsiveness of nm23-transfected melanoma cells. Cell 1991; 65:25–35.
222. Leone A, McBride O, Weston A, et al. Somatic allelic deletion of nm23 in human cancer. Cancer Res 1991; 51:2490-2493.
223. Leppert M, Dobbs M, Scambler P, et al. The gene for familial polyposis coli maps to the long arm of chromosome 5. Science 1987; 238:1411.
224. Levine A, Momand J. Tumor suppressor genes: T he p53 and retinoblastoma sensitivity genes and gene product. Biochim Biophys Acta 1990; 1032:119–136.
225. Levine AJ, Momand J, Finlay CA. The p53 tumor suppressor gene. Nature 1991; 351:453–456.
226. Lew DJ, Dulic V, Reed SI. Isolation of three novel human cyclins by rescue of G1 cyclin (Cln) function in yeast. Cell 1991; 66:1197–1206.
227. Lewin B. Driving the cell cycle: M phase kinase, its partners and substrates. Cell 1990; 61:743–752.
228. Li FP. Cancer families: Human models of susceptibility to neoplasia—the Richard and Hinda Rosenthal Foundation Award Lecture. Cancer Res 1988; 48:5381–5386.
229. Lillie JW, Green M, Green MR. An adenovirus E1A protein region required for transformation and transcriptional repression. Cell 1986; 46:1043–1051.
230. Lillie JW, Loewenstein PM, Green MR, et al. Functional domains of adenovirus type 5 E1A proteins. Cell 1987; 50:1091-1110.
231. Lin BTY, Gruenwald S, Morla AO, et al. Retinoblastoma cancer suppressor gene product is a substrate of the cell cycle regulator cdc2 kinase. EMBO J 1991; 10:857–864.
232. Linzer DI, Levine AJ. Characterization of a 54K dalton cellular SV40 tumor antigen present in SV40-transformed cells and uninfected embryonal carcinoma cells. Cell 1979; 17:43–52.
233. Linzer DI, Maltzman W, Levine AJ. The SV40 A gene product is required for the production of a 54,000 MW cellular tumor antigen. Virology 1979; 98:308–318.
234. Liotta L, Steeg P. Clues to the function of nm23 and Awd proteins in development, signal transduction, and tumor metastasis. J Natl Cancer Inst 1990; 82:1170–1172.
235. Liotta L, Steeg PS, Stetler-Stevenson WG. Tumor metastasis and angiogenesis: An imbalance of positive and negative regulation. Cell 1991; 64:327–336.
236. Longo L, Pandolfi P, Biondi A, et al. Rearrangements and aberrant expression of the retinoic acid receptor α gene in acute promyelocytic leukemias. J Exp Med 1990; 172:1571–1575.

237. Ludlow JW, DeCaprio JA, Huang C-M, et al. SV40 large T antigen binds preferentially to an underphosphorylated member of the retinoblastoma susceptibility gene product family. Cell 1989; 56:57–65.
238. Ludlow JW, Shon J, Pipas JM, et al. The retinoblastoma susceptibility gene product undergoes cell cycle-dependent dephosphorylation and binding to and release from SV40 large T. Cell 1990; 60:387–396.
239. Lumpkin CJ, McClung J, Pereira-Smith O, et al. Existence of high abundance antiproliferative mRNAs in senescent human diploid fibroblasts. Science 1986; 232:393–395.
240. Lynch H. Frequency of hereditary nonpolyposis colorectal carcinoma (Lynch syndromes I and II). Gastroenterology 1986; 90:486–492.
241. Ma J, Ptashne M. A new class of yeast transcriptional activators. Cell 1987; 51:113–119.
242. Malkin D, Jolly K, Barbier N, et al. Germline mutations of the p53 tumor-suppressor gene in children and young adults with second malignant neoplasms. N Engl Med 1992; 326:1309–1315.
243. Malkin D, Li F, Strong L, et al. Germ line p53 mutations in a familial syndrome of breast cancer, sarcomas, and other neoplasms. Science 1990; 250:1233–1238.
244. Marshall CJ. Tumor suppressor genes. Cell 1991; 64:313-326.
245. Martin GA, Viskochil D, Bollag G, et al. The GAP-related domain of the neurofibromatosis type 1 gene product interacts with *ras* p21. Cell 1990; 63:843–849.
246. Matsunaga E. Genetics of Wilm's tumor. Hum Genet 1981; 57:231–246.
247. Matsushime H, Roussel MF, Ashmun RA, et al. Colony-stimulating factor 1 regulates novel cyclins during the G1 phase of the cell cycle. Cell 1991; 65:701–713.
248. Mattei M-G, de The H, Mattei J-F, et al. Assignment of the human hap retinoic acid receptor RAR beta gene to the p24 gene of chromosome 3. Human Genet 1988; 80:189–190.
249. Mecklin J. Frequency of hereditary colorectal carcinoma. Gastroenterology 1987; 93:1021–1025.
250. Meek D, Eckhardt W. Phosphorylation of p53 in normal and simian virus 40-transformed NIH 3T3 cells. Mol Cell Biol 1988; 8:461–465.
251. Meek DW, Simon S, Kikkawa U, et al. The p53 tumor suppressor protein is phosphorylated at serine 389 by casein kinase II. EMBO J 1990; 9:3253–3260.
252. Mercer WE, Avignolo C, Baserga R. Role of the p53 protein in cell proliferation as studied by microinjection of monoclonal antibodies. Mol Cell Biol 1984; 4:276–281.
253. Mercer WE, Shields MT, Amin M, et al. Negative growth regulation in a glioblastoma tumor cell line that conditionally expresses human wild-type p53. Proc Natl Acad Sci USA 1990; 87:6166–6170.
254. Mihara K, Cao X-R, Yen A, et al. Cell cycle-dependent regulation of phosphorylation of the human retinoblastoma gene product. Science 1989; 246:1300–1303.
255. Miller R, Fraumeni J, Manning M. Association of Wilms' tumor with aniridia, hemihypertrophy and other congenital abnormalities. N Engl J Med 1964; 270:922–927.

256. Miller W, Kakizuka A, Frankel S, et al. Reverse transcription polymerase chain reaction for the rearranged retinoic acid receptor alpha clarifies diagnosis and detects minimal residual disease in acute promyelocytic leukemia. Proc Natl Acad Sci USA 1992; 89:2694–2698.
257. Miller W, Warrell R, Frankel S, et al. Novel retinoic acid receptor-alpha transcripts in acute promyelocytic leukemia responsive to all-*trans*-retinoic acid. J Natl Cancer Inst 1990; 82:1932–1933.
258. Milner J, Milner S. SV40–53K antigen: A possible role for 53K in normal cells. Virology 1981; 112:785–788.
259. Milner J, Watson J. Addition of fresh medium induces cell cycle and conformation changes in p53, a tumor-suppressor protein. Oncogene 1990; 11:1683–1690.
260. Mitchell P, Tjian R. Transcriptional regulation in mammalian cells by sequence-specific DNA binding proteins. Science 1989; 245:371–378.
261. Mittnacht S, Weinberg RA. G1/S phosphorylation of the retinoblastoma protein is associated with an altered affinity for the nuclear component. Cell 1991; 3:381–393.
262. Moran E. A region of SV40 large T antigen can substitute for a transforming domain of the adenovirus E1A products. Nature 1988; 334:168–170.
263. Moran E, Zerler B, Harrison TM, et al. Identification of separate domains in the adenovirus E1A gene for immortalization activity and the activation of virus early genes. Mol Cell Biol 1986; 6:3470–3480.
264. Moses HL, Yang EY, Pietenpol JA. TGF-β stimulation and inhibition of cell proliferation: New mechanistic insights. Cell 1990; 63:245–247.
265. Mowat M, Cheng A, Kimura N, et al. Rearrangements of the cellular p53 gene in erythroleukemic cells transformed by Friend virus. Nature 1985; 314:633–636.
266. Mudryj M, Devoto SH, Hiebert SW, et al. Cell cycle regulation of the E2F transcription factor involves an interaction with cyclin A. Cell 1991; 65:1243–1253.
267. Munger K, Werness B, Dyson N, et al. Complex formation of human papillomavirus E7 proteins with the retinoblastoma tumor suppressor gene product. EMBO J 1989; 8:4099–4105.
268. Munroe D, Rovinski B, Bernstein A, et al. Loss of highly conserved domain on p53 as a result of gene deletion during Friend virus-induced erythroleukemia. Oncogene 1988; 2:621-624.
269. Nelson L, Spaeth G, Nowinski T, et al. Aniridia. A review. Surv Opthalmol 1984; 28:621–642.
270. Nervi C, Vollberg T, George M, et al. Expression of nuclear retinoic acid receptors in normal tracheobronchial cells and in lung carcinoma cells. Experimental Cell Res 1991; 195:163–170.
271. Nevins JR. Mechanisms of viral-mediated transactivation of transcription. Adv Virus Res 1989; 37:35–83.
272. Nigro JM, Baker SJ, Preisinger AC, et al. Mutations in the p53 gene occur in diverse human tumour types. Nature 1989; 342:705–708.
273. Nishisho I, Nakamura Y, Miyoshi Y, et al. Mutations of chromosome 5q21 genes in FAP and colorectal cancer patients. Science 1991; 253:665–669.

274. Noda M, Kitayama H, Matsuzaki T, et al. Detection of genes with a potential for suppressing the transformated phenotype associated with activated *ras* genes. Proc Natl Acad Sci USA 1989; 86:162–166.
275. Noda M, Selinger Z, Scolnick E, et al. Flat revertants isolated from Kirsten sarcoma virus-transformed cells are resistant to the action of specific oncogene. Proc Natl Acad Sci USA 1983; 80:5602–5606.
276. Okamato M, Sasaki M, Sugio K, et al. Loss of constitutional heterozygosity in colon carcinoma from patients with familial polyposis coli. Nature (London) 1988; 331:273.
277. Oren M. The p53 cellular tumor antigen: Gene structure, expression and protein properties. Biochem Biophys Acta 1985; 823:67–78.
278. Oren M, Levine AJ. Molecular cloning of a cDNA specific for the murine p53 cellular tumor antigen. Proc Natl Acad Sci USA 1983; 80:56–59.
279. Oren M, Maltzman W, Levine AJ. Post-translational regulation of the 54K cellular tumor antigen in normal and transformed cells. Mol Cell Biol 1981; 1:101–110.
280. Orkin S, Goldman D, Sallan S. Development of homozygosity for chromosome 11p markers in Wilms' tumor. Nature (London) 1984; 309:172–174.
281. Parada LF, Land H, Weinberg RA. Tumorigenic conversion of primary embryo fibroblasts requires at least two cooperating oncogenes. Nature 1983; 304:596–602.
282. Parada LF, Land H, Weinberg RA, et al. Cooperation between gene encoding p53 tumour antigen and *ras* in cellular transformation. Nature 1984; 312:649–651.
283. Pelletier J, Breuning W, Kashtan C, et al. Germline mutations in the Wilms' tumor suppressor gene are associated with abnormal urogenital development in Denys-Drash syndrome. Cell 1991; 67:437–447.
284. Pelletier J, Bruening W, Li F, et al. WT1 mutations contribute to abnormal genital system development and hereditary Wilms' tumour. Nature 1991; 353:431–434.
285. Pelletier J, Schalling M, Buckler A, et al. Expression of the Wilms' tumor gene WT1 in the murine urogenital system. Genes Dev 1991; 5:1345–1356.
286. Pennica D, Goeddel GV, Hayflick JS, et al. The amino acid sequence of murine p53 determined from a cDNA clone. Virology 1984; 134:477–482.
287. Pereira-Smith OM, Smith JR. Genetic analysis of indefinite division in human cells: Identification of four complementation groups. Proc Natl Acad Sci USA 1988; 16:6042–6046.
288. Peto P, Roe F, Lee P, et al. Cancer and ageing in mice and man. Br J Cancer 1975; 32:411–426.
289. Pietenpol JA, Holt JT, Stein RW, et al. Transforming growth factor beta 1 suppression of c-*myc* gene transcription: role in inhibition of keratinocyte proliferation. Proc Natl Acad Sci USA 1990; 87:3758–3762.
290. Pietenpol JA, Munger K, Howley PM, et al. Factor-binding element in the human c-*myc* promoter involved in transcriptional regulation by transforming growth factor beta 1 and by the retinoblastoma gene product. Proc Natl Acad Sci USA 1991; 88:10227–10231.
291. Pietenpol JA, Stein RW, Moran E, et al. TGF-β1 inhibition of c-*myc*

transcription and growth in keratinocytes is abrogated by viral transforming proteins with pRB binding domains. Cell 1990; 61:777–785.
292. Pines J, Hunter T. Human cyclin A is adenovirus E1A-associated protein p60 and behaves differently from cyclin B. Nature 1990; 346:760–763.
293. Pines J, Hunter T. p34cdc2: The S and M kinase? New Biologist 1990; 2:389–401.
294. Ping A, Reeve A, Law D, et al. Genetic linkage of Beckwith-Wiedemann syndrome to 11p15. Am J Hum Genet 1989; 44:720–723.
295. Plutzky J, Neel B, Rosenberg R. Isolation of a novel SRC homology 2 (SH2) containing tyrosine phosphatase. Proc Natl Acad Sci USA 1992; 89:1123–1127.
296. Plutzky J, Neel B, Rosenberg R, et al. Chromosomal localization of an SH2-containing tyrosine phosphatase (PTPN6). Genomics 1992; 13:869–872.
297. Ponder B. Inherited predisposition to cancer. TIG 1990; 6:213–218.
298. Ponder BA. Gene losses in human tumours. Nature 1988; 335:400–402.
299. Porteous D, Bickmore W, Christie S, et al. HRAS-1-selected chromosome transfer generates markers that colocalize aniridia-and genitourinary dysplasia-associated translocation breakpoints and the Wilms' tumor gene within 11p13. Proc Natl Acad Sci USA 1987; 84:5355–5359.
300. Pritchard-Jones K, Fleming S, Davidson D, et al. The candidate Wilms' tumor gene is involved in genitourinary development. Nature 1990; 346:194–197.
301. Puisieux A, Lim S, Groopman J, et al. Selective targeting of p53 gene mutational hotspots in human cancers by etiologically defined agents. Cancer Res 1991; 51:6185–6189.
302. Ralston R, Bishop JM. The protein products of the *myc* and *myb* oncogenes and adenovirus E1A are structurally related. Nature 1983; 306:803–806.
303. Rastinejad F, Polverini P, Bouck N. Regulation of the activity of a new inhibitor of angiogenesis by a cancer suppressor gene. Cell 1989; 56:345–355.
304. Rauscher FI, Morris J, Tournay O, et al. Binding of the Wilms' tumor locus zinc finger protein to the EGR-1 consensus sequence. Science 1990; 250:1259–1262.
305. Raycroft L, Schmidt J, Yoas K, et al. Analysis of p53 mutants for transcriptional activity. Mol Cell Biol 1991; 11:6067–6074.
306. Raycroft L, Wu H, Lozano G. Transcriptional activation by wild-type but not transforming mutants of the p53 anti-oncogene. Science 1990; 249:1049–1051.
307. Reeve A, Housiaux P, Gardner R, et al. Loss of a Harvey *ras* allele in sporadic Wilms' tumor. Nature (London) 1984; 309:174–176.
308. Reeve AE, Sih SA, Raizis AM, et al. Loss of allelic heterozygosity at a second locus on chromosome 11 in sporadic Wilms' tumor cells. Mol Cell Biol 1989; 9:1799–1803.
309. Reich N, Levine A. Growth regulation of a cellular tumour antigen, p53, in nontransformed cells. Nature 1984; 308:199–201.
310. Reich NC, Oren M, Levine AJ. Two distinct mechanisms regulate the levels of a cellular tumor antigen, p53. Mol Cell Biol 1983; 3:2143–2150.

311. Riccardi V, Sujansky E, Smith A, et al. Chromosomal imbalance in the aniridia-Wilms' tumor association: 11p interstitial deletion. Pediatrics 1978; 61:604–610.

312. Riccardi VM, Hittner HM, Francke U, et al. The aniridia-Wilms' tumor association: The critical role of chromosome band 11p13. Cancer Genet Cytogenet 1990; 2:131–137.

313. Robbins PD, Horowitz JM, Mulligan RC. Negative regulation of human c-*fos* expression by the retinoblastoma gene product. Nature 1990; 346:668–671.

314. Rodrigues NR, Rowan A, Smith MEF, et al. p53 mutations in colorectal cancer. Proc Natl Acad Sci USA 1990; 87:7555–7559.

315. Rose EA, Glaser T, Jones C, et al. Complete physical map of the WAGR region of 11p13 localizes a candidate Wilms' tumor gene. Cell 1990; 60:495–508.

316. Rosengard AM, Krutzsch HC, Shearn A, et al. Reduced *nm23/awd* protein in tumor metastasis and aberrant *Drosphilia* development. Nature 1989; 342:177–180.

317. Rotter V, Wolf D. Biological and molecular analysis of p53 cellular-encoded tumor antigen. Adv Cancer Res 1984; 43:113-141.

318. Rovinski B, Benchimol S. Immortalization of rat embryo fibroblasts by the cellular p53 oncogene. Oncogene 1988; 2:445-452.

319. Rovinski B, Munroe D, Peacock J, et al. Deletion of 5'-coding sequences of the cellular p53 gene in mouse erythroleukemia: A novel mechanism of oncogene regulation. Mol Cell Biol 1987; 7:847–853.

320. Royer-Pokora B, Ragg S, Heckl-Ostreicher B, et al. Direct pulsed field gel electrophoresis of Wilms' tumors shows that DNA deletions in 11p13 are rare. Genes, Chromosomes, Cancer 1991; 3:89–100.

321. Ruley HE. Adenovirus early region 1A enables viral and cellular transforming genes to transform primary cells in culture. Nature 1983; 304:602–606.

322. Rustgi A, Dyson N, Bernards R. Amino-terminal domains of c-*myc* and N-*myc* proteins mediate binding to the retinoblastoma gene product. Nature 1991; 8:541–544.

323. Sager R. Genetic suppression of tumor formation. Adv Cancer Res 1985; 44:43–68.

324. Sager R. Genetic suppression of tumor formation: A new frontier in cancer research. Cancer Res 1986; 46:1573–1580.

325. Sager R. Tumor suppressor genes: The puzzle and the promise. Science 1989; 246:1406–1412.

326. Sarnow P, Ho Y, Williums J, et al. Adenovirus E1B-58kd tumor antigen and SV40 large tumor antigen are physically associated with the same 54 kd cellular protein in transformed cells. Cell 1982; 28:387.

327. Sasaki M, Okamoto M, Sato C, et al. Loss of constitutional heterozygosity in colorectal tumors from patients with familial polyposis coli and those with nonpolyposis colorectal carcinoma. Cancer Res 1989; 49:4402–4406.

328. Sato T, Akiyama F, Sakamoto G, et al. Accumulation of genetic alterations and progression of primary breast cancer. Cancer Res 1991; 51:5794–5799.

329. Saxon PJ, Srivatsan ES, Stanbridge EJ. Introduction of human chromosome 11 via microcell transfer controls tumorigenic expression of HeLa cell. EMBO J 1986; 5:3461–3466.

330. Schaefer R, Iyer J, Iten E, et al. Partial reversion of the transformed phenotype in HRAS-transfected tumorigenic cells by transfer of a human gene. Proc Natl Acad Sci USA 1988; 85:1590-1594.

331. Scheffner M, Munger K, Byrne J, et al. The state of the p53 and retinoblastoma genes in human cervical cancer. Proc Natl Acad Sci USA 1991; 88:5523–5527.

332. Scheffner M, Werness B, Huibregtse J, et al. The E6 oncoprotein encoded by human papillomavirus types 16 and 18 promotes the degradation of p53. Cell 1990; 63:1129–1136.

333. Schmid M, Haaf T, Grunert D. 5-azacytidine-induced undercondensations in human chromosomes. Hum Genet 1984; 67:257-263.

334. Schneider JF, Fisher F, Goding CR, et al. Mutational analysis of the adenovirus E1A gene: The role of transcriptional regulation in transformation. EMBO J 1987; 6:2053–2060.

335. Seshadri T, Campisi J. Repression of c-fos transcription and an altered genetic program in senescent human fibroblasts. Science 1990; 247:205–209.

336. Shen S-H, Bastien L, Posner B, et al. A protein tyrosine phosphatase with sequence similarity to the SH2 domain of the protein tyrosine kinases. Nature 1991; 352:736–738.

337. Sherman M. Retinoids and Cell Differentiation. Boca Raton, CRC Press 1986; p. 198.

338. Shew J, Chen P, Bookstein R, et al. Deletion of a splice donor site ablates expression of the following exon and produces an unphosphorylated RB protein unable to bind SV40 T antigen. Cell Growth Diff 1990; 1:17–25.

339. Shew J, Lin BT, Chen P, et al. C-terminal truncation of the retinoblastoma gene product leads to functional inactivation. Proc Natl Acad Sci USA 1990; 87:6–10.

340. Shobat OM, Greenberg M, Reisman D, et al. Inhibition of cell growth mediated by plasmids encoding p53 antisense. Oncogene 1987; 1:277–283.

341. Sidransky D, Mikkelson T, Schwechheimer K, et al. Clonal expansion of p53 mutant cells is associated with brain tumour progression. Nature 1992; 355:846–847.

342. Sidransky D, Tokino T, Hamilton S, et al. Identification of ras oncogene mutations in the stool of patients with curable colorectal tumors. Science 1992; 256:102–105.

343. Sidransky D, Von Eschenbach A, Tsai Y, et al. Identification of p53 gene mutations in bladder cancers and urine samples. Science 1991; 252:706–709.

344. Skuse GR, Rowley PT. Tumor suppressor genes and inherited predisposition to malignancy. Semin Oncol 1989; 16:128–137.

345. Smith DH, Ziff EB. The amino-terminal region of the adenovirus serotype 5 E1A protein performs two separate functions when expressed in primary baby rat kidney cells. Mol Cell Biol 1988; 8:3882–3890.

346. Solomon E, Borrow J, Goddard AD. Chromosome aberrations and cancer. Science 1991; 254:1153–1160.

347. Solomon E, Voss R, Hall V, et al. Chromosome 5 allele loss in human colorectal carcinomas. Nature 1987; 328:616–619.
348. Sparkes R, Murphree A, Lingua R, et al. Gene for hereditary retinoblastoma assigned to human chromosome 13 by linkage to esterase D. Science 1983; 219:971.
349. Sparkes R, Sparkes M, Wilson M, et al. Regional assignment of genes for human esterase D and retinoblastoma to chromosome band 13q14. Science 1980; 208:1042.
350. Stanbridge E, Wilkinson J. Dissociation of anchorage independence from tumorigenicity in human cell hybrids. Int J Cancer 1980; 26:1–8.
351. Stanbridge EJ. Suppression of malignancy in human cells. Nature 1976; 260:17–20.
352. Stanbridge EJ. Genetic analysis of human malignancy using somatic cell hybrids in nude mice. Cancer Res 1988; 41:573-580.
353. Stanbridge EJ, Flandermeyer RR, Daniels D, et al. Specific chromosome loss associated with the expression of tumorigenicity in human cell hybrids. Somatic Cell Genet 1981; 7:699–712.
354. Stanbridge EJ, Wilkinson J. Analysis of malignancy in human cells: Malignant and transformed phenotypes are under separate genetic control. Proc Natl Acad Sci USA 1978; 75:1466–1469.
355. Steeg P, Bevilacqua G, Kopper L, et al. Evidence for a novel gene associated with low tumor metastatic potential. J Natl Cancer Inst 1988; 80:200–204.
356. Stein GH, Beeson M, Gordon L. Failure to phosphorylate the retinoblastoma gene product in senescent human fibroblasts. Science 1990; 249:666–669.
357. Stoler A, Bouck N. Identification of a single chromosome in the normal human genome essential for suppression of hamster cell transformation. Proc Natl Acad Sci USA 1985; 82:570–574.
358. Sturzbecher H-W, Addison C, Jenkins J. Characterization of mutant p53-*hsp* 72/73 protein-protein complexes by transient expression in monkey COS cells. Mol Cell Biol 1988; 8:3740-3747.
359. Sturzbecher H-W, Chumakov P, Welch W, et al. Mutant p53 proteins bind p53 *hsp* 72/73 cellular heat-shock-related proteins in SV40-transformed monkey cells. Oncogene 1987; 1:201-211.
360. Sugawara O, Oshimura M, Koi M, et al. Induction of cellular senescence in immortalized cells by human chromosome 1. Science 1990; 247:707–710.
361. Sukhatme VP, Cao X, Chang L, et al. A zinc finger-encoding gene coregulated with c-*fos* during growth and differentiation and after cellular depolarization. Cell 1988; 53:37–43.
362. Sumegi J, Uzvolgyi E, Klein G. Expression of the RB gene under the control of the MuLV LTR suppresses tumorigenicity of WERI-RB-27 retinoblastoma cells in immunodefective mice. Cell Growth Differ 1990; 1:247–250.
363. Szekely L, Uzvolgyi E, Jiang W-Q, et al. Subcellular localization of the retinoblastoma protein. Cell Growth Differ 1991; 2:287–295.
364. T'Ang A, Varley JM, Chakraborty S, et al. Structural rearrangement of the retinoblastoma gene in human breast cancer. Science 1988; 242:263–266.

365. T'Ang A, Wu K, Hashimoto T, et al. Genomic organization of the human retinoblastoma gene. Oncogene 1989; 4:401–407.

366. Takahashi R, Hashimoto T, Xu H-J, et al. The retinoblastoma gene functions as a growth and tumor suppressor in human bladder carcinoma cells. Proc Natl Acad Sci USA 1991; 88:5257–5261.

367. Templeton DJ, Park SO, Lanier L, et al. Nonfunctional mutants of the retinoblastoma protein are characterized by defects in phosphorylation, viral oncoprotein association and nuclear tethering. Proc Natl Acad Sci USA 1991; 88:3033–3037.

368. Toguchida J, Ishizaki K, Sasaki MS, et al. Preferential mutation of paternally derived RB gene as the initial event in sporadic osteosarcoma. Nature 1989; 338:156–158.

369. Toguchida J, Yamaguchi T, Dayton S, et al. Prevalence and spectrum of germline mutations of the p53 gene among patients with sarcoma. N Engl J Med 1992; 326:1301–1308.

370. Ton C, Huff V, Call K, et al. Smallest region of overlap in Wilms' tumor deletions uniquely implicates an 11p13 zinc finger gene as the disease locus. Genomics 1991; 10:293–297.

371. Trent JM, Stanbridge EJ, McBride HL, et al. Tumorigenicity in human melanoma cell lines controlled by introduction of human chromosome 6. Science 1990; 247:568–571.

372. Tsai L, Harlow E, Meyerson M. Isolation of the human cdk2 gene that encodes the cyclin A-and adenovirus E1A-associated p33 kinase. Nature 1991; 353:174–177.

373. van den Elsen P, Houweling A, van der Eb AJ. Expression of region E1B of human adenovirus in the absence of region E1A is not sufficient for complete transformation. Virology 1983; 128:377–390.

374. van Heyningen V, Bickmore WA, Seawright A, et al. Role for the Wilms' tumor gene in genital development. Proc Natl Acad Sci USA 1990; 87:5383–5386.

375. van Heyningen V, Boyd P, Seawright A, et al. Molecular analysis of chromosome 11 deletions in aniridia-Wilms' tumor syndrome. Proc Natl Acad Sci USA 1985; 82:8592–8596.

376. Viskochil D, Buchberg AM, Xu G, et al. Deletions and a translocation interrupt a cloned gene at the neurofibromatosis type 1 locus. Cell 1990; 61:187–192.

377. Vogelstein B, Fearon ER, Hamilton SR, et al. Genetic alterations during colorectal-tumor development. N Engl J Med 1988; 319:525–532.

378. Vogelstein B, Fearon ER, Kern SE, et al. Allelotype of colorectal carcinomas. Science 1989; 244:207.

379. Wallace MR, Marchuk DA, Andersen LB, et al. Type 1 neurofibromatosis gene: Identification of a large transcript disrupted in three NF1 patients. Science 1990; 249:181–186.

380. Wallet V, Mutzel R, Troll H, et al. *Dictyoselium* nucleoside diphosphate kinase highly homologous to *nm23* and *awd* proteins involved in mammalian tumor metastasis and *Drosophila* development. J Natl Cancer Inst 1990; 18:1199-1202.

381. Wang EH, Friedman PN, Prives C. The murine p53 protein blocks

replication of SV40 in vitro by inhibiting the initiation functions of SV40 large T antigen. Cell 1989; 57:379–392.

382. Warrell R, Frankel S, Miller W, et al. Differentiation therapy of acute promyelocytic leukemia with tretinoin (all-*trans*-retinoic acid). N Engl J Med 1991; 324:1385–1393.

383. Weinberg R. The retinoblastoma gene and cell growth control. Trends Biochem Sci 1990; 15:199–202.

384. Weissman BE, Saxon PJ, Pasquale SR, et al. Introduction of a normal human chromosome 11 into a Wilms' tumor cell line controls its tumorigenic expression. Science 1987; 236:175–180.

385. Weissmann BE, Stanbridge EJ. Complementation of the tumorigenic phenotype in human cell hybrids. J Natl Cancer Inst 1983; 70:667–672.

386. Werness BA, Levine AJ, Howley PM. Association of human papillomavirus types 16 and 18 E6 proteins with p53. Science 1990; 248:76–79.

387. Whang-Peng J, Kao-Shan S, Lee E, et al. Specific chromosome defects associated with human small cell lung cancer: Deletion of 3p (14–23). Science 1982; 215:181–182.

388. Whyte P, Buchkovich K, Horowitz JM, et al. Association between an oncogene and an anti-oncogene: The adenovirus E1A proteins bind to the retinoblastoma gene product. Nature 1988; 334:124–129.

389. Whyte P, Ruley H, Harlow E. Two regions of the adenovirus early region 1A proteins are required for transformation. J Virol 1988; 62:257–265.

390. Whyte P, Williamson N, Harlow E. Cellular targets for transformation by the adenovirus E1A proteins. Cell 1989; 56:67-75.

391. Wiggs J, Nordenskjold M, Yandell D, et al. Prediction of the risk of hereditary retinoblastoma, using DNA polymorphisms within the retinoblastoma gene. N Engl J Med 1988; 318:151–157.

392. Wigler M. GAPs in understanding Ras. Nature 1990; 346:696-697.

393. Wolf D, Harris N, Rotter V. Reconstitution of p53 expression in a nonproducer Ab-MuLV-transformed cell line by transfection of a functional p53 gene. Cell 1984; 38:119–126.

394. Wolf DS, Admon S, Oren M, et al. Abelson murine leukemia virus-transformed cells that lack p53 protein synthesis express aberrant p53 mRNA species. Mol Cell Biol 1984; 4:552–558.

395. Woodford-Thomas T, Rhodes J, Dixon J. Expression of a protein tyrosine phosphatase in normal and v-*src*-transformed mouse 3T3 fibroblasts. J Cell Biol 1992; 117:401-414.

396. Wrede D, Tidy J, Crook T, et al. Expression of RB and p53 proteins in HPV-positive and HPV-negative cervical carcinoma cell lines. Mol Carcinog 1991; 4:171–175.

397. Xu G, Lin B, Tanaka K, et al. The catalytic domain of the neurofibromatosis type 1 gene product stimulates *ras* GTPase and complements IRA mutants of *S. cerevisiae*. Cell 1990; 63:835–841.

398. Xu H-J, Sumegi J, Hu S-X, et al. Intraocular tumor formation of RB-reconstituted retinoblastoma cells. Cancer Res 1991; 51:4481–4485.

399. Xu HJ, Hu SX, Cagle PT, et al. Absence of retinoblastoma protein expression in primary non-small cell lung carcinomas. Cancer Res 1991; 15:2735–2739.

400. Yandell D, Campbell T, Dayton S, et al. Oncogenic point mutations in

the human retinoblastoma gene: Their application to genetic counseling. N Engl J Med 1989; 321:1659–1695.

401. Yatani A, Okabe K, Polakis P, et al. *ras* p21 and GAP inhibit coupling of muscarinic receptors to atrial K+ channels. Cell 1990; 61:769–776.
402. Yee S-P, Branton P. Detection of cellular proteins associated with human adenovirus type 5 early region 1A polypeptides. Virology 1985; 147:142–153.
403. Yewdell J, Gannon J, Lane D. Monoclonal antibody analysis of p53 expression in normal and transformed cells. J Virol 1986; 59:444–452.
404. Yi T, Cleveland J, Ihle J. Protein tyrosine phosphatase containing SH2 domains: Characterization, preferential expression in hematopoietic cells, and localization to chromosome 12p12–13. Mol Cell Biol 1992; 12:836–846.
405. Yokota J, Akiyama T, Fung YKT, et al. Altered expression of the retinoblastoma (RB) gene in small-cell carcinoma of the lung. Oncogene 1988; 3:471–475.
406. Yunis J, Ransay N. Retinoblastoma and subband deletion of chromosome 13. Am J Dis Child 1978; 132:161–163.
407. Zakut-Houri R, Oren M, Bienz B, et al. A single gene and a pseudogene for the cellular tumour antigene p53. Nature 1983; 306:594–597.
408. Zentella A, Weis FM, Ralph DA, et al. Early gene responses to transforming growth factor-beta in cells lacking growth suppressive RB function. Mol Cell Biol 1991; 11:4952–4958.
409. Zhu X, Dunn JM, Phillips RA, et al. Preferential germline mutation of the paternal allele in retinoblastoma. Nature 1989; 340:312–313.

Chapter 3

Role of *Ras* Proteins in Signal-Transduction

Veeraswamy Manne

Ras genes are found in all eukaryotes and their transforming alleles (*ras* oncogenes) have been implicated in the development of tumors in humans and other animals. *Ras* oncogenes are the most frequently encountered of the known 50 or so of the oncogenes in human cancer with an overall incidence rate of about 15%.[19] This figure may be misleading since wide variations in incidence rate exist among different forms of human neoplasia (Table 1). For example, pancreatic carcinomas (90%) and colon cancers (50%) exhibit the highest incidence of the *ras* oncogene, whereas carcinomas of the breast carry *ras* oncogene very rarely. Notwithstanding the clinical significance of the presence of *ras* oncogenes in human cancer, extensive interest is focused on this gene family because of the notion that understanding the biochemical functions of *ras* proteins would have a major impact on our knowledge of the molecular basis of human neoplasia. This chapter is focused on the biochemical properties of *ras* proteins with an attempt to picture them as signal-transducers in the cell. Several recent reviews have detailed other aspects of the *ras* oncogene family.[8,19–21,40,51,62,91,134,152]

Structural Features

The mammalian *ras* gene family consists of at least three members, H-*ras*, K-*ras*, and N-*ras*, all of which encode highly conserved

From *The Molecular Basis of Human Cancer:* edited by B. Neel, M.D., Ph.D., R. Kumar, Ph.D. © 1993, Futura Publishing Co. Inc., Mount Kisco, NY.

TABLE 1.
Incidence of *ras* Oncogenes in Human Cancer*

Tumor Type	Incidence** (%)	Predominant ras Oncogene(s)
Pancreatic	95	K
Myeloid	70	K, N
Thyroid	67	H, K, N
Colon adenoma	66	K
Thyroid adenoma	50	H, K, N
Colon	47	K
Seminoma	43	K, N
Lung	33	K
Liver	30	N
Ovarian	20	K
Melanoma	19	N
Lymphoid	18	N
Bladder	17	H
Skin (squamous)	14	H
Breast	13	H, K
Renal	13	H
Prostate	13	K
Cervical	11	H
Keratoacanthoma	10	H
Oesophagus	0	
Glioblastoma	0	
Neuroblastoma	0	
Stomach	0	
Gall bladder	0	

*See references.[19,91] **Highest incidence reported among the cases studied. Significant variations exist among different studies.

proteins of ≈189 amino acid residues and Mr 21 kDa termed p21 *ras*. The *ras* genes were first identified as the oncogenic sequences of certain strains of rat sarcoma viruses.[144] Their normal counterparts (cellular *ras* genes or c-*ras*) are highly conserved and have been identified in a wide variety of eukaryotic cells. Four domains essentially define the primary structure of nascent *ras* proteins[4]: a highly conserved amino terminal domain of 85 residues, a moderately conserved middle domain of the next 80 amino acid residues, a highly variable carboxy terminus, and the end sequence of Cys[186]-A-A-X (where A is any aliphatic amino acid and X is a carboxy-terminal amino acid). Figure 1 illustrates these four domains and the structural and functional properties associated with them. Cellular *ras* genes acquire transforming properties by single point

1	85	165	186 189
Highly Conserved	Moderately Conserved	Highly Variable	Conserved End Sequence
Phosphate of 'GNP' binding Y13-259 Antibody binding Effector domain Naturally occuring oncogenic ras point mutations (12,13, 59 & 61) GAP binding domain GTP hydrolysis	Puring ring of 'GNP' binding Experimentally induced and activating ras mutation domain	Sites of palmi-toylation in H and N ras Site of membrane anchorage strength	Recognition sequence for Post- translational processing steps Site of Farnesylation & Carboxy-methylation Site of membrane attachment

Figure 1. *Linear representation of the ras protein. The principal functions of various domains of the ras protein as understood currently are listed below the respective domain.*

mutations within their coding sequences.[44,122,129,151,154] In naturally occurring *ras* oncogenes, mutations are detected in codons 12, 13, 59, and 61.[8] The high incidence of *ras* mutations in a diverse spectrum of human malignancies suggests a role of *ras* in the biochemistry of most cell types in the body. Indeed, it is now believed that the critical function of *ras* is at the junction where many biochemical pathways converge. There are several *ras*-related genes exhibiting limited sequence homology to the *ras* gene family, that include *rap, rac, rho, ral,* and *rab*[8] which by themselves form another gene family.

All known *ras* proteins bind guanine nucleotides with high affinity and specificity[140] and exhibit a weak GTPase activity.[103] The GTPase activity is potentiated by cooperation with the cellular GTPase activating protein (GAP).[156] In addition, *ras* proteins with threonine substitution at position 59 have an autophosphorylating activity.[143] *Ras* proteins are localized in the inner surface of the plasma membrane,[159] and this membrane localization occurs following a complex series of posttranslational modifications (see below) in the C-terminus of *ras* proteins.[58] These activities/properties are crucial to the biological function of *ras* proteins.[58]

Both normal and oncogenic forms of *ras* share similar GTP/GDP binding properties. However, they differ in their ability to hydrolyze bound GTP. The weak GTPase activity of normal *ras* is further reduced tenfold in oncogenic *ras*.[100] Moreover, the oncogenic forms of *ras* are insensitive to GAP which functions to accelerate the slow intrinsic rate of GTP hydrolysis by normal *ras*.[156] Hence, *ras* is biologically active when GTP bound and inactive when GDP bound. Oncogenic forms of *ras* tend to remain GTP bound and constitutively active whereas normal *ras* activity is regulated by its intrinsic GTPase in concert with the action of GAP. Figure 2 depicts a schematic model for the mode of action of *ras* proteins. This model is based on the known biochemical

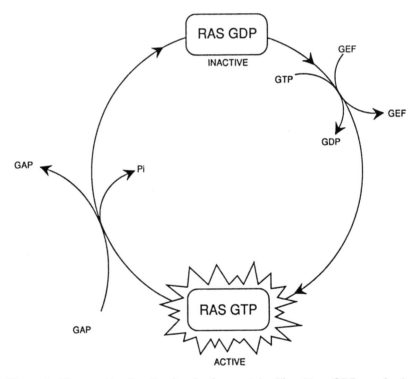

Figure 2. *The operating functional cycle of ras protein. The p21ras.GDP complex is the inactive state and most of the ras protein exists in this form, especially when not generating transmembrane signals. In response to various stimuli p21ras.GTP complex, the functional version, is formed. Conversion of ras.GDP to ras.GTP occurs by exchange of ras-bound GDP to cytosolic GTP mediated by exchange factors. Ras.GTP is reverted to its inactive ras.GDP as GTP is hydrolyzed. GAP protein greatly accelerates the rate of GTP hydrolysis by p21ras. Ras.GTP, the functional state, is short lived and owes its existence to the stimulus. Mechanisms that interfere and prolong the existence of ras.GTP complex result in abnormal functions associated with ras protein.*

and biological properties of *ras* proteins which closely resemble those of well-defined signal-transducing G proteins. The most attractive feature of this model is that it explains the dominant nature and the possible mechanism underlying the function of naturally occurring *ras* mutations in human cancers. The mutant *ras* proteins found in human cancers are constitutively active as a consequence of their reduced intrinsic GTPase activity and their inability to interact with GAP.

The three-dimensional structure of normal and oncogenic form of p21 *ras* protein in GTP as well as GDP bound form were determined.[37,88,121] The structure is composed of five α-helices and six strands of β-sheets interconnected by ten loops (Fig. 3, Table 2). The topological arrangement of the secondary structure elements of p21 *ras* are identical to the GDP-binding domain of EF-Tu (a bacterial protein involved in protein chain elongation), the only other guanine

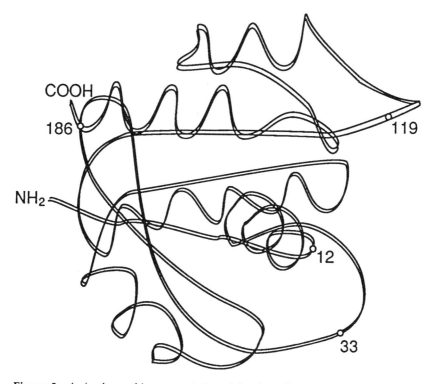

Figure 3. *A simple graphic representation of the three-dimensional backbone structure of ras protein. Location of some critical amino acids, the N-and the C-terminus are indicated. Figure is based on Pai et al.[121]*

TABLE 2.
Secondary Structure Elements of the *ras* Proteins

α-helices		*β-sheets*		*loops*	
#	AAs	#	AAs	#	AAs
1	16–25	1	2–9	1	10–15
2	66–74	2	37–46	2	26–36
3	87–103	3	49–58	3	47–48
4	127–136	4	77–83	4	59–65
5	152–165	5	111–116	5	75–76
		6	141–143	6	84–86
				7	104–110
				8	117–126
				9	137–140
				10	144–151

AA: amino acids. Amino acid residues that form various structures are indicated and based on Pai et al.[121]

nucleotide-binding protein with a known three-dimensional structure. This suggests that all known G proteins could very likely have similar overall architecture. Cellular and mutant *ras* proteins have almost identical structures, and the only significant differences are restricted to loop 4 and in the vicinity of the γ-phosphate.[88]

Membrane localization of *ras* proteins is required for proper biological function and occurs following a series of modifications in the C-terminus of *ras* proteins. All *ras* proteins share a C-terminal sequence known as CAAX box, which consists of a conserved cysteine (C), two aliphatic amino acids (AA), and a carboxy-terminal residue (X). Similar carboxy-terminal motifs have been found in other proteins including various types of *ras*-related molecules, γ-subunit of bovine transducin, and nuclear lamin B. Recent studies have unveiled the biochemical nature of the posttranslational modifications within the CAAX motif of *ras* proteins. They include:

1. farnesylation of the conserved cysteine residue (Cys[186] in mammalian H-*ras*);
2. cleavage of the three carboxy-terminal amino acid residues (AAX); and
3. methylation of the resulting carboxy-terminal farnesyl cysteine (Fig. 4).[24,28,58,64,77]

These posttranslational modifications are sufficient for the interaction with the inner side of the plasma membrane of those *ras*

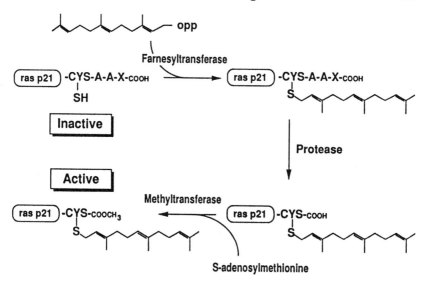

Figure 4. *Various enzymatic steps in C-terminal processing of ras proteins. Some ras proteins, like H-ras, undergo an additional modification, palmitoylation on cysteine(s) upstream of 186, which is not shown in this figure.*

proteins (such as K-*ras*2B) which carry a stretch of basic amino acid residues upstream of the farnesylated cysteine. All other *ras* proteins require palmitoylation of the neighboring cysteine residue(s) to strengthen their association with the plasma membrane.[66] Several lines of evidence suggest that farnesylation (and the subsequent modifications) is essential for *ras* function.[58,66]

The donor of the farnesyl moiety present in *ras* proteins is farnesyl pyrophosphate (FPP), a key intermediate in cholesterol biosynthesis. Inhibiting the synthesis of FPP results in the accumulation of cytosolic *ras* protein that is biologically inactive. Deprivation of mevalonate (a precursor of FPP) in yeast mutants of HMG-CoA reductase (a key enzyme in the pathway leading to the synthesis of cholesterol) restores the normal phenotype to cells that either overexpress the wild type RAS2 gene or carry activated RAS2[val-19] allele.[139] Moreover, inhibitors of HMG-CoA reductase blocked the H-*ras*[val-12] protein-mediated maturation of *Xenopus* oocytes.[139] These results have raised the possibility that inhibitors of FPP (and hence cholesterol) biosynthesis might be used to block the transforming activity of *ras* oncoproteins in human tumors. Unfortunately, the strict requirements of mammalian cells for FPP makes it likely that the concentrations of such inhibitors needed to block *ras* oncogenes may have undesirable toxic effects. Therefore, targeting the *ras* C-terminal modification steps for the development of new drugs for the treatment of tumors (induced by *ras* activation) is considered more logical and promising. Protein farnesyltransferase (FT), the enzyme that catalyzes the transfer of farnesyl from FPP to cys[186] of *ras* proteins is currently the focus of anticancer drug development. FT has been identified and characterized in several laboratories.[101,130,137] The susceptibility of FT to inhibition by CAAX motif tetrapeptides[54,131] strengthens the idea that this enzyme may be effectively inhibited for therapeutic applications.

Functional Aspects

The precise biochemical function of *ras* proteins remains a mystery. However, the high degree of conservation among these proteins throughout eukaryotic evolution suggests that they perform certain fundamental cellular functions. The role of *ras* proteins is not limited to cell proliferation since these proteins are expressed in most cell types including nondividing neuronal cells[87] and in all stages of development of the embryo.[111] No clear correlation exists between proliferation and high level expression of *ras*, since both proliferating and nonproliferating tissues express these proteins at high levels.[56] In addition, *ras* oncogenes can also induce differentiation of PC12 cells, which are of neuronal origin.[116] In yeast, *ras* genes are required for survival[85] and mating.[48] Thus, *ras* proteins participate in a wide variety of biological processes. In the following paragraphs various properties and phenomena associated with the biochemical activities of *ras* will be discussed.

The known biochemical properties of *ras* proteins, namely membrane localization, high affinity guanine nucleotide binding, and weak GTPase activity, are also shared by a family of guanine nucleotide-binding proteins known as the G proteins.[52] The G proteins are multisubunit functional complexes in which the α-subunit binds guanine nucleotides. The α-subunits exhibit sequence homology to *ras* proteins.[50,74] The G proteins are a diverse group that includes polypeptide chain initiation and elongation factors, tubulin, transducin, and G proteins of the eukaryotic adenyl cyclase system.[1] The G proteins of hormone responsive adenyl cyclase and transducin in the visual system are well characterized and are known to act as transmembrane signal-transducers.[53] Gi/Gs, transducin, and *ras* proteins are all membrane localized. Their localization and biological similarity have suggested a function for *ras* proteins in transmembrane signaling.

GTPase activating protein (GAP) is a 100 to 120 kDa protein found in nearly every cell. Recently it has been shown that GAP interacts with *ras* protein and increases the GTPase activity of *ras* by more than 100-fold. Although it is generally accepted that the interaction of GAP with *ras* is physiologically relevant, the exact role of GAP is not well understood. The biochemical activity of GAP[156] indicates that it is a negative regulator of *ras* function. Some data derived from studies using structural mutants of *ras*[138] and other biochemical experiments also point to GAP as at least a part of the effector system of *ras* function.[162] The region comprising amino acids 32–40 of *ras* is conserved in all *ras* proteins. Mutations within this region destroy the transforming ability of oncogenic *ras* protein without affecting GDP/GTP binding, GTP hydrolysis, and plasma membrane localization. This "effector" region, so called because it is presumed to be involved in the interaction of *ras* with its target system, is involved in the binding and interaction of *ras* with GAP. These observations implicate GAP as a negative regulator of *ras* activity and its downstream effector. This notion is appealing conceptually, as the *ras* target effector system generates a signal as it terminates its own ability to produce that signal (Fig. 2).

Saccharomyces cerevisiae contains two *ras* proteins: RAS1 and RAS2, which are structurally and biochemically related to their mammalian counterparts.[35,153] However, yeast RAS proteins appear to have different cellular functions. Yeast RAS1 may indirectly regulate glucose-induced inositol phospholipid turnover,[79] whereas RAS2 participates in the control of adenyl cyclase.[155] Adenyl cyclase is regulated by G proteins[52,53] and, in *S cerevisiae*, RAS2 is apparently the G protein that stimulates the adenyl cyclase signal-transduction pathway.[23] However, *ras* proteins do not operate through the adenyl cyclase system in other eukaryotes. In fact, mammalian cells transformed by viral *ras* exhibit reduced adenyl cyclase activity, and purified *ras* proteins do not affect mammalian adenyl cyclase activity.[9] In addition, human *ras* proteins when microinjected induce maturation of *Xenopus* oocytes without affecting cAMP levels.[16] Interestingly, the adenyl cyclase system coupled to *ras* proteins is not even common to all yeasts, since *ras* proteins in *S pombe* do not affect cAMP levels.[48,112] These findings indicate that the overall role and activity of *ras* may be dictated by the specific interactions with other proteins and that these proteins may be species specific.

Increased membrane ruffling and pinocytosis occur following the interaction of some hormones and mitogens with their receptors. Binding of growth factors such as EGF[60], PDGF,[34] NGF[30], and insulin[55] to target cells results in such membrane activity. The proposed role of *ras* proteins in the transduction of mitogenic signals across the membrane is consistent with the observed induction of membrane ruffling and pinocytosis when *ras* proteins are microinjected into quiescent fibroblasts.[6] The molecular mechanisms by which *ras* proteins alter membrane dynamics are at present unknown. However, this parallel in the action of *ras* and growth factors has suggested that growth factor signals may be transduced through *ras*.

Phospholipase A_2 catalyzes hydrolysis of fatty acid ester bonds at the 2 position of various phospholipids, producing arachidonate and lysophospholipids. Prostaglandins, leukotrienes, and thromboxanes, which are collectively referred to as eicosanoids, are metabolites derived from arachidonate. These eicosanoids are powerful regulators of several physiological responses.[63,105] Stimulation of phospholipase A_2 activity has been implicated in cell proliferation initiated by serum and other growth factors. Synthesis of lysophospholipids, the products of phospholipase A_2, was found to be stimulated following microinjection of oncogenic *ras* proteins.[7] It is not clear whether the stimulation of phospholipase A_2 by *ras* is indirect or direct. However, a G protein has been implicated in the regulation of Ca^{2+}-dependent phospholipase A_2 activity.[18] Thus the apparent stimulatory effect of *ras* proteins on phospholipase A_2 activity fits well with multiple biological processes ascribed to *ras*. However, there are reports of decreased levels of PLC A_2, arachidonate and prostaglandin E2 in NIH3T3 cells transfected with C-*ras* or oncogenic EJ-*ras* compared to control cells.[11] Moreover, these NIH3T3 cells expressing the transfected *ras* proteins show decreased prostaglandin E2 and arachidonate production in response to PDGF.[11] Such dilemmas may stem from the differences in different experimental systems.

Cells and tissues exposed to hormones, neurotransmitters, or growth factors exhibit a large increase in inositol lipids turnover.[13,15,95] Stimulation of polyphosphoinositide (PPI) metabolism has been implicated in the initiation of cell proliferation by serum and other growth factors.[102,104,114] Agonist occupation of receptors results in the hydrolysis of phosphatidylinositol 4,5-biphosphate (PIP_2) by phosphoinositide phospholipase C (PI-PLC) to generate diacylglycerol (DAG) and inositol triphosphate (IP$_3$). Both IP$_3$ and DAG appear to function as second messengers. The pathway driven by IP$_3$ leads to changes in the concentrations of free calcium, an important intracellular signal for cell proliferation.[22] DAG controls the other signal pathway by stimulating protein kinase C (PKC). PKC appears to be the major endogenous receptor for the phorbol esters,[25] which act by stimulating protein phosphorylation through this enzyme. As a consequence of PKC-mediated protein phosphorylation, the Na$^+$/H$^+$ antiporter which extrudes protons in exchange for sodium is activated. The resulting fall in the intracellular level of hydrogen ions and the increase in calcium appear to be important steps in initiating cellular proliferation.[106,132] The mechanism by which these changes contribute to the onset of DNA synthesis probably involves stimulation of protein phosphorylation by specific kinases, one of the earliest biochemical changes recorded when cells are stimulated with growth factors. Some of the targets of protein phosphorylation are believed to be transcription factors, and these are often the products of proto-oncogenes.

The pathways leading to the formation of PIP$_2$, and production and degradation of IP$_3$ and DAG, are all potential targets for extensive regulation. Some of the proteins that participate in this cascade system could be encoded by cellular proto-oncogenes.[14] For example, v-*sis* encodes a protein that is homologous to PDGF, which stimulates phosphoinositide metabolism.[38] Also, the v-*erb*-B protein has a very similar structure to a segment of the receptor for EGF,[43] which also stimulates phosphoinositide metabolism.[136] Moreover, phosphoinositide based second messengers are produced immediately following the exposure of cells to IL-2[45] and IL-3.[46] Transformed cells exhibit enhanced phosphatidylinositol (PI) turnover as compared to normal cells.[36] Thus there is a clear connection among PI turnover, cell proliferation, growth factors, and proto-oncogenes. The possibility that proto-oncogene products play a role in PI turnover has recently been strengthened by studies indicating that cells transformed by v-*fes* or v-*fms* oncogenes contained significantly higher activities of a guanine nucleotide-activated PIP$_2$-PLC as compared to the nontransformed parental cell-line.[76]

Many recent studies have focused on a possible role of *ras* proteins in the PI signaling pathway. Transformation of Balb3T3 cells with the H-*ras* oncogene inhibits the adenyl cyclase response to α-adrenergic agonists while increasing muscarinic agonist dependent hydrolysis of PPIs.[26] The steady state levels of DAG and IP$_2$ + IP$_3$

were found to be elevated in H, K, and N-*ras*-transformed cells (NIH3T3) as compared with their normal counterparts.[47] Another study reported expression of oncogenic *ras* either in stably transformed NIH3T3 cells or transiently in COS-1 cells and elevation of the basal rate of IP production.[65] This effect was specific to the action of the oncoprotein, since overexpression of the normal protein or the expression of various mutant proteins did not affect the IP levels. In a separate study, DAG levels were found elevated in K-*ras*-transformed NRK cells compared to nontransformed NRK cells.[125] It was also shown that the expression of N-*ras* in NIH3T3 cells leads to the coupling of certain growth factor receptors, especially bombesin, gastrin-releasing peptide, and bradykinin, to stimulate inositol phosphate production.[158] Increased N-*ras* protein concentration has been correlated with increased bombesin stimulated inositol phosphate production, implying that increased efficiency of coupling of the bombesin receptor to inositol phosphate production is related to the concentration of N-*ras*. This increased efficiency of coupling is not due to altered levels of receptors for bombesin[158] and carbamoylcholine.[27] The underlying hypothesis encompassing these studies is that *ras* protein may be the putative G protein which couples the receptors of certain growth factors to the stimulation of PIP_2-PLC.[158] A similar enhanced stimulation of IP formation to bradykinin was observed in NIH3T3 cells transformed by K-*ras* and viral H-*ras*[123] and in rat-1 cells transformed by all three types of *ras* genes.[41] However, these studies find that *ras*-induced bradykinin responsiveness is due to an increase in the number of receptors and not directly related to coupling of receptor to PIP_2-PLC by *ras*.

In contrast to the above systems where increased steady state levels of DAG and IP and increased growth factor/hormone receptor coupling to the PPI system are shown in *ras*-transformed cells, there are reports of desensitization of PDGF coupling to PI hydrolysis as a result of EJ-*ras* transformation of NIH3T3 cells,[11,123,142] and it is concluded that the transforming potential of activated forms of *ras* protein does not result from persistent activation of PI-PLC and that *ras* proteins cannot substitute for G protein that couples the receptors to PI-PLC.[142,163] On the other hand, Wakelam et al.[158] reported significant PDGF stimulation of IP formation in N-*ras*-transformed NIH3T3 cells. It is not clear whether the differences are due to the use of different *ras* genes. In any case, some growth factors may use another pathway independent of PI turnover. For example, EGF neither stimulates PI turnover nor potentiates the action of bombesin in normal NIH3T3 or N-*ras*-transformed NIH3T3 cells.[158]

Other studies found that some of the *ras*-induced (transformation) changes in PI metabolism are also produced by transformation by membrane associated (*trk*, *met*, or *src*) and cytoplasmic (*mos* or *raf*) kinase oncogenes.[2] Similar results were obtained in NIH3T3 cells expressing oncogenic *ras* and v-*mos* but not proto-oncogenic *ras* protein.[96] This study also showed desensitization of the Ca^{2+} mobilizing system to serum growth factors as a result of oncogenic *ras* and v-*mos* expression. Yet another study showed that in a cell-free system, normal but not surprisingly oncogenic *ras* protein increased by threefold the formation of IP_3.[82]

Studies employing the technique of scrape loading *ras* protein into Swiss 3T3 cells, thus eliminating the problem of distinguishing primary versus secondary effects associated with most of the studies that examined the connection of *ras* and PI metabolism, have shown that oncogenic *ras* causes rapid activation of PKC without PI hydrolysis[107,127] and results in down regulation of agonist-stimulated IP production.[126] Although these results may explain some of the differences seen by various authors, the relation of PI metabolism with *ras* function is controversial.

In the last few years GTP-binding proteins have been implicated in the regulation of PLC. In light of the strong experimental evidence implicating a G protein in PPI turnover[117] and the influence, whether direct or indirect, of *ras* on the PI system, it is tempting to link *ras* and the G protein of the PPI system. In fact, it has been proposed that *ras* protein may actually be the G protein that couples the receptors of certain growth factors to the stimulation of PI-PLC.[158] However, recent results suggest that *ras* does not directly activate PI-PLC.

The enzyme(s) that catalyzes the phosphodiesteric cleavage of phosphoinositides plays a crucial role in the initiation of cell responses based on PI system. Characterization of these enzymes is central to understanding the dynamics of inositol lipid based second messenger production by the cell. In recent years, several enzymes that degrade phosphoinositides have been purified and characterized.[33,39,61,69,70] In general, these PLCs are soluble enzymes, require Ca^{2+} for activity, and are present in a wide variety of tissues. In most tissues, PLC is present in multiple forms. At present it is unclear which, if any, of these PLCs is the receptor-coupled enzyme involved in agonist based PI hydrolysis. Extensive data accumulated on agonist-elicited PI metabolism predict that the receptor-coupled enzyme should be specific to PIP_2, since many different cells respond with specific hydrolysis of PIP_2 with no significant changes in PIP and PI. In addition, the PIP_2-PLC activity should be Ca^{2+}-independent, G protein regulated, and membrane associated. However, none of the PLCs characterized to date satisfies all of these criteria, although evidence clearly suggests that such a PIP_2-PLC exists in a number of cell types. Recently PLCs that show specificity toward PIP and PIP_2 have been identified and resolved from the nonspecific PLC that acts on all three phosphoinositides.[98] One of these PLC enzymes has been highly purified and shown to be specific for PPIs.[99] This PPI-specific PLC exhibits maximum activity in the presence of physiological Mg^{2+} concentrations without any added Ca^{2+}. Thus this enzyme fulfills the two most important criteria attributed to receptor-controlled PI-PLC.

Several lines of evidence point to the possibility that the transmembrane signaling system based on *ras* proteins is connected to certain other receptor pathways. In cells transformed by *ras* the GDP-binding activity of *ras* proteins is stimulated by EGF.[81] In addition, *ras*-transformed cells produce elevated levels of TGFα, an EGF-like growth factor. These observations suggest some biochemical interaction between *ras* proteins and the EGF receptor pathway. Cells transformed by growth factor receptor-derived oncogenes such as *fms* or plasma membrane-associated kinases such as *fes* and *src* cannot enter S phase when microinjected with monclonal antibody Y13–259 specific for p21 *ras* protein. However, this antibody has no effect on cells transformed by *mos* and *raf* oncogenes, the products of which are located in the cytoplasm.[147] These results indicate that *ras* proteins are intermediates in signal-transduction from certain receptors and membrane-associated molecules to cytoplasmic proteins. Differentiation of PC12 cells into neuron-like cells occurs upon infection with retroviruses containing *ras*,[116] transfection with the activated N-*ras* gene,[57] or microinjection with oncogenic or normal (provided in the form complexed to nonhydrolyzable GTPγS) *ras* proteins.[7,135] Other studies have shown that microinjection of PC12 cells with monoclonal antibody Y13–259 inhibits neurite formation induced by NGF[59] and basic fibroblast growth factor[3] but not by cAMP.[59] These results indicate that *ras*-induced differentiation of PC12 cells is similar to that induced by NGF, but clearly proceeds through a mechanism independent of cAMP.

Although it is generally accepted that DAG generated in response to agonist stimulation in most cell types is derived from phosphoinositides, there are indications that phosphatidylcholine (PC) or some other lipid is the source of a proportion of the newly generated DAG in at least some cell types.[17,73,109] Some investigators have reported elevated levels of DAG without a corresponding increase in inositol phosphates in *ras*-transformed cells.[11,12,90,118,123,160] These findings imply that lipids other than phosphoinositides are the major sources of elevated DAG in *ras*-transformed cells. Increased PC and phosphatidylethanolamine (PE) breakdown observed in *ras*-transformed cells indicate that PC and PE could be the source of DAG elevated in these cells. However, the significance of the increase in PC breakdown is in question following the observation of choline kinase activity in *ras*-transformed cells.[94] Confusing matters further, the increased PC breakdown in cells containing oncogenic *ras* itself appears to be a result of PKC activation.[126] There are also suggestions that increased DAG content in *ras*-transformed cells may be partly due to the defect of DAG kinase translocation from cytosol to membrane.[86] Nonetheless, it is interesting to note that a GTP-binding protein has been implicated in coupling purinergic receptors of a PC-specific PLC in rat liver plasma membranes.[75] It remains to be determined whether the *ras* protein activates either directly or indirectly a PLC specific to PC and PE through its function as a G protein.

As mentioned earlier, one of the signal-transduction pathways based on PI turnover involved in cellular proliferation proceeds through PKC.[115] PKC activates the Na^+/H^+ antiporter[157] which causes a rapid intracellular alkalization and initiation of DNA synthesis. Microinjection of *ras* oncoproteins into NIH3T3 cells results in DNA synthesis[148] and elevation of intracellular pH.[59] These results indicate that PKC is probably activated as a consequence of *ras*-induced second messenger (DAG) generation. Moreover, it was shown that phorbol esters, which downregulate PKC, inhibit the mitogenic function of *ras* protein, and this inhibition can be overcome by microinjection of PKC.[89,124] Together, these results strongly suggest that whatever second messenger *ras* protein generates in response to proliferative stimuli is connected to PKC. An 80 kDa protein is an ubiquitous substrate for PKC. The phosphorylation of this substrate is significantly increased in *ras*-transformed cells and correlates closely with increases in DAG concentration in these cells.[160] On the other hand, *ras*-transformed cells are slightly refractory to the phosphorylation of an 80 kDa protein stimulated by phorbol esters. These results indicate that transformation by *ras* results in partial activation and downregulation of PKC, probably as a consequence of elevated cellular DAG. The transforming effects of ras require activation of PKC, a conclusion supported by observation that the total amount of PKC is reduced with a concomitant loss of 80 kDa PKC substrate in a ras-resistant cell-line expressing high levels of K-ras proteins.[83]

There are indications that ras proteins generate PKC-independent signals in addition to PKC-dependent signals. Morphological transformation, increase in cell motility, and increases in c-myc expression seem to occur in a PKC-independent fashion.[49,93] In addition, mitogenic signals emanating from certain growth factors like PDGF and EGF which operate independent of functional PKC[31,107] but are known to be dependent on functional ras[110,163] could be operating through this PKC-independent pathway. At present, the nature of the PKC-independent signal-transduction pathway remains obscure. However, these signals might feed into nuclear transcription through a TGACTCT promoter element called ras-responsive element.[119,120] Despite bearing some resemblance to TGAGTCAG AP1 consensus sequence, this element responds more effectively to ras than to fos/jun and is recognized by a 120 kDa protein.[119] The involvement of the products of c-raf and c-mos proto-oncogenes which are serine/threonine kinases in this pathway remains to be examined in view of the observation that ras-transformed cells contain constitutively activated c-raf kinase.[108]

The well-documented involvement of ras in the differentiation of PC12 cells has been discussed previously. Similarly, cultured human medullary thyroid carcinoma cells (MTC) derived from an endocrine tumor differentiate upon introduction of oncogenic H-ras[113] by transfection. The decreased cellular proliferation, DNA synthesis, and differentiation-inducing effects of ras on PC12 and MTC cells may have a role in normal neuroendocrine differentiation.[113] Other studies indicate that activated ras induces 1) growth arrest as in murine Schwann cells and rat embryo fibroblasts;[68], 2) malignant transformation and plasmacytoid differentiation of human lymphoblasts;[141] and 3) steroidogenesis in primary granulosa cells transfected with SV40[4]. In marked contrast, activated ras oncogenes are shown to block differentiation of myoblasts[149] and mammary epithelial cells.[5] Thus, ras could participate in positive as well as negative control of differentiation.

The activities of known G proteins are controlled by transmembrane receptors or other ancillary proteins that catalyze GDP/GTP exchange. This results in replacement of GDP with GTP in the G.GDP complex to form active G.GTP complex. Recently, three groups have described a protein that is capable of stimulating GDP/GTP exchange on *ras* proteins.[42,72,161] The physiological importance of this *ras* upstream process is beyond any question and underscored by the observation that *ras* neutralizing antibody Y13–259 specifically inhibits this exchange.[67] The product of CDC25 acts as GDP/GTP exchange factor for yeast *ras* proteins.[78] In addition, the carboxy-terminal portion of the SCD25 gene product can also catalyze in vitro exchange of guanine nucleotides bound to *ras* proteins.[32]

The two major second messenger producing systems, one related to cAMP and the other to IP_3 and DAG, do not appear to be mutually exclusive in all tissues. In platelets, agonist-induced phosphoinositide breakdown is blocked concurrently and progressively by increasing amounts of cAMP.[133,164] There are indications that cAMP probably interferes with the enzymes that supply PIP_2. Alternatively, in several systems, stimulation of the phosphoinositide pathway potentiates the adenyl cyclase pathway.[71,150] The PKC pathway seems to mediate these effects[10,145] probably by facilitating the interaction between Gs and adenyl cyclase or by inactivating Gi by phosphorylation.[84] Finally, the two systems can operate independently as in hepatocytes where phosphoinositide turnover is induced by α-adrenergic stimulators or by cAMP.[80]

Future Directions

Identification of the effector system that is regulated by *ras* is a major task now being undertaken by several laboratories. The *ras* protein seems to participate in multiple biological processes that are apparently distinct for each cell type. How does it exert these multiple but disparate functions? Are the effector systems and the second messengers involved different or the same? Is there a unique second messenger system that might disrupt proliferative functions in growing cells as well as specialized functions in differentiated cells? The PPI system-based second messengers, IP_3 and DAG, which are proposed as signal-bifucation messengers, appear to be unique in their role in a variety of biological processes such as cell proliferation and specialized responses of differentiated cells. The enzyme that breaks down these phosphoinositides is probably of central importance in various biological functions and subject to extensive regulation. The importance of this phosphoinositide phosphodiesterase is comparable to that of adenyl cyclase which converts ATP into cAMP and serves as a major trans-membrane signaling system since cAMP controls many activities of eukaryotic as well as prokaryotic cells. Phosphoinositide phospho-diesterase has not been extensively studied and should be the focus of future research to understand the mechanism of generation of IP_3 and DAG. Notwithstanding the biological similarities between *ras* and G proteins, it remains to be determined whether *ras*, like G, acts to regulate PIP_2-PLC. Answers to these questions await detailed character-ization of the phosphoinositide phosphodiesterase.

References

1. Allende JE. The binding, hydrolysis and release of GTP and GDP as a mechanism that regulates the reversible association of macromolecules. A comparison of four different systems. Arch Biol Med Exp 1982; 15:347–355.
2. Alonso T, Morgon RO, Marvizon JC, et al. Malignant transformation by *ras* and other oncogenes produces common alterations in inositol lipid signalling pathways. Proc Natl Acad Sci USA 1988; 85:4271–4275.
3. Altin JG, Wetts R, Bradshaw RA. Microinjection of a p21ras antibody into PC12 cells inhibits neurite outgrowth induced by nerve growth factor and basic fibroblast growth factor. Growth Factors 1991; 4:145–155.
4. Amsterdam A, Zauberman A, Meir G, et al. Cotransfection of granulosa cells with simian virus 40 and Ha-*ras* oncogene generates stable lines capable of induced steroidogenesis. Proc Natl Acad Sci USA 1988; 85:7582–7586.
5. Andres AC, Vandervalk MA, Schonenberg CAS, et al. Ha-*ras* and c-*myc* oncogene expression interferes with morphological and functional differ-entiation of mammary epithelial cells in single and double transgenic mice. Genes Dev 1988; 2:1486-1495.
6. Bar-Sagi D, Feramisco JR. Induction of membrane ruffling and fluid-phase pinocytosis in quiescent fibroblasts by *ras* proteins. Science 1986; 233:1061–1068.
7. Bar-Sagi D, Feramisco JR. Microinjection of the *ras* oncogene protein into PC12 cells induces morphological differentiation. Cell 1985; 42:841–848.
8. Barbacid M. *Ras* genes. Ann Rev Biochem 1987; 56:779-827.
9. Beckner SK, Hattori S, Shih TY. p21 does not function as a regulatory component of adenylate cyclase. Nature 1985; 317:71-72.
10. Bell JD, Buxton ILO, Brunton LL. Enhancement of adenylate cyclase activity in S49 lymphoma cells by phorbol esters. Putative effect of C-kinase on α-GTP-catalytic subunit interaction. J Biol Chem 1985; 260:2625–2628.
11. Benjamin CW, Tarpley WG, Gorman RR. Loss of platelet-derived growth factor-stimulated phospholipase activity in NIH3T3 cells expressing the EJ-*ras* oncogene. Proc Natl Acad Sci USA 1987; 84:546–550.
12. Benzamin CW, Conner JA, Tarpley WG, et al. NIH-3T3 cells transformed

by the EJ-*ras* oncogene exhibit reduced platelet-derived growth factor-mediated Ca^{2+} mobilization. Proc Natl Acad Sci USA 1988; 85:4345–4349.

13. Berridge MJ, Irvine RF. Inositol trisphosphate, a novel second messenger in signal transduction. Nature 1984; 312:315-321.

14. Berridge MJ. Oncogenes, Inositol lipids and cellular proliferation. Bio/technology 1984; 1:541–546.

15. Berridge MJ. Inositol trisphosphate and diacylglycerol as second messengers. Biochem J 1984; 220:345–360.

16. Birchmeier C, Brock D, Wigler M. RAS proteins can induce meiosis in Xenopus oocytes. Cell 1985; 43:615–621.

17. Bocckino SB, Blackmore PF, Exton JH. Stimulation of 1,2-diacylglycerol accumulation in hepatocytes by vasopressin, epinephrine, and angiotensin II. J Biol Chem 1985; 260:14201-14207.

18. Bokoch GM, Gilman AG. Inhibition of receptor-mediated release of arachidonic acid by pertussis toxin. Cell 1984; 39:301–308.

19. Bos JL. *Ras* oncogenes in human cancer: A review. Cancer Research 1989; 49:4682–4689.

20. Bourne HR, Sanders DA, McCormick F. The GTPase superfamily: A conserved switch for diverse cell functions. Nature 1990; 348:125–131.

21. Bourne HR, Sanders DA, McCormick F. The GTPase superfamily: Conserved structure and molecular mechanism. Nature 1991; 349:117–127.

22. Boynton AL, Whitfield JF, Isaacs RJ, et al. Control of 3T3 cell proliferation by calcium. In Vitro 1974; 10:12–17.

23. Brock D, Samiy N, Fasano O, et al. Differential activation of yeast adenylate cyclase by wild type and mutant RAS proteins. Cell 1985; 41:763–769.

24. Casey PJ, Solski PA, Der CJ, et al. p21[ras] is modified by a farnesyl isoprenoid. Proc Natl Acad Sci USA 1989; 86:8323-8327.

25. Castagna M, Takai Y, Kaibuchi K, et al. Direct activation of calcium-activated, phospholipid-dependent protein kinase by tumor-promoting phorbol esters. J Bio Chem 1982; 257:7847-7851.

26. Chiarugi V, Porciatti F, Pasquali F, et al. Transformation of balb/3T3 cells with EJ/T24/H-*ras* oncogene inhibits adenylate cyclase response to β-adrenergic agonist while increases muscarinic receptor dependent hydrolysis of inositol lipids. Biochem Biophys Res Commun 1985; 132:900–907.

27. Chiarugi VP, Pasquali F, Vannucchi S. Point-mutated p21[ras] couples a muscarinic receptor to calcium channels and polyphosphoinositide hydrolysis. Biochem Biophys Res Commun 1986; 141:591–596.

28. Clarke S, Vogel JP, Deschenes RJ, et al. Posttranslational modification of the Ha-*ras* oncogene protein: Evidence for a third class of protein carboxyl methyltransferases. Proc Natl Acad Sci USA 1988; 85:4643–4647.

29. Cockroft S, Gomperts BD. Role of guanine nucleotide binding protein in the activation of polyphosphoinositide phosphodiesterase. Nature 1985; 314:534–536.

30. Connolly JL, Greene LA, Viscarello RR, et al. Rapid, sequential changes in surface morphology of PC12 pheochromocytoma cells in response to nerve growth factor. J Cell Biol 1979; 82:820–827.

31. Coughlin SR, Lee WMF, Williams PW, et al. c-*myc2* gene expression is stimulated by agents that activate protein kinase C and does not account for the mitogenic effect of PDGF. Cell 1985; 43:243–251.

32. Crechet JB, Poullet P, Mistou MY, et al. Enhancement of the GDP-GTP exchange of RAS proteins by the carboxy-terminal domain of SCD2N. Science 1990; 248:866–868.

33. Creutz CE, Dowling GG, Kyger EM, et al. Phosphatidylinositol-specific phospholipase C activity of McCormick granule-binding proteins. J Biol Chem 1985; 260:7171–7173.

34. Davies PF, Ross R. Mediation of pinocytosis in cultured arterial smooth muscle and endothelial cells by platelet-derived growth factor. J Cell Biol 1978; 79:663–671.

35. DeFeo-Jones D, Scolnick EM, Koller R, et al. *ras*-related gene sequences identified and isolated from *Saccharomyces cerevisiae*. Nature 1983; 306:707–709.

36. Deringer H, Friis RR. Changes in phosphatidylinositol metabolism correlated to growth state of normal and rous sarcoma virus-transformed Japanese quail cells. Cancer Res 1977; 37:2979-2984.

37. deVos A, Tong L, Milburn MV, et al. Three-dimensional structure of an oncogene protein: Catalytic domain of human c-H-*ras* p2N. Science 1988; 239:888–893.

38. Doolittle RF, Hunkapillar MW, Hood LE, et al. Simian sarcoma virus onc gene, v-*sis*, is derived from the gene (or genes) encoding a platelet-derived growth factor. Science 1983; 221:275-277.

39. Downes CP, Mitchell RH. The polyphosphoinositide phosphodiesterase of erythrocyte membranes. Biochem J 1981; 198:133–140.

40. Downward J. The *ras* superfamily of small GTP-binding proteins. Trends Biochem Sci 1990; 15:469–472.

41. Downward J, Gunzburg JD, Riehl R, et al. p21^{ras}-induced responsiveness of phosphatidylinositol turnover to bradykinin is a receptor number effect. Proc Natl Acad Sci USA 1988; 85:5774–5778.

42. Downward J, Riehe R, Wu L, et al. Identification of a nucleotide exchange promoting activity for p21^{ras}. Proc Natl Acad Sci USA 1990; 87:5998–6002.

43. Downward J, Yarden Y, Mayes E, et al. Close similarity of epidermal growth factor receptor and v-*erb*-B oncogene protein sequences. Nature 1984; 307:521–527.

44. Eva A, Aaronson SA. Frequent activation of c-*kis* as a transforming gene in fibrosarcomas induced by methylcholanthrene. Science 1983; 220:955–956.

45. Farrar WL, Anderson WB. Interleukin-2 stimulates association of protein kinase C with plasma membrane. Nature 1985; 315:233-235.

46. Farrar WL, Thomas TP, Anderson WB. Altered cytosol/membrane enzyme redistribution on interleukin-3 activation of protein kinase C. Nature 1985; 315:235–237.

47. Fleischman LF, Chahwala SB, Cantley L. *ras*-transformed cells: Altered levels of phosphatidylinositol 4,5-bisphosphate and catabolites. Science 1986; 231:407–410.

48. Fukui Y, Kozasa T, Kaziro Y, et al. Role of a *ras* homolog in the life cycle of *Schizosaccharomyces pombe*. Cell 1986; 44:329–336.

49. Gauthier-Rouviere C, Fernandez A, Lamb NJC. *ras*-induced c-*fos* expression and proliferation in living rat fibroblasts involves C-kinase activation and the serum response element pathway. EMBO J 1990; 9:171–180.
50. Gay NJ, Walker JE. Homology between human bladder carcinoma oncogene product mitochondrial ATP-synthase. Nature 1983; 301:262–264.
51. Gibbs JB, Marshall MS. The *ras* oncogene—an important regulatory element in lower eucaryotic organisms. Microbiol Rev 1989; 53:171–185.
52. Gilman AG. G proteins and dual control of adenylate cyclase. Cell 1984; 36:577–579.
53. Gilman AG. G proteins: Transducers of receptor generated signals. Ann Rev Biochem 1987; 56:615–649.
54. Goldstein JL, Brown MS, Stradley SJ, et al. Nonfarnesylated tetrapeptide inhibitors of protein farnesyltransferase. J Biol Chem 1991; 266:15575–15578.
55. Goshima K, Masuda A, Owaribe K. Insulin-induced formation of ruffling membranes of KB cells and its correlation with enhancement of amino acid transport. J Cell Biol 1984; 98:801-809.
56. Goyette M, Petropoulos CJ, Shank PR, et al. Expression of a cellular oncogene during liver regeneration. Science 1983; 219:510–512.
57. Guerrero I, Wong H, Pellicer A, et al. Activated N-*ras* gene induces neuronal differentiation of PC12 rat pheochromocytoma cells. J Cell Physiol 1986; 129:71–76.
58. Gutierrez L, Magee AI, Marshall CJ, et al. Post-translational processing of p21^{ras} is two-step and involves carboxyl-methylation and carboxy-terminal proteolysis. EMBO J 1989; 8:1093–1098.
59. Hagag N, Lacal JC, Graber M, et al. Microinjection of *ras* p21 induces a rapid rise in intracellular pH. Mol Cell Biol 1987; 7:1984–1988.
60. Haighler HT, McKanna JA, Cohen S. Rapid stimulation of pinocytosis in human carcinoma cells A-431 by epidermal growth factor. J Cell Biol 1979; 83:82–90.
61. Hakata H, Kambayashi J, Kosaki G. Purification and characterization of phosphatidylinositol-specific phospholipase C from bovine platelets. J Biochem 1982; 92:929–935.
62. Hall A. The cellular functions of small GTP-binding proteins. Science 1990; 249:635–640.
63. Hammarstrom S. Biosynthesis and biological actions of prostaglandins and thromboxanes. Arch Biochem Biophys 1982; 214:431–445.
64. Hancock JF, Magee AI, Childs JE, et al. All *ras* proteins are polyisoprenylated but only some are palmitoylated. Cell 1989; 57:1167–1177.
65. Hancock JF, Marshall CJ, McKay IA, et al. Mutant but not normal p21^{ras} elevates inositol phospholipid breakdown in two cell systems. Oncogene 1988; 3:187–193.
66. Hancock JF, Paterson H, Marshall CJ. A polybasic domain or palmitoylation is required in addition to the CAAX motif to localize p21^{ras} to the plasma membrane. Cell 1990; 63:133–139.
67. Hattori S, Clanton DJ, Satoh T, et al. Neutralizing monoclonal antibody against *ras* oncogene product p21 which impairs guanine nucleotide exchange. Mol Cell Biol 1987; 7:1999-2002.

68. Hirakawa T, Ruley HE. Rescue of cells from *ras* oncogene-induced growth arrest by a second, complementing, oncogene. Proc Natl Acad Sci USA 1988; 85:1519–1523.

69. Hirasawa K, Irwine RF, Dawson RMC. Heterogeneity of the calcium-dependent phosphoinositide phosphodiesterase in rat brain. Biochem J 1982; 205:437–442.

70. Hofmann SL, Majerus PW. Identification and properties of two distinct phosphatidylinositol-specific phospholipase C enzymes from sheep seminal vesicular glands. J Biol Chem 1982; 257:6461-6469.

71. Hollingsworth EB, Daly JW. Accumulation of inositol phosphates and cyclic AMP in guinea-pig cerebral cortical preparations. Effects of norepinephrine, histamine, carbamylcholine and 2-chloroadenosine. Biochim Biophys Acta 1985; 847:207–216.

72. Huang YK, Kung HF, Kamata T. Purification of a factor capable of stimulating the guanine nucleotide exchange reaction of *ras* proteins and its effect on *ras*-related small molecular mass G proteins. Proc Natl Acad Sci USA 1990; 87:8008-8012.

73. Hughes BP, Ryr K, Pickford LB, et al. A transient increase in diacylglycerols is associated with the action of vasopressin in hepatocytes. Biochem J 1984; 222:535–540.

74. Hurley JB, Simon MI, Teplow DB, et al. Homologies between signal-transducing G proteins and *ras* gene products. Science 1984; 226:860–862.

75. Irving HR, Exton JH. Phosphatidylcholine breakdown in rat liver plasma membrane. Role of guanine nucleotides and p_2-purinergic agonists. J Biol Chem 1987; 262:3440–3443.

76. Jackowski S, Rettenmier CW, Sherr CJ, et al. A guanine nucleotide dependent phosphatidylinositol-4,5-diphosphate phospholipase C in cells transformed by v-*fms* and v-*fes* oncogenes. J Biol Chem 1986; 261:4978–4985.

77. Jackson JH, Cochrane CG, Bourne JR, et al. Farnesol modification of Kirsten-*ras* exon 4B protein is essential for transformation. Proc Natl Acad Sci USA 1990; 87:3042-3046.

78. Jones S, Vignais ML, Broach JR. The CDC25 protein of *Saccharomyces cerevisiae* promotes exchange of guanine nucleotides bound to *ras*. Mol Cell Biol 1991; 11:2641-2646.

79. Kaibuchi K, Miyajima A, Arai KI, et al. Possible involvement of *ras*-encoded proteins in glucose-induced inositol phospholipid turnover in *Saccharomyces cerevisiae*. Proc Natl Acad Sci USA 1986; 83:8172–8176.

80. Kaibuchi K, Takai Y, Ogawa Y, et al. Inhibitory action of adenosine 3',5'-monophosphate on phosphatidylinositol turnover: Difference in tissue response. Biophys Res Commun 1982; 104:105–112.

81. Kamata T, Feramisco JR. Epidermal growth factor stimulates guanine nucleotide binding activity and phosphorylation of *ras* oncogene proteins. Nature 1984; 310:147–150.

82. Kamata T, Kung HF. Effects of *ras*-encoded proteins and platelet-derived growth factor on inositol phospholipid turnover in NRK cells. Proc Natl Acad Sci USA 1988; 85:5799–5803.

83. Kamata T, Sullivan NF, Wooten MW. Reduced protein kinase C activity in

a *ras*-resistant cell line derived from Ki-MSV transformed cells. Oncogene 1987; 1:37–46.

84. Katada T, Gilman A, Watanabe Y, et al. Protein kinase C phosphorylates the inhibitory guanine-nucleotide-binding regulatory component and apparently supresses its function in hormonal inhibition of adenyl cyclase. Eur J Biochem 1985; 151:431–437.

85. Kataoka T, Powers S, McGill C, et al. Genetic analysis of yeast *Saccharomyces cerevisiae* RAS1 and RAS2 genes. Cell 1984; 37:437–445.

86. Kato H, Kawai S, Takenawa T. Disappearance of diacylglycerol kinase translocation in *ras*-transformed cells. Biochem Biophys Res Commun 1988; 154:959–966.

87. Kerr IB, Lee FD, Quintanilla M, et al. Immunocytochemical demonstration of p21 *ras* family oncogene product in normal mucosa and in premalignant and malignant tumors of the colorectum. Br J Cancer 1985; 52:695–700.

88. Krengel U, Schlichting I, Scherer A, et al. Three-dimensional structures of H-*ras* p21 mutants: Molecular basis for their inability to function as signal switch molecules. Cell 1990; 62:539–548.

89. Lacal JC, Fleming TP, Warren BS, et al. Involvement of functional protein kinase C in the mitogenic response to the H-*ras* oncogene product. Mol Cell Biol 1987; 7:4146–4149.

90. Lacal JC, Moscat J, Aaronson SA. Novel sources of 1,2-diacylglycerol elevated in cells transformed by Ha-*ras* oncogene. Nature 1987; 330:269–271.

91. Lemoine N. *Ras* oncogenes in human cancer. In: Molecular Biology of Cancer Genes, Sluyser M, ed. England, Ellis Horwood Limited 1990; pp. 82–118.

92. Litosch I, Wallis C, Fain JN. 5-Hydroxytryptamine stimulates inositol phosphate production in a cell-free system from brownfly salivary glands. Evidence for a role of GTP in coupling receptor activation to phosphoinositide breakdown. J Biol Chem 1985; 260:5464–5471.

93. Lloyd AC, Paterson HF, Morris JDH, et al. p21$^{H\text{-}ras}$ induced morphological transformation and increases in c-*myc* expression are independent of functional protein kinase C. EMBO J 1989; 8:1099–1104.

94. Macara I. Elevated phosphocholine concentration in *ras*-transformed NIH3T3 cells arises from increased choline kinase activity, not from phosphatidylcholine breakdown. Mol Cell Biol 1989; 9:325–328.

95. Majerus PW, Newfeld EJ, Wilson DB. Production of phosphoinositide-derived messengers. Cell 1984; 37:701–703.

96. Maly K, Doppler W, Oberhuber H, et al. Desensitization of the Ca^2+-mobilizing system to serum growth factors by Ha-*ras* and v-*mos*. Mol Cell Biol 1988; 8:4212–4216.

97. Manne V, Kung HF. Characterization of phosphoinositide-specific phospholipase C from human platelets. Biochem J 1987; 243:763–771.

98. Manne V. Identification of polyphosphoinositide-specific phospholipase C from human platelet extract. Oncogene 1987; 2:49–54.

99. Manne V. A novel candidate for receptor-coupled phospholipase C purified from human platelets. Oncogene 1988; 3:579–585.

168   THE MOLECULAR BASIS OF HUMAN CANCER

100. Manne V, Bekesi E, Kung HF. Ha-*ras* proteins exhibit GTPase activity: Point mutations that activate Ha-*ras* gene products result in decreased GTPase activity. Proc Natl Acad Sci USA 1985; 82:376–380.
101. Manne V, Roberts D, Tobin A, et al. Identification and preliminary characterization of protein cysteine farnesyltransferase. Proc Natl Acad Sci USA 1990; 87:7541-7545.
102. Marz JL. A new view of receptor action. Science 1984; 224:271–274.
103. McGrath JP, Capon DJ, Goeddel DV, et al. Comparative biochemical properties of normal and activated human *ras* protein. Nature 1984; 310:644–649.
104. Mitchell RH, Receptor-controlled phosphatidylinositol 4,5-biphosphate hydrolysis in the control of rapid receptor-mediated cellular responses and of cellular proliferation. In: Molecular Mechanisms of Transmembrane Signalling, Cohen P, Houslay MD, eds. Amsterdam, Elsevier 1985; pp. 3–56.
105. Moncada S, Vane JR. Pharmacology and endogenous roles of prostaglandin endoperoxides, thromboxane A2, and prostacyclin. Pharm Rev 1978; 30:293–331.
106. Moolenaar WH, Mummery CL, Van der Saag PT, et al. Rapid ionic events and the initiation of growth in serum-stimulated neuroblastoma cells. Cell 1981; 23:789–798.
107. Morris JDH, Price B, Lloyd AC, et al. Scrape-loading of swiss 3T3 cells with *ras* protein rapidly activates protein kinase C in the absence of phosphoinositide hydrolysis. Oncogene 1989; 4:27–31.
108. Morrison D, Kaplan D, Rapp U, et al. Signal transduction from membrane to cytoplasm: Growth factors and membrane-bound oncogene products increase *raf*-1 phosphorylation and associated protein kinase activity. Proc Natl Acad Sci USA 1988; 85:8855–8859.
109. Muir JG, Murray AW. Bombesin and phorbol ester stimulate phosphatidylcholine hydrolysis by phospholipase C: Evidence for a role of protein kinase C. J Cell Physiol 1987; 130:382–391.
110. Mulcahy LS, Smith MR, Stacey DW. Requirement for *ras* protooncogene function during serum-stimulated growth of NIH3T3 cells. Nature 1985; 313:241–243.
111. Muller R, Slamon DJ, Adamson ED, et al. Transcription of c-onc genes c-*ras*[ki] and c-*fms* during mouse development. Mol Cell Biol 1983; 3:1062–1069.
112. Nadin-Davis SA, Nasim A, Beach D. Involvement of *ras* in sexual differentiation but not in growth control in fission yeast *Schizosaccharomyces cerevisiae*. EMBO J 1986; 5:2963-2972.
113. Nakagawa T, Marby M, Bustros AD, et al. Introduction of v-Ha-*ras* oncogene induces differentiation of cultured human medullary thyroid carcinoma cells. Proc Natl Acad Sci USA 1987; 84:5923–5927.
114. Nishizuka Y. Protein kinases in signal transduction. Trends Biochem Sci 1984; 9:163–171.
115. Nishizuka Y. Studies and perspectives of protein kinase C. Science 1986; 233:305–312.
116. Noda M, Ko M, Ogura A, et al. Sarcoma viruses carrying *ras* oncogenes

induce differentiation-associated properties in a neuronal cell line. Nature 1985; 318:73–75.

117. Oberdisse E, Lapetina EG. GDPβS enhances the activation of phospholipase C caused by thrombin in human platelets: Evidence for involvement of an inhibitory GTP-binding protein. Biochem Biophys Res Commun 1987; 144:1188–1196.

118. Olinger PL, Gorman RR. NIH-3T3 cells expressing high levels of the c-*ras* proto-oncogene display reduced platelet derived growth factor-stimulated phospholipase activity. Biochem Biophys Res Commun 1988; 150:937–941.

119. Owen RD, Ostrowski MC. Transcriptional activation of a conserved sequence element by *ras* requires a nuclear factor distinct from c-*fos* and c-*jun*. Proc Natl Acad Sci USA 1990; 87:3866–3870.

120. Owen RD, Bortner DM, Ostrowski MC. *ras* oncogene activation of a VL30 transcriptional element is linked to transformation. Mol Cell Biol 1990; 10:1–9.

121. Pai EF, Kabsch W, Krengel U, et al. Structure of the guanine-nucleotide-binding domain of the Ha-*ras* oncogene product p21 in the triphosphate conformation. Nature 1989; 341:209–214.

122. Parada LF, Weinberg RA. Presence of a kirsten murine sarcoma virus in cells transformed by 3-methylcholanthrene. Mol Cell Biol 1983; 3:2298–2301.

123. Parries G, Hoebel R, Racker E. Opposing effects of a *ras* oncogene on growth factor-stimulated phosphoinositide hydrolysis: Desensitization to platelet-derived growth factor and enhanced sensitivity to bradykinin. Proc Natl Acad Sci USA 1987; 84:2648–2652.

124. Pasti G, Lacal JC, Warren BS, et al. Loss of mouse fibroblast cell response to phorbol esters restored by microinjected protein kinase C. Nature 1986; 324:375–377.

125. Preiss J, Loomis CR, Bishop WR, et al. Quantitative measurement of sn-1,2-diacylglycerols present in platelets, hepatocytes and *ras*-and *sis*-transformed normal rat kidney cells. J Biol Chem 1986; 261:8597–8600.

126. Price B, Morris JDC, Marshall CJ, et al. Scrape-loaded p21[ras] down-regulates agonist-stimulated inositol phosphate production by a mechanism involving protein kinase C. Biochem J 1989; 260:157–161.

127. Price B, Morris J, Marshall C, et al. Stimulation of phosphatidylcholine hydrolysis, diacylglycerol release, and arachidonic acid production by oncogenic *ras* is a consequence of protein kinase C activation. J Biol Chem 1989; 264:16638–16643.

128. Rebecchi MJ, Rosen OM. Stimulation of polyphosphoinositide hydrolysis by thrombin in membranes from human fibroblasts. Biochem J 1987; 245:49–57.

129. Reddy EP, Reynolds RK, Santos E, et al. A point mutation is responsible for the acquisition of transforming properties by the T24 human bladder carcinoma oncogene. Nature 1982; 300:149-152.

130. Reiss Y, Goldstein JL, Seabra MC, et al. Inhibition of purified p21[ras] farnesyl:protein transferase by Cys-AAX tetrapeptides. Cell 1990; 62:81–88.

131. Reiss Y, Stradley SJ, Gierasch LM, et al. Sequence requirement for peptide recognition by rat brain p21^{ras} protein farnesyltransferase. Proc Natl Acad Sci USA 1991; 88:732-736.

132. Rozengurt E. Stimulation of DNA synthesis in quiescent cultured cells: Exogenous agents, internal signals and early events. Curr Top Cell Reg 1980; 17:59–88.

133. Sano K, Takai Y, Yamanishi J, et al. A role of calcium-activated phospholipid-dependent protein kinase in human platelet activation. J Biol Chem 1983; 258:2010–2013.

134. Santos E, Nebreda AR. Srtuctural and functional properties of *ras* proteins. FASEB J 1989; 3:2151–2163.

135. Satoh T, Nakamura S, Kaziro Y. Induction of neurite formation in PC12 cells by microinjection of proto-oncogenic Ha-*ras* protein preincubated with guanosine-5''-O-(3-thiotriphosphate). Mol Cell Biol 1987; 7:4553–4556.

136. Sawyer ST, Cohen S. Enhancement of calcium uptake and phosphatidylinositol turnover by epidermal growth factor in A431 cells. Biochemistry 1981; 20:6280–6286.

137. Schaber MD, O'Hara MB, Garsky VM, et al. Polyisoprenylation of *ras* in vitro by a farnesyl-protein transferase. J Biol Chem 1990; 265:14701–14704.

138. Schaber MD, Garsky VM, Boylaw D, et al. *Ras* interaction with the GTPase activating protein (GAP). Proteins 1989; 6:306–315.

139. Schafer WR, Kim R, Sterne R, et al. Genetic and pharmacological supression of oncogenic mutations in RAS genes of yeast and humans. Science 1989; 245:379–385.

140. Scolnick EM, Papageorge AG, Shih TY. Guanine nucleotide-binding activity as an assay for the *src*-protein of rat-derived murine sarcoma virus. Proc Natl Acad Sci USA 1979; 76:5355–5359.

141. Seremetis S, Inghirami G, Ferraro D, et al. Transformation and plasmacytoid differentiation of EBV-infected human B lymphoblasts by *ras* oncogenes. Science 1989; 243:660-663.

142. Seuwen K, Lagavde A, Pouyssegur J. Deregulation of hamster fibroblast proliferation by mutated *ras* oncogenes is not mediated by constitutive activation of phosphoinositide-specific phospholipase C. EMBO J 1988; 7:161–168.

143. Shih TY, Papageorge AG, Stokes PE, et al. Guanine nucleotide-binding and autophosphorylating activities associated with the p21 protein of harvey murine sarcoma virus. Nature 1980; 287:686–691.

144. Shih TY, Williams DR, Weeks MO, et al. Comparison of the genomic organization of kirsten and harvey sarcoma viruses. J Virol 1978; 27:45–55.

145. Sibley DR, Jeffs RA, Daniel K, et al. Phorbol diester treatment promotes enhanced adenylate cyclase activity in frog erythrocytes. Arch Biochem Biophys 1986; 244:373–381.

146. Smith CD, Lane BC, Kusaka I, et al. Chemoattractant receptor-induced hydrolysis of phosphatidylinositol 4,5-biphosphate in human polymorphonuclear leukocyte membranes: Requirement for a guanine nucleotide regulatory protein. J Biol Chem 1985; 260:5875–5878.

147. Smith MR, DeGudicibus SJ, Stacey DW. Requirement for c-*ras* proteins during viral oncogene transformation. Nature 1986; 320:540–543.
148. Stacey DW, Kung HF. Transformation of NIH3T3 cells by microinjection of Ha-*ras* p21 protein. Nature 1984; 310:508-511.
149. Sternberg EA, Spizz G, Perry ME, et al. A *ras*-dependent pathway abolishes activity of a muscle-specific enhancer upstream from the muscle creatine kinase gene. Mol Cell Biol 1989; 9:594–601.
150. Sugden D, Vanecek J, Kelin DC, et al. Activation of protein kinase C potentiates isoprenaline-induced cyclic AMP accumulation in rat pineal-ocytes. Nature 1985; 314:359–361.
151. Tabin CJ, Bradley SM, Bargmann CI, et al. Mechanism of action of a human oncogene. Nature 1982; 300:143–149.
152. Tamanoi F. Yeast RAS genes. Biochim Biophys Acta 1988; 948:1–15.
153. Tamanoi F, Walsh M, Kataoka T, et al. A product of yeast RAS2 gene is a guanine nucleotide binding protein. Proc Natl Acad Sci USA 1984; 81:6924–6928.
154. Taparowsky E, Suard Y, Fasano O, et al. Activation of the T24 bladder carcinoma transforming gene is linked to a single amino acid change. Nature 1982; 300:762–765.
155. Toda T, Uno I, Ishikawa T, et al. In yeast RAS proteins are controlling elements of adenylate cyclase. Cell 1985; 40:27-36.
156. Trahey M, McCormick F. A cytoplasmic protein stimulates normal N-*ras* p21 GTPase, but does not affect oncogenic mutants. Science 1987; 238:542–545.
157. Vara F, Schneider JA, Rozengurt E. Ionic responses rapidly elicited by activation of protein kinase C in quiescent swiss 3T3 cells. Proc Natl Acad Sci USA 1985; 82:2384–2388.
158. Wakelam MJO, Davies SA, Housley MD, et al. Normal p21[N-ras] couples bombesin and other growth factor receptors to inositol phosphate production. Nature 1986; 323:173–176.
159. Willumsen BM, Christensen A, Hubbert NL, et al. The p21[ras] C-terminus is required for transformation and membrane association. Nature 1984; 310:583–586.
160. Wolfman A, Macara IG. A cytosolic protein catalyzes the release of GDP from p21[ras]. Science 1990; 248:67–69.
161. Wolfman A, Macara I. Elevated levels of diacylglycerol and decreased phorbolester sensitivity in *ras*-transformed fibroblasts. Nature 1987; 325:359–361.
162. Yatani A, Okabe K, Polakis P, et al. *ras* p21 and GAP inhibit coupling of muscarinic receptors to atrial K+ channels. Cell 1990; 61:769–776.
163. Yu CY, Tsai MH, Stacey DW. Cellular *ras* activity and phospholipid metabolism. Cell 1988; 52:63–71.
164. Zavoico GB, Feinstein MB. Cytoplasmic Ca^{2+} in platelets is controlled by cyclic AMP: Antagonism between stimulators and inhibitors of adenylate cyclase. Biochem Biophys Res Commun 1984; 120:579–585.

Chapter 4

Protein-Serine/Threonine Kinases: *Mos* and *Raf*

Friedrich Propst, Stephen M. Storm, Ulf R. Rapp

Phosphorylation on serine and threonine residues is one of the most commonly used mechanisms to control the biological activity of proteins in eukaryotic cells. Among the fundamental cellular processes regulated by serine/threonine phosphorylation are the metabolism of nutrients, the function of the cytoskeleton, gene transcription, DNA replication, and cell division.

Protein-serine/threonine kinases are positioned at crucial control points in the cellular response to changes in the environment and in the execution of intracellular programs. They function in the transmission of intra- and extracellular signals controlling cell growth, differentiation, and function. The protein-serine/threonine kinases involved in the regulation of these processes comprise a family of proteins with distinctive structural features.[19] In particular, characteristic amino acid sequence motifs in the catalytic domains can be used to identify new family members and to predict their specificity toward serine and threonine rather than tyrosine. In addition to the catalytic domain, most if not all protein kinases contain regulatory domains through which the activity of each kinase can be regulated by a variety of mechanisms. These include phosphorylation on tyrosine, serine, or threonine residues by other kinases, binding of regulatory proteins, and binding of small molecules such as second messengers. Once activated, a given kinase can phosphorylate a number of different

From *The Molecular Basis of Human Cancer:* edited by B. Neel, M.D., Ph.D., R. Kumar, Ph.D. © 1993, Futura Publishing Co. Inc., Mount Kisco, NY.

proteins on serine and/or threonine, provided the phospho-acceptor residue is within a short, specific amino acid sequence. This stretch of about five amino acids determines at least in part the substrate specificity of each kinase.

The fact that protein-tyrosine and protein-serine/threonine kinases can directly or indirectly regulate the activity of other regulatory proteins, for example other protein kinases or transcription factors, has two important consequences: first, an extracellular or intracellular signal is usually transduced along a certain pathway, in which several steps involve a protein kinase. During transduction the primary signal can be amplified considerably. Second, since the activity of some protein kinases can be regulated by more than one other kinase and/or by several different regulatory proteins, these proteins form a regulatory network of converging and interdependent signal-transduction pathways. This has important implications for our understanding of how certain protein-serine/threonine kinases participate in the control of cell growth and differentiation and how their activation can lead to oncogenic transformation or other alterations in normal cell function.

Among several genes coding for protein-serine/threonine kinases suspected to be involved in growth control, so far only three, *mos*, *raf*, and *pim*-1 have been identified as oncogenes (Fig. 1). This might reflect a special position of these kinases in the regulatory network, suggesting that many receptors for diverse extracellular growth regulatory signals share a few second messenger kinase systems for signal-transduction. On the other hand, *mos*, *raf*, and *pim*-1 might be the only genes coding for protein-serine/threonine kinases that fulfill all the conditions imposed on the activation to a dominant transforming gene. Activation requires that mutations in the gene can lead to either deregulated expression of the kinase (for example, overexpression or expression in the wrong cell type) or expression of a mutant form that is no longer subject to down regulation of its activity or has altered substrate specificity. Another constraint is that the activated kinase must not interfere with fundamental controls of cell division and metabolism in a way detrimental to the cell. *mos* and *raf* are among the most potent transforming genes known to date. In this chapter we will review studies undertaken over the last decade to elucidate their normal function, their place in the regulatory network, the mechanisms by which they transform cells, and their possible role in the development of human tumors.

Considerably less is known about *pim*-1. This gene is frequently activated in murine T-cell lymphomas where it appears to cooperate

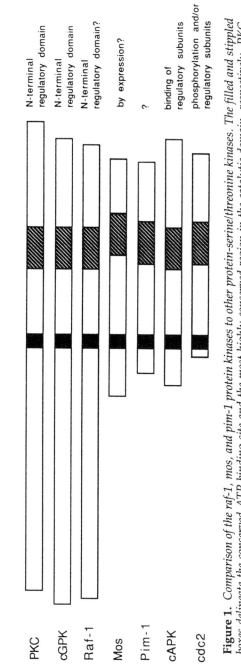

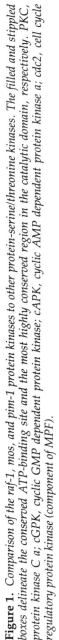

Figure 1. *Comparison of the raf-1, mos, and pim-1 protein kinases to other protein-serine/threonine kinases. The filled and stippled boxes delineate the conserved ATP-binding site and the most highly conserved region in the catalytic domain, respectively. PKC, protein kinase C α; cGPK, cyclic GMP dependent protein kinase; cAPK, cyclic AMP dependent protein kinase α; cdc2, cell cycle regulatory protein kinase (component of MPF).*

with other oncogenes such as *myc* to cause tumorigenic transformation. *pim*-1 codes for a 34 kDa polypeptide with an amino acid sequence related to but clearly distinguishable from the sequences of all other oncogenic protein kinases (Fig. 1).[19] Its protein-serine/ threonine kinase activity has only recently been established.[72]

The *mos* Proto-Oncogene

General Aspects of the *mos* Proto-Oncogene

The *mos* oncogene was first identified as the transforming gene of the Moloney murine sarcoma virus.[75] This acutely transforming retrovirus was isolated by Moloney from a rhabdomyosarcoma obtained after infection of a mouse with Moloney murine leukemia virus, and probably arose by genetic recombination between the leukemia virus and a mouse genomic sequence, the *mos* proto-oncogene. Moloney murine sarcoma virus causes the rapid formation of fibrosarcomas at the site of injection, with frequent regression of the primary tumor in adult animals.[75]

The cloning of the viral transforming sequences, the viral *mos* oncogene, led to the isolation and characterization of the cellular *mos* homologs of human, monkey, mouse, rat, chicken, and frog.[52,70,75] In all species examined thus far, *mos* appears to be a single copy gene without introns. It codes for a protein 37–39 kDa in size with an ATP-binding site and a catalytic domain characteristic of protein kinases. *Mos* is localized on the long arm of human chromosome 8 near the centromere at band q11-q12.[86] In the mouse genome, *mos* is localized on chromosome 4 also near the centromere.[10,56,87] The expression of the *mos* proto-oncogene has been most extensively studied in the mouse. Early studies revealed that the highest levels of *mos* mRNA are found in male and female germ cells, in particular haploid spermatids and growing and maturing oocytes.[55] Subsequently, *mos* transcripts have been detected in the testes and ovaries of all species examined including primates, indicating an evolutionary conserved function in germ cell differentiation. In the mouse, *mos* RNA is also expressed in embryos and in some adult tissues including brain, kidney, and epididymis at low levels, but in most adult tissues *mos* expression has not been detected. The *mos* protein has been detected in oocytes of frog[70] and mouse[51] and evidence for protein expression in male germ cells and somatic tissues has also been reported.[22,23]

Structural analysis of *mos* transcripts found in the few *mos* expressing tissues revealed that different promoters are utilized in a tissue-specific manner, suggesting a stringent and tissue-specific control of *mos* RNA expression. Additional elements of control are exerted at the levels of translation and degradation of *mos* RNA and protein. For example, in differentiating oocytes, the *mos* protein is translated from previously transcribed and stored mRNA during a limited and precisely defined period followed by rapid degradation of *mos* RNA and/or protein.[51,93] These observations suggest that the *mos* protein kinase might be regulated at the level of expression rather than by binding of regulatory molecules or posttranslational modifications. However, the latter cannot be ruled out at present and needs further investigation.

The biochemical activities of the *mos* protein kinase have been studied using viral or cellular *mos* proteins expressed in *E coli* or in eukaryotic cells.[75] It was shown that *mos* proteins have an ATP-dependent and probably sequence unspecific DNA-binding domain which is located in the N-terminal half of the protein. As predicted from the amino acid sequence, *mos* proteins have protein-serine kinase activity first detected as autoophosphorylation activity directed toward certain serines in the polypeptide. In oocytes *mos* proteins were shown to be phosphorylated and it is possible that this is the result of autophosphorylation or phosphorylation by another kinase. The effect of phosphorylation on the kinase activity or other biochemical properties of *mos* proteins is not clear. The *mos* protein kinase can phosphorylate the intermediate filament protein vimentin,[77] the cell cycle regulatory protein cyclin B2,[68] and tubulin[98] in vitro. The significance of phosphorylation of these proteins for normal function and transforming activity of *mos* are discussed below.

The Normal Function of *mos*

The distinctive pattern of expression during mouse development and in certain adult tissues suggests that *mos* might play a role not only in the differentiation and function of male and female germ cells but also in cells of the nervous system and other somatic cell types. However, to date the function of *mos* has been studied in some detail only in oocyte maturation. This was greatly facilitated by the cloning of the frog homolog of *mos*,[70] which allowed the investigation of *mos* function in frog eggs, a system that is well characterized and accessible to experimental manipulation. Aspects of the function of *mos* in oocyte maturation have also been studied in the mouse with results similar to those obtained in the frog.[49,51,97] Considering the fact that *mos* is probably expressed in the oocytes of all vertebrates,[55] the results described below might be of general significance.

Fully grown oocytes prior to maturation contain four complements of the genome and are arrested at the prophase of the first meiotic division (Fig. 2). Upon induction of maturation by agents that vary between species, oocytes resume meiosis, enter metaphase 1, complete the first meiotic division, and proceed to the metaphase of the second meiotic division where they are again arrested. Sperm penetration triggers exit from metaphase 2 and completion of the second meiotic division. Entry into metaphase 1 and 2, respectively, requires the activation of a pre-existing but inactive metaphase promoting factor (MPF), a protein complex consisting of a protein-serine/threonine kinase called cdc2 and the cell cycle regulatory protein cyclin B2. It has been demonstrated that *mos* is necessary for progesterone-induced maturation of frog oocytes and sufficient to activate and stabilize MPF, and thus plays a key role in the regulation of meiosis.[14,15,69-71,93] Upon stimulation of oocytes with progesterone, previously transcribed and stored *mos* mRNA is translated to give rise to the *mos* protein kinase. This is sufficient to activate MPF and leads to the resumption of meiosis and entry into metaphase 1. Activation of MPF could be achieved by phosphorylation of the cyclin B2 compo-

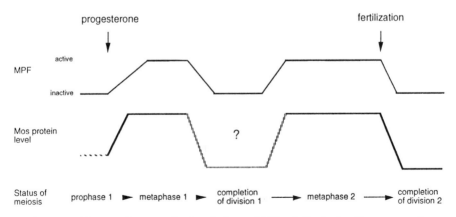

Figure 2. *Mos protein expression in relation to MPF activity during Xenopus oocyte meiotic maturation. This figure was adapted from Sagata N, Watanabe N, Vande Woude GF, et al. The c-mos proto-oncogene product is a cytostatic factor responsible for meiotic arrest in vertebrate eggs. Nature 1989; 342:512–518.*

nent of MPF by the *mos* kinase.[68] To exit metaphase and complete the first meiotic division it is necessary that MPF is inactivated or degraded. At present it is not clear whether this requires inactivation or degradation of the *mos* protein. After the completion of meiosis 1, reactivation of MPF leads to entry into metaphase 2. However at this stage, active MPF is stabilized and the oocytes are arrested at metaphase 2 by a cytostatic factor (CSF), the active component of which is the *mos* protein kinase.[71] Stabilization of MPF could be mediated by *mos* through phosphorylation of cyclin B2[68] and/or by phosphorylation of tubulin.[98] The latter could lead to a change in the properties of the microtubuli in the meiotic spindle and microtubuli-associated MPF. The oocytes remain arrested until sperm penetration triggers inactivation of MPF, exit from metaphase 2, and chromosome partition. At this point the *mos* protein is rapidly degraded. Degradation is induced by influx of calcium ions upon fertilization and appears to be mediated through the calcium dependent protease calpain.[71,93]

The results summarized above demonstrate that *mos* has an important function in the regulation of vertebrate meiosis. This function is dependent on the serine/threonine kinase activity (measured in vitro as autophosphorylation activity) of the *mos* protein.[15,94] During oocyte maturation the multiple functions of MPF and the microtubuli might be regulated by the phosphorylation of cyclin and tubulin by the *mos* protein kinase. Additional effects of *mos* might be mediated by the phosphorylation of vimentin[77] and/or of other as yet unidentified target proteins. The cell cycle of somatic cells is subject to control by MPF in a way similar to the MPF regulation of meiosis. However, there is no direct evidence to date that *mos* might be involved in the regulation of somatic cell mitosis. Consistent with the function of *mos* in the meiotic arrest of oocytes, the presence of the *mos* protein kinase after fertilization prevents embryonic cell division by metaphase arrest.[14,71] This observation might explain the previously noted toxicity of high levels of *mos* protein in mouse fibroblasts,[75] but also raises the problem of how to reconcile the normal function of *mos* with its potent transforming activity.

Oncogenic Transformation by Activated *mos* Genes

The *mos* gene was originally discovered because of its ability to cause tumorigenic transformation of primary skeletal muscle cells and fibroblasts in mice.[75] Subsequent studies to elucidate the mechanism by which *mos* transforms cells were predominantly carried out in mouse or rat cell-lines employing morphological transformation, loss of contact inhibition, and anchorage independent growth as assay criteria.

It was established that *mos* does not have to be altered by mutation to become a transforming gene. Elevated expression of the mouse or chicken *mos* proto-oncogene is sufficient to cause transformation of NIH3T3 fibroblasts. The transforming activity of the mouse and chicken homologs is comparable to that of viral *mos* genes isolated from different Moloney murine sarcoma virus strains, whereas the human and frog homologs appear to have lower activity in this system.[15,75,94] Interestingly, the transforming activity of the *mos* proteins from different species correlates with their respective autophosphorylation activity in vitro,[94] and mutational analysis has shown that the protein-serine/threonine kinase activity of *mos* is essential for its transforming function.[78]

Transformation by *mos* leads to several cell biological changes, most of which are also observed when cells are transformed by *ras* or other oncogenes. These changes include production of tumor growth factors and plasminogen activator,[75] abrogation of the requirement of platelet-derived growth factor for cell growth,[96] downregulation of the collagen alpha2[1] promoter,[74] desensitization of the glucocorticoid response,[25,57] changes in the intracellular pH and calcium concentration,[12,39] and alterations in the protein expression pattern.[18,31,42] Expression of *mos*, like expression of several other oncogenes, increases the activity of at least two transcription factors, AP1 and PEA3. Both AP1 and PEA3 were shown to be coded for by proto-oncogenes. AP1 is a heterodimeric protein complex consisting of one *fos* and one *jun* polypeptide,[67] and PEA3 is coded for by the proto-oncogenes *ets*-1 and -2.[91]

Consistent with a function of *fos* in mediating *mos*-induced transformation, mutant cells resistant to *fos*-induced transformation are also resistant to *mos*.[95] In contrast, cells resistant to the transforming activity of *ras* are susceptible to *mos* transformation.[48] Likewise, the injection of anti*ras* antibodies into cells can prevent transformation by *ras* and certain membrane bound receptor oncogenes, but not transformation by *mos*.[80] These experiments suggest that in one signal-transduction pathway that can stimulate cell growth *mos* acts upstream of *fos*, *jun*, and *ets*, but independently or downstream of *ras*.

The latter is suggested by results obtained in frog oocytes where insulin-induced maturation, believed to be mediated by *ras*, is dependent on expression of the *mos* protein.[70]

Little is known about the molecular mechanism by which *mos* transforms cells. It is conceivable that *mos* acts by phosphorylating cyclin,[68] tubulin,[98] or vimentin.[77] However, at present it is not clear whether the transforming mechanism is in any way related to the finding that the viral, mouse, and chicken *mos* proteins which are highly active in inducing frog oocyte maturation also have high transforming activity in NIH3T3 cells, whereas the human homolog is 10-to 100-fold less active in both systems.[94] On the other hand, the metaphase arrest induced by *mos* in oocytes would preclude tumorigenic transformation. It is possible that at very low levels of *mos* protein characteristically found in *mos*-transformed fibroblasts,[75] the *mos* kinase has different effects and does not cause metaphase arrest. Alternatively, *mos* might affect fibroblasts in a different manner because of differences in the set of proteins expressed in these cells. There is no evidence to date that the *mos* kinase expressed in transformed cells is turned off at any particular stage in the fibroblast cell cycle.

The Role of *mos* in Human Tumor Development

Overexpression of the mouse *mos* proto-oncogene in transgenic mice causes harderian gland hyperplasia (Heath and Propst, in preparation), pheochromocytomas, and medullary thyroid tumors.[74a] In addition, rearrangement of the *mos* gene has been implicated in the development of murine plasmacytomas.[75] In contrast, despite considerable efforts over the past eight years, no consistent amplification, rearrangement, or overexpression of the human *mos* gene has been found in human tumors. On the other hand, a rare allele of the *mos* locus, present in < 3% of the population, and distinguishable by a restriction fragment length polymorphism, was found in the DNA of patients with breast tumors, esophageal carcinomas, and melanoma,[11] and in cell-lines derived from leukemic donors.[11] However, the biological significance of this observation is not clear. Very recent studies, prompted by the findings in *mos* transgenic mice, suggest that *mos* might be expressed in human pheochromocytomas and thyroid tumors in patients suffering from multiple endocrine neoplasia syndrome (MEN 2).[74a]

Animal Models to Study *mos* Function and Oncogenicity

In addition to transforming fibroblasts, the deregulated expression of *mos* can have biological consequences as diverse as the immortalization of endothelial cells,[13] dedifferentiation and tumorigenic transformation of thyroid epithelial cells,[16] altered differentiation of carcinoma cells,[73] and induction of differentiation of monocytes to macrophages.[37] Probably the most dramatic manifestation of the pleiotropic effects of *mos* are the various phenotypes observed in transgenic mice that carry copies of the mouse *mos* proto-oncogene linked to a strong viral promoter and overexpress the gene in a variety of tissues. Together with the results obtained in frog oocytes the transgenic phenotypes clearly demonstrate the necessity of precise regulation of *mos* expression. The phenotypes studied thus far include the development of cataracts due to a failure of eye lens cells to differentiate properly[29]; axonal degeneration and inflammatory infiltrates in the brain[54]; behavioral phenotypes such as circling, head bobbing, and hyperactivity[54]; lack of hair cells in the inner ear[54]; harderian gland hyperplasia (Heath and Propst, in preparation); and thyroid medullary tumors and pheochromocytomas.[74a] The possible use of these mice as a model system to study tumor development will be discussed in Ch. 10. The value of *mos* transgenic mice as a model system for neurodegenerative disease is currently under investigation.

Perhaps one of the most interesting aspects of the pleiotropic effects of *mos* overexpression is the mechanism by which *mos* can cause apparently unrelated phenotypes. A major question is whether *mos* causes these phenotypes by phosphorylating many different target proteins or a limited number of ubiquitously expressed target proteins which in turn have different effects depending on the cell type in which they occur. It is remarkable that from the three substrates for the *mos* protein kinase identified thus far, two, tubulin and cyclin B2, are ubiquitously expressed proteins and the third, vimentin, is expressed in many cell types. Thus, it is possible that *mos* causes a variety of phenotypes by interacting with very few protein substrates. Supporting evidence comes from studies of vimentin overexpression in transgenic mice which causes a phenotype similar to *mos* overexpression.[8] On the other hand, it is likely that phosphorylation of tubulin in neurons that have permanently withdrawn from the cell cycle has different effects than it does in oocytes. Thus, *mos* transgenic mice might permit the analysis of the pleiotropic functions of vimentin, tubulin, and cyclin in different cell types. In any case they constitute a valuable system to study pleiotropic effects of a regulatory protein-serine/threonine kinase.

The *raf* Proto-Oncogene

General Aspects of the *raf* Proto-Oncogenes

The v-*raf* oncogene was first identified as the transforming gene of the murine sarcoma virus 3611-MSV, which was obtained from experiments aimed at the isolation of new transforming retroviruses by growth of murine leukemia virus (MuLV) in chemically-transformed mouse cells.[62,64] The history and pathogenicity of the virus has been reviewed.[59] Subsequent screening with the v-*raf* oncogene led to the identification of a family of related cellular genes.[59] Three active members of the *raf* family have been identified to date, A-*raf*-1, B-*raf*, and c-*raf*-1, and all three of these genes have been found in man, mouse, and chicken.[59] They are dispersed over different chromosomes and have been mapped to sites that are frequently altered in human tumors.[83] *raf* genes are differentially expressed in tissues, such that A-*raf*-1 transcripts are present together with the ubiquitous c-*raf*-1 in urogenital tissues, whereas B-*raf* is most abundant in cerebrum and testis.[84] *raf* genes encode cytosolic phosphoproteins of similar size (72/74 kDa for c-*raf*-1; 68 kDa for A-*raf*-1, and 74 kDa for B-*raf*)[35,59] that function as serine/threonine-specific protein kinases (Table 1).[59,79]

raf family genes are highly conserved in evolution, allowing identification of homologous genes from *C elegans*[17] and *Drosophila*,[40] as well as a structurally similar protein from maize.[90] The distantly related gene from *C elegans* apparently encodes a transmembrane serine-kinase receptor, raising the possibility that this receptor class may also exist in mammals. A cognate *raf* gene from *Drosophila*, D-*raf*-1, encodes an intracellular serine/threonine kinase. Genetic analysis of D-*raf*-1 demonstrated that the enzyme is essential for normal cell proliferation of cells in somatic and germ line tissues as well as for normal development.[47] Indeed, consistent with the data from the mammalian system, analysis of D-*raf* function in develop-

TABLE 1.
Summary of *raf* Oncogene Characteristics

1. Three active genes in man, *c-raf-1*, B-*raf*, and A-*raf-1*.
2. Distantly related to protein kinase C.
3. *c-raf-1* on chromosome 3p25, site altered in many epithelial neoplasias, marker for von Hippel-Lindau disease, loss of *c-raf-1* heterozygosity in small-cell lung tumor and renal cancer. A-*raf*-on Xp11.2-11.4, B-*raf* on 7q33–36. *c-raf-1* and A-*raf-1* have pseudogenes, *c-raf-2* and A-*raf-2*; *c-raf-2* marks Huntington's chorea. D-*raf-1* on X chromosome and D-*raf-2* on chromosome 2 in *Drosophila melanogaster*. D-*raf-1* essential for normal cell proliferation and several developmental pathways.
4. Expression: *c-raf-1* ubiquitous, A-*raf-1* urogenital tissues, B-*raf* cerebrum and testis.
5. *c-raf-1*, A-*raf-1*, and B-*raf* encode 74, 68, and 72 kDa proteins, respectively, predominantly found in the cytoplasm, with associated serine/threonine kinase activity.
6. Function in signal-transduction independent of *Ras*.
7. Fraction of activated *c-raf-1* enters nucleus.
8. Synergize in transformation with *Myc*. Involved in the transcriptional control of *fos*, *jun*, TGF-a, etc. *Raf* response elements include AP1/PEA3 motifs.
9. Oncogenic activation can be achieved by truncation, N-terminal extension, or site-specific mutation. ENU-induced murine lung tumors and lymphomas contain consistent *c-raf-1* point mutations, and vaccination with purified *Raf* doubles tumor latency.

ment tentatively places the enzyme in a signal-transduction cascade initiated by receptor-class PTKs that regulate gene expression programs.[1] In the mammalian system, developmental effects of *c-raf-1* are unknown; however, *raf-1* kinase has been shown to affect, in combination with *myc*, lineage determination in the B/myeloid cell lineages.[53]

The Normal Function of *raf*

raf kinases are inactive in quiescent cells. The ubiquitous *c-raf-1* kinase is positively regulated by tyrosine and serine phosphorylations that are initiated by activated growth factor receptor kinases[44,45,58] (see below). Structure/function analysis of *raf-1* suggested a model for allosteric regulation that is reminiscent of PKC (Fig. 1).[63] *Raf* family protein kinases show homology with PKC family enzymes in the kinase domain as well as in the N-terminal, cysteine-rich negative regulatory domain.[5] When activated forms of the c-*raf*-1 gene were expressed in *E coli*, the purified protein had kinase activity in vitro and induced DNA synthesis as well as morphological transformation upon microinjection into quiescent NIH3T3 cells.[81] Thus activated *raf* is an intracellular mitogen.

Raf-1 kinase is a candidate downstream effector of mitogen signal-transduction, since *raf* oncogenes overcome growth arrest resulting from a block of cellular *ras* activity due either to a cellular mutation (*ras* revertant cells) or microinjection of anti*ras* antibodies.[59] *Raf* functions downstream of *ras* in a converging signal-transduction pathway as judged from experiments with *raf* antisense RNA and dominant negative mutant constructs and with *raf* revertant cells.[34] Moreover, mitogen treatment of a variety of cell types activates *raf*-1 kinase activity (see below) and induces a transient translocation of the activated enzyme to the perinuclear area and the nucleus as demonstrated for NIH3T3 cells and brain tissue.[43,50,63] Cells containing activated *raf* have an altered transcription pattern[20] and *raf* oncogenes behave as transcriptional activators for AP1/PEA3-dependent promoters in transient transfection assays.[26,27,92] Conversely, *raf* revertant cells are blocked in induction of a subset of early growth response genes (*fos*, *jun*-B, EGR-1) by TPA and serum.[34a]

Growth Factor Regulation

Growth factor regulation of *raf*-1 kinase activity has been reviewed elsewhere.[58] Briefly, more than a dozen receptor systems have been examined for *raf*-1 coupling leading to the following central findings: All strong mitogens stimulated *raf*-1 kinase activity, and this stimulation was paralleled by increased *raf*-1 phosphorylation leading to a characteristic shift in apparent molecular weight.[2,3,7,9,36,44,45,76,88]

Depending upon the receptor system, the entire pool of cellular *raf*-1 is activated within 5 to 20 minutes, and returns to ground levels within 30 to 120 minutes in the absence of stimulation.[2,3,7, 9,36,44,45,76,88] The type of *raf*-1 phosphorylation that was detected early after receptor activation differed, depending on the receptor system. Direct tyrosine phosphorylation was first reported for *raf*-1 activation by a transmembrane PTK receptor, the receptor for platelet-derived growth factor (PDGF-R).[45] The evidence for direct PDGF-R/*raf*-1 coupling via direct tyrosine phosphorylation is derived mainly from use of an insect cell overexpression system; however, the stoichiometry of this reaction in Balb3T3 cells was exceedingly low (<1%). Genetic analysis will therefore be required to determine to what degree the PDGF-R depends on this route for raf-1 recruitment. Examination of a close relative of PDGF-R, the CSF-1R, did not show any evidence of a role for tyrosine phosphorylation in raf-1 activation and correlated instead with increased phosphorylation on serine residues by as yet unidentified serine kinase(s).[3]

Similarly, representatives of the other three structural classes of transmembrane PTK receptors, the insulin receptor,[7,36] epidermal growth factor receptor (EGF-R),[2] and fibroblast growth factor receptor (FGF-R) (Dell et al., in preparation) activated raf-1 kinase concomitant with increased phosphorylation on serine residues. Moreover, in the case of the insulin receptor, the stimulated raf-1 kinase activity was shown to be resistant to tyrosine phosphatase,[36] and an insulin-regulated raf kinase has now been partially purified.[38a]

In contrast, stimulation of a murine T-cell line, CT10, through the interleukin 2 receptor (IL-2R)[88] or of murine myeloid cell-lines FDC-P1, 32D, or DA-3 by interleukin 3 (IL-3) or GM-CSF[9] leads to rapid (1 to 2 min) and sustained (>15 min) phosphorylation of raf-1 on tyrosine at high stoichiometry (30%–50% at 15 min) that again correlated with an increase in raf-1 kinase activity. Both the IL-2R and IL-3R are kinase negative transmembrane receptors consisting of multiple subunits that trigger rapid phosphorylation of intracellular proteins on both tyrosine and serine residues. The intervening intracellular PTKs are unknown, although there is some evidence in the case of the IL-2R chain for ligand-dependent association and activation of lck PTK (Taniguchi et al., personal communication).

Rapid tyrosine phosphorylation and kinase activation of raf-1 was also observed upon crosslinking of another kinase negative transmembrane receptor class molecule, CD4, and in this case the intervening intracellular PTK was clearly demonstrated to be lck.[86a] CD4 crosslinking induced lck activation, and raf-1 tyrosine phosphorylation was very rapid (30" maximum), limited to 1%–5% of cellular raf-1 and transient with return to groundstate after 5 minutes. At the earliest time of raf-1 activation, increased phosphorylation on serine residues was present, in addition to tyrosine phosphorylation.

From this comparison it appears that PKC-independent (after long-term TPA treatment) serine phosphorylation is the predominant mode of raf-1 coupling for transmembrane PTK receptors, and tyrosine phosphorylation may be characteristic of kinase negative receptors that work via intracellular PTKs. In fact, since it was recently shown that activated PDGF-R associates with and activates intracellular PTKs,[38] the small fraction of raf-1 has come from PDGF-R activated PTKs. The examples presented so far suggest multiple independent routes for raf-1 activation by phosphorylation, although they do not completely exclude raf-1 tyrosine phosphorylation at very low stoichiometry as a uniform priming mechanism for raf-1 recruitment. That possibility appeared remote in a third study that used a murine T-cell hybridoma cell-line, 2B4, stimulated through the T-cell receptor or Thy-1[76] which led to raf-1 activation entirely dependent on PKC. While these findings are not necessarily representative of events in primary T cells, they illustrate the existence of multiple receptor regulated raf-1 activating protein kinases.

raf-1 in Activated Receptor Complexes

Several transmembrane PTKs have been shown to oligomerize upon ligand binding and to display binding sites for second messenger class enzymes, due to conformational changes of their intracellular domains.[89] Raf-1 has been identified as one of the components of such multi-enzyme complexes in the case of the PDGF and EGF receptors, although the fraction of cellular raf-1 present in complexes was very low (~1%) and has yet to be confirmed for the PDGF-R.[2,3,45]

As described above, tyrosine phosphorylation of raf-1 did not accompany receptor association in the case of the EGF-R bound raf-1. For the kinase negative IL-2, IL-3, and GM-CSF receptors, less is known about ligand-induced assemblies of second messenger complexes. These receptors tend to be made up of multiple subunits even before activation that may facilitate rapid signal transmission. However, for one of the kinase negative transmembrane receptors, CD4, there are data on the formation of receptor complexes. CD4 crosslinking is followed by the rapid and transient association and kinase activation of lck as well as raf-1, which becomes tyrosine phosphorylated in the process.[86a]

What may be the physiological significance of complex formation? Since most components of the complexes appear to be substrates for intrinsic or associated receptor PTKs, why are they not released immediately following phosphorylation? For substrates that are retained in the complex, it appears likely that there is a binding domain involved that lies outside the substrate pocket of the PTK and the phosphorylation site of the substrate. We are in the process of defining interaction sites for PDGF-R binding to *raf*-1 using the baculovirus overexpression system. The role of binding may be to facilitate access to PDGF-R and/or membrane-associated substrates of *raf*-1. Alternatively, it may be that *raf*-1 requires multiple modifications by enzymes present in the complex for maximal stimulation. The apparent inclusion of intracellular PTKs in activated transmembrane receptor PTK complexes makes for a curious reunion of members representing three generations of the evolutionarily closely related oncogene protein kinase superfamily. Their joint presence may indicate that signal-transduction from the most recently evolved transmembrane PTKs[19,41] to the cell interior and the nucleus utilizes previously established connections represented by intracellular PTKs and *src* superfamily protein-serine/threonine kinases such as *raf*-1.

raf-1 Dependence of Growth Factor Regulated Proliferation

As described above, there are multiple pathways that lead to receptor-initiated *raf*-1 activation. Is there also redundancy in pathways that connect activated receptors with proliferation? This question has been addressed in NIH3T3 cells stimulated to proliferate by serum, *ras* oncogenes, or TPA.[34] Expression of *raf*-1 antisense RNA or a kinase-negative point mutant of *raf*-1 blocked serum stimulated growth of NIH3T3 cells. Stable low v-*raf* and *raf*-1 expressers were obtained when v-*raf*-transformed NIH3T3 cells were used as target cells, and these were tested for their ability to respond with DNA synthesis to treatment with TPA or serum. The response to both inducers was inhibited in parallel to the decrease in *raf*-1 protein levels. Previous experiments that tested the ability of *raf* family oncogenes to overcome a block of cellular *ras* function had established that v-*raf* works independently of *ras* and suggested that it acts as a downstream effector of *ras* that in turn controls the signal flow of membrane-associated PTKs and PKC.[63] Inhibition by antisense RNA or a kinase inactive mutant blocked proliferation and transformation by Ki-and Ha-*ras* oncogenes. We conclude that *raf* functions as an essential signal transducer downstream of serum growth factor receptors, PKC, and *ras*.

A second line of investigation on the effect of blocked *raf*-1 function on membrane-initiated proliferation utilized *raf*-1 revertant cells.[34a] The pattern of cross-resistance of these cells toward PTK, *ras*, and other oncogenes was identical to the one obtained with *raf*-1 blocking constructs. The revertant cells also showed that a subset of normally growth factor-inducible immediate early genes including *fos*, *jun*-B, and EGR-1[85] were partially or completely resistant to induction by serum or TPA, indicating a critical role for *raf*-1 in their regulation. Moreover, the v-*raf*-transformed phenotype could be restored by transfection with c-*fos*.

In conclusion, the combined studies on *raf*-1 inhibition in NIH3T3 cells demonstrate that *raf*-1 is an essential link in the proliferation-inducing signal-transduction chain of growth factor in serum or of TPA. But is it sufficient?

Effects of Activated *raf*-1 on Growth Factor Dependence

NIH3T3 cells transformed by the v-*raf* oncogene in 3611-MSV or by activated versions of c-*raf* could not be growth arrested by removal of serum.[34a] This suggested that activated *raf*-1 was sufficient to replace the need for growth factors in serum, although the contribution of secondary transformation-associated changes could not be excluded. Such a contribution was eliminated in microinjection experiments with expression vector-derived *raf*-1 proteins that demonstrated acute induction of DNA synthesis by active *raf*-1 kinase.[81] However, in murine myeloid FDC-P1 and 32D cells that specifically depend on IL-3 for growth, v-*raf* did not, by itself, induce rapid growth factor independence, in contrast to the *abl* oncogene and other ectopic PTKs (see above). Nevertheless, v-*raf* clearly contributed to IL-3 independence since its presence dramatically accelerated abrogation by v-*myc* in either cell-line.[87a] The combination of v-*raf* with v-*myc* was as effective as expression of ectopic PTKs for IL-3 abrogation. Therefore it appears that in IL-3-dependent cell-lines, minimally two signaling pathways had to be triggered by the receptor-associated or ectopic PTKs, one leading to c-*myc* induction and the other leading to *raf*-1 activation. It is possible that other cells, especially from primary cultures, require activation of additional parallel pathways that recruit positive or inactivate negative regulators of growth. However, such primary cells also often require multiple qualitatively distinct stimuli for proliferation, not all of which may involve growth factor receptor activation.

Effector Functions of *raf*-1

The data described so far on regulation of *raf*-1 strongly support the idea of convergence in growth factor signal-transduction. But what happens downstream of *raf*-1, what are the substrates of *raf*-1, and what processes do they regulate? It seems likely that there are a number of distinct substrates for *raf*-1 that mediate the diverse effects that *raf* transformation has on cell physiology, although some of this diversity may result instead from pleiotropic effects of *raf*-1 substrate(s). *Raf*-induced changes include effects on lipid metabolism,[30] morphology,[59] stability of the differentiated state,[53] and immediate early gene expression.[34a]

There is good evidence that at least one substrate of *raf*-1 is *raf*-1 itself (Kolch and Rapp, unpublished data). Determination of *raf*-1 autophosphorylation site(s) should perhaps provide some clues as to *raf*-1-specific target sequences. The presence of *raf*-1 in activated growth factor receptor complexes points to other components in these transient multienzyme systems as potential substrates. The notion that growth factor-regulated signal flow may involve a kinase cascade retracing steps in the evolutionary ladder of the *src* superfamily of genes points to *mos* as a potential *raf*-1 substrate through which a tie-in with mitosis may be achieved.[71] Finally, the observation that activated *raf*-1 synergizes with c-*myc* and regulates transcription of immediate early genes prompted us to speculate that *raf* alters the activity of transcription factors via direct or indirect effects on their state of phosphorylation.[61] Consistent with this hypothesis, we have observed phosphorylation of *jun*, but not *fos* (Rauscher, Curran, and Rapp, unpublished observation), *myc* or *myb* (Lurcher and Rapp, unpublished observation) in vitro. Because of the apparent association of an activated *raf*-1 with DNA in the nucleus, it has to be considered that some substrate phosphorylations actually occur in transcription complexes. These possibilities are currently under investigation. So far, most of the work on *raf* family protein-serine/threonine kinases has focused on the ubiquitous *raf*-1 isozyme.

If *raf*-1 is a pivotal switch enzyme controlling the flow of membrane-initiated proliferation signals, what may be the role of the other *raf* isozymes? Their restricted expression in specialized tissues suggests that they do not represent backup systems for *raf*-1. Since truncated versions of all three *raf* genes transform NIH3T3 cells, they probably share some common substrates. However, it seems likely that they differ in the range of receptor systems through which they may be regulated since A-*raf* was apparently not being activated by the PDGF-R (Morrison and Rapp, unpublished observation). The convergence model for growth inducing signal-transduction onto a few cytosolic protein-serine/threonine kinases including *raf*-1 raises questions about the consequence of such an arrangement for growth factor receptor-specific signaling and the risk of cancer. If most growth factor receptors activate PTKs that overlap in their substrate specificity, how may receptor-specific instructions be conveyed? We already know that not all transmembrane PTKs make contact with the full set of candidate second messengers that have so far come to light (PI kinase, PLCγ, MAP2 kinase, GAP, *raf*-1). For example, PLCg is not being phosphorylated by the CSF-1R, and PI kinase is not being activated by the EGF-R.[89] This pattern eliminates both enzymes as essential components of proliferation signal-transduction in the cell types tested, and at the same time illustrates that there probably is a combination of common second messengers characteristic for individual receptor classes, reminiscent of the combinatorial nature of transcriptional enhancer function.

Moreover, the differentiated state of the cell will contribute to the specificity of the growth factor response through provision of partially cell type-specific sets of substrates and target genes. In terms of cancer risk, converging signaling pathways for proliferation control are clearly disadvantageous. This converging nature of signal-transduction allows ectopically-expressed unique growth factor receptors and intracellular PTKs to hook up with central enzymes such as *raf*-1 in virtually all cells and therefore must be largely responsible for the huge target size for individual cell carcinogenesis that is evident from the ever increasing number of cancer genes. Our hope now is that we can take advantage of this shortcoming by developing growth inhibitory drugs for pivotal enzymes such as *raf*-1 that control the transforming ability of most peripheral oncogenes.

Oncogenic Transformation by Activated *raf* Genes

The c-*raf*-1 gene can be converted into an oncogene by N-terminal fusion, truncation,[21,82,92] or by the site-specific mutation.[21,92] The minimal transforming version of the c-*raf*-1 gene consists only of the kinase domain. No point mutations within this domain are required for its transforming function and constitutive kinase activity. These data are consistent with a structure/function model for allosteric regulation of *raf* kinase that is reminiscent of PKC, and involves removal, mutation, or modification of an N-terminal negative regulatory domain for activation. The rules for activation are the same for all *raf* isozymes, and activated versions of A-and B-*raf* transform NIH3T3 cells with an efficiency comparable to equivalent versions of c-*raf*-1. These combined data suggest that *raf* transformation results from continuous signaling within the normal *raf* pathway, and not from acquisition of new substrate specificities. Growth factor abrogation experiments with *raf* oncogenes alone or in combination with *myc* showed that the presence of activated *raf* provides the cell with one (of perhaps no more than two,[63,66]) essential[34] activated signaling pathway.

The Role of *raf* in Human Tumor Development

This subject has recently been reviewed.[83] As yet there is no convincing case for mutational activation of any of the *raf* genes in human tumors. However, constitutive activation of *raf*-1 kinase, overexpression of *raf*-1 protein, and loss of one allele of c-*raf*-1 frequently occur in certain lung and renal cancers. Moreover, our recent finding of consistent c-*raf*-1 point mutations in a mouse model for the induction of lung and T-cell tumors (see below) emphasizes the need for examination of c-*raf*-1 in human tumors at the level of point mutations.

Animal Models to Study *raf* Function and Oncogenicity

In normal rat liver *raf*-1 RNA levels increase approximately fourfold 20 hours following a partial hepatectomy, and this increase in message coincides with peak DNA synthesis.[6] Diethylnitrosamine-induced rat liver tumors promoted with phenobarbital exhibited elevated levels of *raf*-1 mRNA in approximately 85% of either neoplastic nodules or hepatocellular carcinomas.[24] However, in these tumors *raf* expression did not correlate with histone H4 expression, nor did *raf*-1 expression relate to the malignancy of the tumors tested. This indicates that in these tumors *raf* overexpression is not simply a product of or required for increased DNA synthesis or proliferation, and suggests that *raf* may be playing another role in these tumors. Induction of *raf* expression appears to be specific for *raf*-1 as levels of A-*raf* were not altered.

The oncogenically active v-*raf*, derived from mouse c-*raf*-1, is capable of transforming a variety of cell-lines in vitro and inducing a defined spectrum of tumors in vivo. Newborn mice inoculated intraperitoneally with the v-*raf* expressing 3611-MSV develop fibrosarcomas, erythroblastosis, and occasionally erythroleukemia.[33,60,64] One hundred percent of inoculated animals develop one or more of these malignancies with a latency period of 4 to 8 weeks. The first detectable lesions in these mice are clusters of malignant fibroblasts on the diaphragm, which metastasize throughout the peritoneal cavity and invade the spleen. In addition to the above mentioned tumors, histologic examination of these animals revealed that 3611-MSV inoculation also results in foci of pancreatic cancer cells, which are seen throughout the parenchyma. These tumors are detectable as early as 15 days following injection of 3611-MSV. Susceptibility to 3611-MSV-induced tumorigenesis is highest for newborns and rapidly decreases as mice become weanlings. It has been demonstrated that this resistance of older mice to 3611-MSV-induced erythroleukemias is controlled by a different genetic locus or loci that is responsible for resistance to *raf/myc*-induced lymphomas.[32] Additionally, chickens infected with either the v-*myc* expressing MC29 or MH2 which expressed v-*myc* and the avian homolog of v-*raf*, v-*mil*, develop pancreatic carcinomas.[4] The difference in tumor spectrums induced by *raf* and *myc* expressing retroviruses suggest that the preferred *myc* targets (lymphoid) differ from the preferred *raf* targets (erythroid, fibroblast) in the rate limiting pathways through which their growth is normally controlled.[46,61]

Consistent Point Mutations in c-*raf*-1 in Transplacentally-Induced Mouse Lung and T-cell Tumors

The original isolation of 3611-MSV involved inoculation of newborn NFS mice with a particular cell culture-derived transforming virus stock. The tumor bearing mouse from which the transforming virus was reisolated had developed a large lung tumor in addition to a peritoneal tumor.[64] This observation prompted the development of a lung tumor induction model for the evaluation of a potential role of raf-1 in this tumor type. Transplacental injection of ENU resulted in the development of lung adenocarcinomas in nearly 100% of the F1 mice, and development of lymphomas in approximately 70%. We have determined that exposure to ENU on day 16 of gestation produces optimal lung tumor induction. This is in agreement with other studies which examined the effect of developmental time of exposure on tumor formation.[28]

The lung tumors generated have been classified as papillary lung adenocarcinomas, and are histologically indistinguishable from their human counterparts, thus making them clinically relevant.[61,65] The lymphomas have been determined to be invasive T-cell lymphomas by lineage-specific cell surface markers. F1 animals die from these tumors with a median age of approximately 20 weeks. Although this one time exposure to ENU in utero causes rapid tumor induction, even faster tumorigenesis was achieved by using a tumor promoter in conjunction with the carcinogen. When BHT was administered intraperitoneally on a weekly basis beginning at 3 weeks of age, the median age for death resulting from these tumors decreased from 20 to roughly 12 weeks of age in comparison to unpromoted animals (p<.005). Promotion with BHT did not affect the tumor spectrum but merely increased the rate of genesis, as again nearly all developed lung adenocarcinomas and approximately 70% acquired T-cell lymphomas.

Vaccination of animals exposed to both carcinogen and promoter with purified raf protein resulted in a dramatic increase in tumor latency, as determined by length of time until moribund. The impact of this vaccination can be summarized as follows. Animals receiving ENU, BHT, and a control vaccine (BSA) showed the same rate of tumorigenesis as those receiving ENU and BHT alone. Animals exposed to ENU, BHT, and vaccinated with raf protein had a death curve nearly identical to those receiving only ENU. In fact there is no statistical difference between the two groups. Thus, vaccination with purified raf protein has a definite biological effect in this system in that it nearly doubles the length of time required for animals to succumb to lung tumors and, in effect, cancels out the promoter's influence.[61,65]

RNAse protection analysis of c-raf suggested the presence of a mutant raf allele in these tumors. Examination of 18 lung tumors revealed the presence of an extra band, when compared to the completely protected fragment from an untreated F1 mouse. The size of this fragment corresponded to an alteration roughly in the region of the exon 14/15 junction. In each case tumors expressed one normal and one mutant allele at equivalent levels. Subsequent amplification of this region via PCR and sequencing revealed that indeed these tumors contained point mutations in c-*raf*-1. In each tumor examined a mutation was found within a small stretch (approximately 20 amino acids) in the catalytic domain of the kinase (Rapp and Storm, unpublished observation). The biological activity of these mutated c-*raf*-1 genes is currently being evaluated.

References

1. Ambrosio L, Mahowald AP, Perrimon N. Requirement of the *Drosophila raf* homologue for torso function. Nature 1989; 342:288–291.
2. App H, Hazan R, Zilberstein A, et al. EGF stimulates association with c-*raf* and its kinase activity in living cells. Mol Cell Biol 1991; 11:913–919.
3. Baccarini M, Sabatini DM, App H, et al. Colony stimulating factor-1 (CSF-1) stimulates temperature-dependent phosphorylation and activation of the *raf*-1 protooncogene product. EMBO J 1990; 9:3649–3657.
4. Beard JW. Biology of avian retroviruses. In: Viral Oncology, Klein G, ed. New York, Raven Press 1980; 79.
5. Beck TW, Huleihel M, Gunnell M, et al. The complete coding sequence of the human A-*raf*-1 oncogene and transforming activity of a human A-*raf* carrying retrovirus. Nucleic Acids Res 1987; 15:595–609.
6. Beer DG, Neveu MJ, Paul DL, et al. Expression of the c-*raf* proto-oncogene, gamma-glutamyltranspeptidase, and gap junction protein in rat liver neoplasms. Cancer Res 1988; 48:1610–1617.
7. Blackshear PJ, Haupt DM, App H, et al. Insulin activates the *raf*-1 protein kinase. J Biol Chem 1990; 265:12131–12134.
8. Capetanaki Y, Smith S, Heath JP. Overexpression of the vimentin gene in transgenic mice inhibits normal lens cell differentiation. J Cell Biol 1989; 109:1653–1664.
9. Carroll MP, Clark-Lewis I, Rapp UR, et al. Interleukin-3 and granulocyte-macrophage colony stimulating factor mediate rapid phosphorylation and activation of cytosolic c-*raf*. J Biol Chem 1990; 265:19812–19817.
10. Dandoy F, De Maeyer-Guignard J, De Maeyer E. Linkage analysis of the murine *mos* proto-oncogene on chromosome 4. Genomics 1989; 4:546–551.
11. Dietrich KD, Fourney RM, Aubin RA, et al. A rare c-*mos* RFLP in normal (noncancerous) fibroblasts from two related cancer patients. Nucleic Acids Res 1989; 17:1273.
12. Doppler W, Jaggi R, Groner B. Induction of v-*mos* and activated Ha-*ras* oncogene expression in quiescent NIH 3T3 cells causes intracellular alkalinisation and cell-cycle progression. Gene 1987; 54:147–153.
13. Faller DV, Kourembanas S, Ginsberg D, et al. Immortalization of human endothelial cells by murine sarcoma viruses, without morphologic transformation. J Cell Physiol 1988; 134:47–56.

14. Freeman RS, Kanki JP, Ballantyne SM, et al. Effects of the v-*mos* oncogene on Xenopus development: Meiotic induction in oocytes and mitotic arrest in cleaving embryos. J Cell Biol 1990; 111:533–541.

15. Freeman RS, Pickham KM, Kanki JP, et al. Xenopus homolog of the *mos* proto-oncogene transforms mammalian fibroblasts and induces maturation of Xenopus oocytes. Proc Natl Acad Sci USA 1989; 86:5805–5809.

16. Fusco A, Portella G, Di Fiore PP, et al. A *mos* oncogene-containing retrovirus, myeloproliferative sarcoma virus, transforms rat thyroid epithelial cells and irreversibly blocks their differentiation pattern. J Virol 1985; 56:284–292.

17. Georgi LL, Albert PS, Riddle DL. *daf-1*, a C. elegans gene controlling dauer larva development, encodes a novel receptor protein kinase. Cell 1990; 61:635–645.

18. Giancotti V, Pani B, D'Andrea P, et al. Elevated levels of a specific class of nuclear phosphoproteins in cells transformed with v-*ras* and v-*mos* oncogenes and by cotransfection with c-*myc* and polyoma middle T genes. EMBO J 1987; 6:1981–1987.

19. Hanks SK, Quinn AM, Hunter T. The protein kinase family: Conserved features and deduced phylogeny of the catalytic domains. Science 1988; 241:42–52.

20. Heidecker G, Cleveland JL, Beck T, et al. Role of *raf* and *myc* oncogenes in signal transduction. In: Genes and Signal Transduction in Multistage Carcinogenesis, Colburn N, ed. New York, Marcel Dekker, Inc 1989; pp. 339–374.

21. Heidecker G, Huleihel M, Cleveland JL, et al. Mutational activation of c-*raf*-1 and definition of the minimal transforming sequence. Mol Cell Biol 1990; 10:2503–2512.

22. Herzog NK, Ramagli LS, Khorana S, et al. Evidence for somatic cell expression of the c-*mos* protein [corrected] [published erratum appears in Oncogene 1990 Apr,5(4):623]. Oncogene 1989; 4:1307–1315.

23. Herzog NK, Singh B, Elder J, et al. Identification of the protein product of the c-*mos* proto-oncogene in mouse testes. Oncogene 1988; 3:225–229.

24. Hsieh LL, Hsiao WL, Peraino C, et al. Expression of retroviral sequences and oncogenes in rat liver tumors induced by diethylnitrosamine. Cancer Res 1987; 47:3421–3424.

25. Jaggi R, Salmons B, Muellener D, et al. The v-*mos* and H-*ras* oncogene expression represses glucocorticoid hormone-dependent transcription from the mouse mammary tumor virus LTR. EMBO J 1986; 5:2609–2616.

26. Jamal S, Ziff E. Transactivation of c-*fos* and beta-actin genes by *raf* as a step in early response to transmembrane signals. Nature 1990; 344:463–466.

27. Kaibuchi K, Fukumoto Y, Oku N, et al. Activation of the serum response element and 12-O-tetradecanoylphorbol-13-acetate response element by the activated c-*raf*-1 protein in a manner independent of protein kinase C. J Biol Chem 1989; 264:20855–20858.

28. Kauffman SL. Susceptibility of fetal lung to transplacental 1-ethyl-1-nitrosourea: Its relation to epithelial proliferation. J Nat Cancer Inst 1976; 57:821.

29. Khillan JS, Oskarsson MK, Propst F, et al. Defects in lens fiber differentia-

tion are linked to c-*mos* overexpression in transgenic mice. Genes Dev 1987; 1:1327–1335.

30. Kiss Z, Rapp UR, Anderson WB. Phorbol ester stimulates the synthesis of sphingomyelin in NIH 3T3 cells. A diminished response in cells transformed with human A-*raf* carrying retrovirus. FEBS Lett 1988; 240:221–226.

31. Klemenz R, Hoffmann S, Werenskiold AK. Serum-and oncoprotein-mediated induction of a gene with sequence similarity to the gene encoding carcinoembryonic antigen. Proc Natl Acad Sci USA 1989; 86:5708–5712.

32. Klinken SP, Hartley JW, Fredrickson TN, et al. Susceptibility to *raf* and *raf/myc* retroviruses is governed by different genetic loci. J Virol 1989; 63:2411–2414.

33. Klinken SP, Rapp UR, Morse HC 3d. *raf/myc*-infected erythroid cells are restricted in their ability to terminally differentiate. J Virol 1989; 63:1489–1492.

34. Kolch W, Heidecker G, Lloyd P, et al. *Raf*-1 protein kinase is required for growth of NIH3T3 cells induced by serum, TPA, and *ras* oncogenes. Nature 1991; 349:426–428.

34a. Kolch W, Heidecker G, Troppmain J, et al. *Raf* revertant cells resist transformation by non-nuclear oncogenes and are deficient in the induction of early response genes by TPA and serum. Oncogene 1993; 8:361–370.

35. Kolch W, Weissinger E, Mischak H, et al. Probing structure and function of the *raf* protein kinase domain with monoclonal antibodies. Oncogene 1990; 5:713–720.

36. Kovacina KS, Yonezawa K, Brautigan DL, et al. Insulin activates the kinase activity of the *raf*-1 proto-oncogene by increasing its serine phosphorylation. J Biol Chem 1990; 265:12115–12118.

37. Kurata N, Akiyama H, Taniyama T, et al. Dose-dependent regulation of macrophage differentiation by *mos* mRNA in a human monocytic cell line. EMBO J 1989; 8:457–463.

38. Kypta RM, Goldberg Y, Ulug ET, et al. Association between the PDGF receptor and members of the *src* family of tyrosine kinases. Cell 1990; 62:481–492.

38a. Lee R, Rapp UR, Blackshear PJ. Evidence for one or more *Raf*-1 kinases activated by insulin and polypeptide growth factors. J Biol Chem 1991; 266:10351–10357.

39. Maly K, Doppler W, Oberhuber H, et al. Desensitization of the Ca2+-mobilizing system to serum growth factors by Ha-*ras* and v-*mos*. Mol Cell Biol 1988; 8:4212–4216.

40. Mark GE, MacIntyre RJ, Digan ME, et al. *Drosophila* melanogaster homologs of the *raf* oncogene. Mol Cell Biol 1987; 7:2134–2140.

41. Mark GE, Rapp UR. Primary structure of v-*raf*: Relatedness to the *src* family of oncogenes. Science 1984; 224:285–289.

42. Mayo JK, Sampson KE, Adams LD, et al. Increased amount of a 25-kilodalton phosphoprotein after v-*mos* transfection of CHO cells. Mol Cell Biol 1988; 8:4685–4691.

43. Mihaly A, Olah Z, Kuhnt U, et al. Transient increase of *raf*-protein-kinase-like immunoreactivity in the dentate gyrus during long term potentiation. Neurosci Lett 1990; 116:45–50.

44. Morrison DK, Kaplan DR, Escobedo JA, et al. Direct activation of the serine/threonine kinase activity of *raf*-1 through tyrosine phosphorylation by the PDGF beta-receptor. Cell 1989; 58:649–657.

45. Morrison DK, Kaplan DR, Rapp U, et al. Signal transduction from membrane to cytoplasm: Growth factors and membrane-bound oncogene products increase *raf*-1 phosphorylation and associated protein kinase activity. Proc Natl Acad Sci USA 1988; 85:8855–8859.

46. Morse HC 3rd, Rapp UR. Tumorigenic activity of artificially activated c-oncogenes. In: Cellular Oncogene Activation, Klein G, ed. New York, Marcel Dekker, Inc 1988; pp. 335–364.

47. Nishida Y, Hata M, Ayaki T, et al. Proliferation of both somatic and germ cells is affected in the *Drosophila* mutants of *raf* proto-oncogene. EMBO J 1988; 7:775–781.

48. Noda M, Selinger Z, Scolnick EM, et al. Flat revertants isolated from Kirsten sarcoma virus-transformed cells are resistant to the action of specific oncogenes. Proc Natl Acad Sci USA 1983; 80:5602–5606.

49. O'Keefe SJ, Wolfes H, Kiessling AA, et al. Microinjection of antisense c-*mos* oligonucleotides prevents meiosis II in the maturing mouse egg. Proc Natl Acad Sci USA 1989; 86:7038–7042.

50. Olah Z, Komoly S, Nagashima N, et al. Cerebral ischemia induces transient intracellular redistribution and intranuclear translocation of the *raf* proto-oncogene product in hippocampal pyramidal cells. Exp Brain Res 1991; 84:403–10.

51. Paules RS, Buccione R, Moschel RC, et al. Mouse *mos* protooncogene product is present and functions during oogenesis. Proc Natl Acad Sci USA 1989; 86:5395–5399.

52. Paules RS, Propst F, Dunn KJ, et al. Primate c-*mos* protooncogene structure and expression: Transcription initiation both upstream and within the gene in a tissue specific manner. Oncogene 1988; 3:59–68.

53. Principato M, Cleveland JL, Rapp UR, et al. Transformation of murine bone marrow cells with combined v-*raf*-v-*myc* oncogenes yields clonally related mature B cells and macrophages. Mol Cell Biol 1990; 10:3562–3568.

54. Propst F, Rosenberg MP, Cork LC, et al. Neuropathological changes in transgenic mice carrying copies of a transcriptionally activated *mos* protooncogene. Proc Natl Acad Sci USA 1990; 87:9703–9707.

55. Propst F, Rosenberg MP, Vande Woude GF. Proto-oncogene expression in germ cell development. Trends Genet 1988; 4:183–187.

56. Propst F, Vande Woude GF, Jenkins NA, et al. The *mos* proto-oncogene maps near the centromere on mouse chromosome 4. Genomics 1989; 5:118–123.

57. Qi M, Hamilton BJ, DeFranco D. v-*mos* oncoproteins affect the nuclear retention and reutilization of glucocorticoid receptors. Mol Endocrinol 1989; 3:1279–1288.

58. Rapp UR. Role of *raf*-1 serine/threonine protein kinase in growth factor signal transduction. Oncogene 1991; 6:495–500.

59. Rapp UR, Cleveland JL, Bonner TI, et al. The *raf* oncogenes. In: The

Oncogene Handbook, Curran T, Reddy EP, Skalka A, eds. The Netherlands, Elsevier Science Publishers 1988; pp. 213–253.

60. Rapp UR, Cleveland JL, Fredrickson TN, et al. Rapid induction of hemopoietic neoplasms in newborn mice by a *raf(mil)/myc* recombinant murine retrovirus. J Virol 1985; 55:23–33.

61. Rapp UR, Cleveland JL, Storm SM, et al. Transformation by raf and *myc* oncogenes. In: Oncogenes and Cancer, Aaronson SA, Bishop J, Sugimura T, et al., eds. Tokyo, Tokyo/VNU Sci 1987; pp. 55–74.

62. Rapp UR, Goldsborough MD, Mark GE, et al. Structure and biological activity of v-*raf*, a unique oncogene transduced by a retrovirus. Proc Natl Acad Sci USA 1983; 80:4218–4222.

63. Rapp UR, Heidecker G, Huleihel M, et al. *raf* family serine/threonine protein kinases in mitogen signal transduction. Cold Spring Harb Symp Quant Biol 1988; 53:173–184.

64. Rapp UR, Reynolds FH Jr, Stephenson JR. New mammalian transforming retrovirus: Demonstration of a polyprotein gene product. J Virol 1983; 45:914–924.

65. Rapp UR, Storm SM, Cleveland JL. Oncogenes: Clinical relevance. Hamatol Bluttransfus 1987; 31:450–459.

66. Rapp UR, Troppmair J, Carroll M, et al. Role of *raf*-1 protein kinase in IL-3 and GM-CSF mediated signal transduction. Curr Top Microbiol Immunol (Berlin) 1990; 129–139.

67. Rauscher FJ 3d, Cohen DR, Curran T, et al. *Fos*-associated protein p39 is the product of the *jun* proto-oncogene. Science 1988; 240:1010–1016.

68. Roy LM, Singh B, Gautier J, et al. The cyclin B2 component of MPF is a substrate for the c-*mos*(xe) proto-oncogene product. Cell 1990; 61:825–831.

69. Sagata N, Daar I, Oskarsson M, et al. The product of the *mos* proto-oncogene as a candidate "initiator" for oocyte maturation. Science 1989; 245:643–646.

70. Sagata N, Oskarsson M, Copeland T, et al. Function of c-*mos* proto-oncogene product in meiotic maturation in Xenopus oocytes. Nature 1988; 335:519–525.

71. Sagata N, Watanabe N, Vande Woude GF, et al. The c-*mos* proto-oncogene product is a cytostatic factor responsible for meiotic arrest in vertebrate eggs. Nature 1989; 342:512–518.

72. Saris CJM, Domen J, Berns A. The *pim*-1 oncogene encodes two related protein-serine/threonine kinases by alternative initiation at AUG and CUG. EMBO J 1991; 10:655–664.

73. Scherdin U, Steffen M, Dietel M, et al. Elevated expression of v-*mos* is correlated with altered differentiation of carcinoma cells. Oncogene 1990; 5:1619–1627.

74. Schmidt A, Setoyama C, de Crombrugghe B. Regulation of a collagen gene promoter by the product of viral *mos* oncogene. Nature 1985; 314:286–289.

74a. Schulz N, Propst F, Rosenberg MP, et al. Phaeochromocytomos and c-cell thyroid neoplasms and transgenic c-*mos* mice: A model for human multiple endocrine neoplasia Type II syndrome. Cancer Res 1992; 52:450–455.

75. Seth A, Vande Woude GF. The *mos* oncogene. In: The Oncogene

Handbook, Curran T, Reddy EP, Skalka A, eds. The Netherlands, Elsevier Science Publishers 1988; pp. 213–253.

76. Siegel JN, Klausner RD, Rapp UR, et al. T-cell antigene receptor stimulation activates the c-*raf* kinase exclusively via serine/threonine phosphorylation. J Biol Chem 1990; 265:18472–18480.

77. Singh B, Arlinghaus RB. Vimentin phosphorylation by p37*mos* protein kinase in vitro and generation of a 50-kDa cleavage product in v-*mos*-transformed cells. Virology 1989; 173:144–156.

78. Singh B, Hannink M, Donoghue DJ, et al. p37*mos*-associated serine/threonine protein kinase activity correlates with the cellular transformation function of v-*mos*. J Virol 1986; 60:1148–1152.

79. Sithanandam G, Kolch W, Duh FM, et al. Complete coding sequence of a human B-*raf* cDNA and detection of a B-*raf* protein kinase with isozyme specific antibodies. Oncogene 1991; 5:1775–1780.

80. Smith MR, DeGudicibus SJ, Stacey DW. Requirement for c-*ras* proteins during viral oncogene transformation. Nature 1986; 320:540–543.

81. Smith MR, Heidecker G, Rapp UR, et al. Induction of transformation and DNA synthesis after microinjection of *raf* proteins. Mol Cell Biol 1990; 10:3828–3833.

82. Stanton VP Jr, Nichols DW, Laudano AP, et al. Definition of the human *raf* amino-terminal regulatory region by deletion mutagenesis. Mol Cell Biol 1989; 9:639–647.

83. Storm SM, Brennscheidt U, Sithanandam G, et al. *Raf* oncogenes in carcinogenesis. CRC Reviews on Cancer 1990; 2:1–8.

84. Storm SM, Cleveland JL, Rapp UR. Expression of *raf* family proto-oncogenes in normal mouse tissues. Oncogene 1990; 5:345–351.

85. Sukhatme VP, Cao XM, Chang LC, et al. A zinc finger-encoding gene coregulated with c-*fos* during growth and differentiation, and after cellular depolarization. Cell 1988; 53:37–43.

86. Testa JR, Parsa NZ, Le Beau MM, et al. Localization of the proto-oncogene *mos* to 8q11–q12 by in situ chromosomal hybridization. Genomics 1988; 3:44–47.

86a. Thompson PA, Ledbetter JA, Rapp UR, et al. The *Raf*-1 serine-threonine kinase is a substrate for the p56*lck* protein tyrosine kinase in human T-cells. Cell Growth and Diff 1991; 2:609–617.

87. Threadgill DW, Womack JE. Regional localization of mouse *abl* and *mos* proto-oncogenes by in situ hybridization. Genomics 1988; 3:82–86.

87a. Troppmain J, Cleveland JL, Askew DS, et al. v-*raf*/v-*myc* synergism in abrogation of IL-3 dependence: v-*raf* suppresses apoptosis. Curr Top Microbiol Immunol 1992; 182:453–460.

88. Turner BC, Rapp UR, App H, et al. Interleukin-1 (IL1) induces phosphorylation and activation of p68–74 *raf* kinase in T-lymphocytes. Proc Natl Acad Sci USA 1991; 88:1227–1231.

89. Ullrich A, Schlessinger J. Signal transduction by receptors with tyrosine kinase activity. Cell 1990; 61:203–212.

90. Walker JC, Zhang R. Relationship of a putative receptor protein kinase from maize to the S-locus glycoproteins of Brassica. Nature 1990; 345:743–746.

91. Wasylyk B, Wasylyk C, Flores P, et al. The c-*ets* proto-oncogenes encode

transcription factors that cooperate with c-*fos* and c-*jun* for transcriptional activation. Nature 1990; 346:191–193.

92. Wasylyk C, Wasylyk B, Heidecker G, et al. Expression of *raf* oncogenes activates the PEA1 transcription factor motif. Mol Cell Biol 1989; 9:2247–2250.

93. Watanabe N, Vande Woude GF, Ikawa Y, et al. Specific proteolysis of the c-*mos* proto-oncogene product by calpain on fertilization of Xenopus eggs. Nature 1989; 342:505–511.

94. Yew N, Oskarsson M, Daar I, et al. *mos* gene transforming efficiencies correlate with oocyte maturation and cytostatic factor activities. Mol Cell Biol 1991; 11:604–610.

95. Zarbl H, Latreille J, Jolicoeur P. Revertants of v-*fos*-transformed fibroblasts have mutations in cellular genes essential for transformation by other oncogenes. Cell 1987; 51:357–369.

96. Zhan X, Goldfarb M. Growth factor requirements of oncogene-transformed NIH 3T3 and BALB/c 3T3 cells cultured in defined media. Mol Cell Biol 1986; 6:3541–3544.

97. Zhao X, Batten B, Singh B, et al. Requirement of the c-*mos* protein kinase for murine meiotic maturation. Oncogene 1990; 5:1727–1730.

98. Zhou R, Oskarsson M, Paules RS, et al. The ability of the c-*mos* product, pp39*mos*, to associate with and phosphorylate tubulin. Science 1991; 251:671–675.

Chapter 5

Nonreceptor Protein Tyrosine Kinases

Marius Sudol

Eighty years ago, Peyton Rous, working at the Rockefeller Institute for Medical Research in New York, provided the first clue to the viral etiology of cancer. In meticulously controlled experiments he showed that a chicken sarcoma could be transmitted to healthy birds by means of a cell-free filtrate prepared from the tumor.[14] The viral nature of tumor formation implicated by Rous' experiments was for some time a matter of controversy, and his discovery was met with disbelief. Subsequent studies, though, identified a transforming retrovirus, named Rous sarcoma virus (RSV), and pointed to a specific viral gene, the viral-*src* (v-*src*) oncogene, as responsible for the induction of neoplasia.[22] An important and interesting development in this field was the realization that the v-*src* gene has a homolog in the chromosomes of normal cells.[2] This normal counterpart is called cellular-*src* (c-*src*) or *src* proto-oncogene. Examining this discovery from the reverse perspective, it was recognized that retroviruses are able to transduce cellular genes that encode proteins involved in controlling the processes of cellular growth and differentiation. All these findings, especially the isolation of transforming viruses and the identification of oncogenes and their proto-oncogenes, have provided a foundation for understanding the molecular basis of cancer.

From *The Molecular Basis of Human Cancer:* edited by B. Neel, M.D., Ph.D., R. Kumar, Ph.D. © 1993, Futura Publishing Co. Inc., Mount Kisco, NY.

The *src* Protein: Structural and Functional Organization of a Nonreceptor Protein Tyrosine Kinase

The *src* gene of RSV encodes a 60-kd phosphoprotein (p60$^{v\text{-}src}$) that exhibits tyrosine-specific protein kinase activity both in vitro and in vivo.[9] At the amino terminus, p60^{src} contains sequences necessary for myristoylation. The second residue of p60^{src} is a conserved glycine that becomes myristoylated. This fatty acid modification anchors the *src* molecule, which does not have any hydrophobic domains, to the cytoplasmic face of cellular membranes. In contrast to protein tyrosine kinases encoded by EGF or insulin receptors, the *src* protein does not span the cellular membrane and does not communicate directly with the extracellular environment. Based on these characteristics, *src* and other tyrosine kinases of similar design are termed nonreceptor type protein tyrosine kinases (NRPTKs), or cytoplasmic tyrosine kinases. The latter term is now less frequently used and was abandoned when David Baltimore and his colleagues at the Whitehead Institute in Massachusetts described one form of the *c-abl* gene product as a nuclear protein.[25,27] For this protein kinase, an amino acid sequence responsible for nuclear localization was found in the carboxyl half of the molecule outside its enzymatic domain.

The NRPTKs can be divided into four families: the *src-*, *abl-*, *fps/fes-*, and *tyk2*-families[8,24] (Table 1). The *src*-family consists of nine closely related enzymes.[5,6] Three of them, *c-src*, *c-yes*, and *c-fgr*, have been identified as normal counterparts of viral oncogenes.[5,6] The remaining members, *fyn*, *lck*, *lyn*, *hck*, *blk*, and *tkl*,† were identified as related genes using DNA probes derived mainly from the *src* and *yes* genes.[5] The canonical structure of a NRPTK of the *src* family is shown in Figure 1. The various structural and functional domains have been defined based largely upon analyses of the *c-src* gene product; other kinases of this family have a similar overall organization.[22,24] At the amino terminus of the *src*-related kinases are the sequences necessary for myristoylation (see above). The extreme amino terminal sequences (approximately 12 to 14 amino acids) are also involved in specific interaction with a membrane receptor that stabilizes the anchorage of a NRPTK to the membrane. Using chemical crosslinking, Marilyn Resh and her col-

---

†See section below entitled "Recent Developments Concerning Nonreceptor Protein Tyrosine Kinases (NRPTKs)."

TABLE 1.
Classification of Nonreceptor Protein Tyrosine Kinases

Kinase	Chromosomal Location	Transcript Size KB	Protein Product	Expression Pattern
c-src*	20q 13.3	5.0h, 3.9 ch	p60	ubiquitous; high in developing neural tissues, platelets, testis, ovary
c-yes	18q 21.3	4.8h, 3.9 ch	p62	ubiquitous; high in adult brain, retina, lung, testis, kidney; low in muscle
c-fgr	1p 36.1	3.0,3.6 h	p55	monocytes, granulocytes, alveolar and splenic macrophages
fyn*	6p 21	2.8, 3.3 h	p59	widely expressed; high in brain, spleen, thymus
lck	1p 32–35	2.3 h	p56	T cells, less in B cells; found in some colon and lung tumor cell-lines
lyn	8q 13-fer	3.2 h	p56	spleen, tonsils, macrophages, monocytes, platelets, B cells; low in T cells
hck*	20q 11–12	2.1 h	p59	hematopoietic tissues, cell-lines of myeloid and B lymphoid lineages
blk	—	2.5 h	p55	specific expression in spleen, B lymphocytes
tkl†	—	3.8 h; 3.8 ch	—	spleen, brain, stomach, colon; not detected in lung, tonsils
c-abl*	9q 34	6, 7 h	p150	widely expressed; enriched in thymus, spleen
arg*	1q 24–25	12 h	—	widely expressed; present in monocytes
c-fps/fes	15q 25–26	2.8 ch	NCP92	bone marrow, spleen, lung cells of granulocyte and macrophage lineage
fer	—	3 h	NCP94	widely expressed; high in brain, eye, kidney, ovary
ferT	—	2.4 m	NCP51	specific expression in spermatogenic cells of testis
tyk2	19p 13.2	4.4 h	p134	hematopoietic, nonhematopoietic cell-lines, tissue expression unknown; cDNA isolated from human T-cell lymphoma cell-line library

Asterisks indicate that multiple forms of the proto-oncogene products exist and they are generated by differential splicing. Tabulation is based on Perlmutter et al[24], Hanafusa[12]; Ramakrishman et al[25]; Cooper[5]; Kruh et al[18]; and Frimbach-Kraft et al.[8] † See section below entitled "Recent Developments Concerning Nonreceptor Protein Tyrosine Kinases (NRPTKs)."

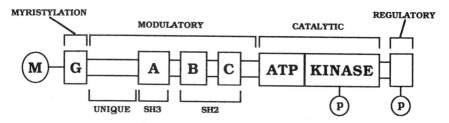

Figure 1. *Schematic representation of a canonical NRPTK from the src family. The structures and functions of the domains delineated here have been deduced from sequence comparisons and from biochemical and genetic data generated mostly for the c-src gene product. Representation of the NRPTK as a linear arrangement of domains is an oversimplification. In fact, accumulating evidence suggests that the amino terminus of the src proto-oncogene is closely apposed to its carboxy-terminus (see text). The three-dimensional organization of these domains awaits results of the crystal structure analysis of a NRPTK. M, myristate; G, glycine; P, phosphorylation sites. Other terms are explained in the text.[22]*

leagues at Princeton University identified a 32 kd membrane protein that acts as the receptor for the myristoyl-*src* protein.[26]† They showed that both the fatty acid and protein components of *src* contribute to receptor recognition and binding. Because myristoylation and membrane association are essential for the transforming activity of p60[v-src] and possibly for the normal function of p60[c-src], knowledge of the structure of the membrane-receptor-*src* complex is important.

The amino acid sequence downstream from the myristoylation and anchor receptor recognition sequences is unique for each of the NRPTKs. These regions, also called "fingerprint domains," are thought to interact with specific cellular substrates. However, based on results obtained with the *lck* kinase,[35] these sequences might also interact with various cellular receptors. In that case, the accessibility or the selection of substrates could be a consequence of a specific interaction with receptors.

Further downstream from each unique region lies a homology domain containing stretches of sequence similarity shared with other NRPTKs and with a number of membrane-associated proteins involved in signal-transduction pathways.[20,23,28] These blocks are termed A, B, and C, or SH3 and SH2 domains. Two of these blocks, one of approximately 50 amino acids (block B) and another of approximately 10 amino acids (block C), are found in all NRPTKs except *tyk2*, and are termed the SH2 domain (for *src* homology 2; SH1 being the kinase domain). The third block of homology, termed A or SH3, is present in the src and abl families but absent in the fps/fes and tyk2 families (Fig. 2).[23] Recently, other gene products have been shown to contain SH2 and/or SH3 domains. These include the crk oncogene and proto-oncogene, GTPase Activator Protein (GAP), phospholipase C, myosinIB, spectrin, and others (Fig. 3).[13,20,21,28] The presence of well conserved SH2 and SH3 motifs in diverse proteins of single-celled and higher eukaryotes suggests a basic function for these domains. A number of experimental results suggest possible roles for SH2 and SH3 domains in cellular processes. Mutations in SH2 domains of NRPTKs produce host range phenotypes which could be explained by assuming the interaction of the SH2 domain with cellular proteins. These proteins may have a modulatory role for NRPTKs because deletions of SH2 or SH3 domains in some proto-oncogenes (see below) activate their oncogenic potential. The SH2 and SH3 domains can function independently since some proteins contain only the SH3 or the SH2 domain (Figs. 2,3). In general, the SH3 domain-containing proteins tend to localize in the cortical cytoplasm, suggesting that this domain recognizes common components in the membrane cytoskeleton.[20,28] Two oxidase factors, p47 and p67, which contain tandem repeats of SH3 domains, are translocated from the cytosol to the membrane skeleton following activation of the oxidative burst in phagocytic cells.[20] Interestingly, their SH3 domains border with proline-rich regions, and similar sequences (SH3 + proline-rich stretch) were found in the ATP-independent actin binding site of nonmuscle myosin. Altogether these findings suggest, but do not prove, that the SH3 domain participates in localizing proteins to the membrane cytoskeleton.

The SH2 domain binds to phosphotyrosine-containing proteins. Initially, this was inferred from studies with the crk oncogene by Hidesaburo Hanafusa and colleagues at the Rockefeller University.[13,20b,21] However, the most direct proof of SH2-phosphotyrosine binding comes from the following experiments. Bacterially expressed SH2 domains of the abl and src oncogenes were shown to bind specifically to phosphotyrosine-containing proteins or to activated and autophosphorylated growth factor receptors, respectively.[1,21] In the case of the abl SH2, there was binding competition from a phosphotyrosine analog rather than phosphoserine (Mayer, B. and Baltimore, D., personal communication). The binding of the src SH2 with EGF and PDGF receptors was detected only in ligand stimulated (hence phosphorylated) receptors.[1] Although these studies were performed in vitro, they strongly suggest that the SH2 domain can

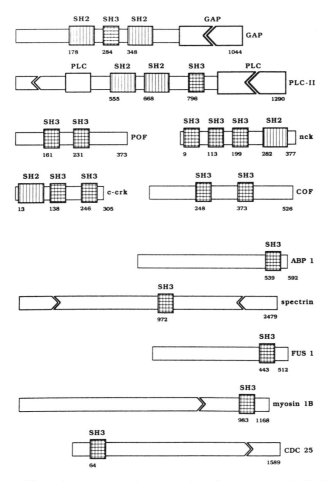

Figure 3. *Schematic structures of proteins that show sequence similarities with NRPTKs. It has been shown that various proteins implicated in signal-transduction and a number of cytoskeletal proteins are related to NRPTKs through their SH2 and SH3 domains. Among these proteins are: GTP-ase Activating Protein, GAP; phospholipase C-II and IV; phagocyte oxidase factor, POF; cytosolic oxidase factor, COF; nck, a protein isolated from a human melanoma library with a monoclonal antibody against a melanoma-associated antigen; c-crk protein; actin binding protein 1, ABP1; alpha-spectrin. Fus1, a membrane protein from yeast that is involved in the catalysis of processes connected with cell wall or plasma membrane fusion; myosin IB, cytoskeletal protein; and CDC25, a yeast regulatory protein involved in the control of the ras/adenylate cyclase pathway. As before, numbers indicate the first amino acid of the homology domain and the last amino acid of the protein.*[19,20,28]

bind to phosphotyrosine residues present on substrates and endogenous kinases, and possibly to regulatory phosphotyrosines of parental molecules. The latter suggestion that the SH2 domains of the *src* family of NRPTKs interact intramolecularly with the regulatory phosphotyrosine located at the carboxy-terminal end (see below) seems attractive.[10,13] This hypothesis is supported by various observations including the isolation of a monoclonal antibody that recognizes an epitope assembled from the amino- and carboxy-terminal sequences of *src* protein.[22] In addition, this conformational model is in agreement with protease resistance data and with the demonstration that a synthetic peptide containing a fragment of the p60[v-src] SH2 domain specifically inhibits *src* kinase activity.[21,29] Implicit in this model is the participation of the SH2 domain in the enzymatic regulation of NRPTKs and its contribution to conformational changes between oncogene and proto-oncogene proteins.

The presence in NRPTKs of conserved SH2 and SH3 domains involved in protein-protein interactions prompts the question of whether these sequences are major players in the molecular processes mediated by these enzymes. Do these domains target NRPTKs to their presumptive substrates? The SH2 and SH3 domains are reminiscent of the protein-binding modules present in transcription factors, and invoke analogous combinatorial models in which heteromeric complexes of NRPTKs with cellular receptors and other signaling molecules bring about the desired specificity of signal transmission as in the case of multicomponent complexes and transcription. The association of the same NRPTK with various cellular receptors and other signaling molecules supports such models (see below).

The most conserved region of the *src*-family of kinases is the carboxy-terminal half. It contains the ATP-binding site, the major site of in vitro tyrosine autophosphorylation, and the catalytic domain which carries the phosphotransferase activity. In the case of the *fyn* kinase, two forms exist which contain different sequences around the ATP-binding sites as a result of alternative splicing.[6] One of the forms is specifically expressed in hematopoietic cells and contains a modified sequence similar to that found in one of the yeast kinases. Both forms are enzymatically active, and the biological significance of this modification is unknown.

At the carboxyl end of the *src* family of NRPTKs, there is a short stretch of conserved amino acids containing the major site of in vivo tyrosine phosphorylation. This modification attenuates kinase activity, whereas its dephosphorylation correlates with the activation of the enzyme.[5]

Cellular, Viral, and Activated NRPTKs

Among NRPTKs, the transforming activation of the c-*src* kinase has been characterized most extensively. In general, the biochemical properties of p60$^{v\text{-}src}$ are similar to those of its cellular homolog, p60$^{c\text{-}src}$, except that the specific kinase activity of the viral protein is significantly elevated as a result of mutations.[14] Transformation by RSV results in a tenfold increase in the level of total cellular phosphotyrosine, suggesting that phosphorylation of cellular substrates by p60$^{v\text{-}src}$ is responsible for the observed neoplastic transformation.[14,22] Multiple amino acid substitutions and an altered carboxy-terminus differentiate p60$^{v\text{-}src}$ from p60$^{c\text{-}src}$ (Fig. 4). The divergence at the carboxy-terminal ends, where 19 amino acids in p60$^{c\text{-}src}$ are replaced by 12 unrelated amino acids in p60$^{v\text{-}src}$, is important because these changes remove the tyrosine whose phosphorylation is implicated in the negative regulation of enzymatic activity.[14] In order to determine which structural differences between the coding sequences of v-*src* and c-*src* are necessary for transformation, chimeric genes containing portions of v-*src* and c-*src* were tested in RSV constructs. These variants transformed normal cells. However, a construct containing the entire c-*src* gene in place of v-*src* was unable to transform cells even though the proto-oncogene protein was present in great excess over endogenous levels. To study the activation of the c-*src* gene, Hidesaburo Hanafusa and coworkers analyzed forward mutations of this gene.[14] When c-*src* was expressed in the RSV vector and passaged in fibroblasts for extended periods of time, tumorigenic variants arose spontaneously. Analysis of the sequence for two such mutants revealed that a single amino acid change in the kinase domain confers transforming ability onto c-*src*. More detailed studies were performed to analyze in vitro mutations affecting the amino-terminal region of c-*src*, some of which also activated the kinase, and to demonstrate that there is a threshold level of p60$^{v\text{-}src}$ required for cell transformation. These studies indicated that both structural and regulatory changes are required to convert the *src* proto-oncogene product into a transforming protein.[14]

Recently, one of the *src*-related genes, *fyn*, for which a viral oncogene is not known, was shown to acquire transforming proper-

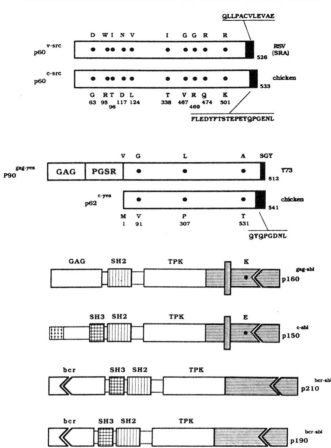

Figure 4. *Schematic representation of changes that convert the cellular NRPTKs to activated enzymes. The best characterized example is the comparison between the v-and c-src gene products which differ in multiple amino acid substitutions and carboxy-terminal peptides (uppermost diagram). Differences between p60ᵛ⁻ˢʳᶜ of the Schmidt-Ruppin strain of RSV and the normal chicken p60ᶜ⁻ˢʳᶜ homolog are depicted in the diagram. For the v-yes protein of the Yamaguchi 73 (Y73) virus and the normal chicken homolog, p62ᶜ⁻ʸᵉˢ, the changes are more complex. In addition to the amino acid substitutions and changes in carboxy-terminal peptides, the v-yes protein contains a viral gag sequence fused in frame to the peptide derived from the 5'noncoding region of c-yes cDNA (proline-, glycine-, serine-, arginine-rich polypeptide; PGSR). This peptide is in turn fused to the coding sequence of c-yes. The v-abl protein of Abelson murine leukemia virus differs from the c-abl protein in one amino acid substitution (indicated by a dot), in a short sequence having a different reading frame (indicated by a crossed rectangle), and the viral-gag sequences which in v-abl are located at the amino terminus of the protein. Two products of the bcr-abl oncogenes expressed in human leukemias are generated by chromosomal translocations as described in the text. Letters indicate amino acids and numbers their position within the protein.[14,27,33]*

ties when propagated in cultured fibroblasts in a retroviral vector.[17,30] Interestingly, in one of the spontaneous transformants a single amino acid change within the kinase domain, and in another a deletion within the SH2 domain, were sufficient to produce a transforming *fyn* protein with an enhanced tyrosine kinase activity.[30] These experiments indicated that a gene isolated by virtue of sequence similarity with the *src* gene has a transforming potential.

As in the case of v-*fps* and v-*yes*, the v-*abl* protein contains virally-derived *gag* sequences that are fused to the amino-terminal domain of the protein.[25,27] The Moloney murine leukemia virus *gag* sequences replace part of the c-*abl* sequence, including the SH3 domain. The SH3 domain appears to be critical for normal c-*abl* function. Analysis of a series of c-*abl* deletion mutants has revealed that constructs lacking the SH3 domain transform NIH3T3 cells and induce lymphomas in mice. In addition to the fusion of *gag*, one amino acid substitution and a frameshift mutation differentiate the v-*abl* oncogene from its proto-oncogene (Fig. 4). More detailed analysis of the viral and in vitro mutagenized c-*abl* genes indicated that the mechanism of activation of the c-*abl* gene involves both quantitative and qualitative alterations. Forms of activated *abl* oncogenes are also found in human leukemias as described below (Fig. 4).

Functional Studies

In the last decade, several experimental approaches have been elected to investigate the function of NRPTKs. One approach has been to correlate the pattern of NRPTK expression in normal tissues with physiological or developmental processes. Although these studies did not provide clear functional clues, they pointed to a number of valuable systems for studying NRPTKs in isolated cells and tissues (e.g., T cells for *lck*, platelets for *src*, cerebellum for *yes*).[9,32,35] Based on the expression results, NRPTKs have been divided into two groups, one that consists of kinases that are expressed ubiquitously, such as *src*, *yes*, *fyn*, and *fer*, and a second that consists of kinases expressed only in one type of cell, such as *lck*, *blk*, and *fer*T. p60^{src} is one of the best characterized tyrosine kinases. However, because of its ubiquitous expression (Table 1), the study of its function has been difficult. Numerous investigations have implicated p60^{c-src} in various cellular processes and the proposed functions usually correlated with the subcellular localization of the protein or the overall function of the analyzed tissue. The variable localization of p60$^{c\text{-}src}$ within cellular compartments[16] complicated the formulation of a unified model of src function and instead suggested pleiotropy. Recently the question of src function was addressed by Philippe Soriano and his colleagues at the Baylor College of Medicine, who employed homologous recombination to generate mice carrying a null mutation inactivating its src gene.[31] The phenotype of homozygous mice was surprising as the animals were abnormal in bone formation and developed osteopetrosis. Interestingly, histologic examination of the brain and platelets, where src is expressed at elevated levels, did not reveal any abnormalities. It is possible that other ubiquitous NRPTKs such as yes and fyn can complement the activity of the mutated src protein in these tissues. In keeping with this reasoning, it would be interesting to determine whether osteoclasts exclusively express c-src or other NRPTKs as well. Generating double or triple mutants with null mutations for various combinations of ubiquitous NRPTKs could produce phenotypes illuminating the roles of these enzymes in normal physiology.

Results of other studies involving activated NRPTKs such as bcr/abl (see below) and v-fps in transgenic animals have yielded some interesting results[27,37] (see Ch. 10). One of the important conclusions coming from the studies of the fps transgene was that the ectopic expression of this oncogene produced tumors only in certain organs, suggesting that only some of the pre-existing cell-specific transduction pathways could be used by the fps oncogene[37] to elicit transformation.

Another approach in studying the function of NRPTKs has been the isolation of substrate proteins of activated kinases, especially substrates of p60$^{v\text{-}src}$. Many cellular proteins that are phosphorylated on tyrosine have been identified in RSV transformed cells.[22] Among these are soluble glycolytic enzymes, and cytoskeletal and calcium-binding proteins.[22] However, most of these proteins are phosphorylated at low stoichiometry, making it difficult to demonstrate that they are direct substrates of p60$^{v\text{-}src}$. In addition, for the putative substrates, it has been difficult to establish whether the phosphorylation on tyrosine has any regulatory function. The most promising results have been obtained by Thomas Parsons' group at the University of Virginia.[22] They generated monoclonal antibodies against affinity purified proteins from RSV transformed cells using antiphosphotyrosine IgG as an affinity reagent. These monoclonal antibodies identified a number of potential substrates which are now being cloned from cDNA expression libraries.[15] The use of kinase positive and transformation defective mutants of RSV should allow the sorting of these proteins into adventitious and target substrates. Other questions have to be considered as well. What are the relevant substrates of cellular kinases? Are these substrates the same as those of viral kinases, differing only in that the stoichiometry of their modification by cellular enzymes is lower? Are substrates of the kinases encoded by partially transforming mutant subsets of the target substrates for fully transforming kinases, or are some novel proteins involved? The definition of target substrates has been the overriding problem for the field of NRPTKs since the first kinase, *src*, was discovered, and it is hoped that recent developments in this area will provide meaningful answers to the above questions.

An intense search for substrates revealed that p60^{c-src} itself is a substrate for a number of kinases, including an undetermined protein kinase that phosphorylates *src* at the carboxy-terminal regulatory tyrosine.[14,22] Two serine kinases, A and C, modify p60^{c-src} at the amino-terminal residues, and another kinase called p34^{cdc2}, or maturation promoting factor phosphorylates the *src* protein at serine and threonine residues as cells enter mitotic divisions.[14,22] These results strengthen our speculations that p60^{c-src} and other ubiquitously expressed NRPTKs may act as effectors of multiple kinases and could be involved in various signaling pathways.

Another functional approach has been to investigate the association of NRPTKs with cellular proteins. With the discovery of receptor protein tyrosine kinases came the concept of NRPTKs as "broken receptors." This notion implicitly suggests an indirect communication of NRPTKs with the outside environment. Since NRPTKs are membrane associated but do not have external domains to communicate with the extracellular milieu, they could serve as amplifiers in cellular signal-transduction networks. This hypothesis, proposed by Tony Hunter of the Salk Institute, was confirmed in the case of the *lck* protein, which was found to interact physically and functionally with receptor molecules.[22,35] p56^{lck} forms a stable complex with the T lymphocyte receptors CD4 and CD8, and is involved in signal coordination between these molecules and components of the T-cell antigen receptor complex during lymphocyte activation. Recently other NRPTKs have been found in complexes with receptors[6] (Fig. 5). In T cells, the *fyn* kinase is complexed with T-cell receptors. In normal fibroblasts, *src*, *yes*, and *fyn* are complexed with the ligand stimulated PDGF receptor.[6] Although the biological significance of this association is not clear and the stoichiometry of interaction is low, one could explain this complex quite simply. In order to transmit its growth signal in fibroblasts, the PDGF receptor kinase uses these three NRPTKs to phosphorylate substrates which it cannot access by itself. An immediate observation emerging from this data is that in different cell types, the same tyrosine kinase, namely *fyn*, can form complexes with different receptors, PDGFR and TCR. The observed high levels of *yes* protein in normal keratinocytes, cells which are devoid of PDGF receptors, further supports this. Possibly, the role of the *yes* proto-oncogene in keratinocytes is different from its role in fibroblasts. It also may form complexes with different receptors as well, as in the case of mouse mast cells, where p62^{c-yes} associates with the high affinity IgE receptor.[6] Crosslinking of the receptor results in the activation of *yes* kinase activity in these cells. Interestingly, crosslinking of the same receptor in rat basophils activates another kinase, p56^{lyn}, which also can be immunoprecipitated with antibodies directed to the receptor. To add to this complexity, the surface IgM receptor was reported to be associated in B cells with p56^{lyn} as well (Fig. 5).[36] Although this scenario gives the impression of random interactions, in all cases described here the association between receptors and kinases seems specific, is stable in the presence of nonionic detergents, and occurs only after receptor activation with the appropriate ligands or with crosslinking antibodies. With the exception of the *lck*/CD4 complex,[6] other interactions described here could be mediated by phosphotyrosine-SH2 binding. Site-directed mutagenesis of the conserved residues in the SH2 domains of NRPTKs could elucidate this possibility.

Recently, other proteins that are involved in signal-transduction pathways have been shown to associate with NRPTKs.[3,11,13,34] Phosphatidylinositol-3 (PI-3) kinase is an enzyme that catalyzes phosphorylation of phosphoinositides and is implicated in the mito-genic response to polypeptide growth factors through its association with the intracellular domain of ligand-associated growth factor receptors. This enzyme also associates with the protein product of the v-*src* oncogene but not with the proto-oncogene protein.[11,13] However, in platelets stimulated with thrombin, the physiological activa-tor of platelet aggregation, p60^{c-src}, and p59^{fyn} become physically associated with PI-3 kinase.[11] These results suggest that transforma-tion by activated NRPTKs can be interpreted as constitutive activation of pathways normally regulated by proto-oncogenic nonreceptor kinases in postmitotic, differentiated cells.[11]

GTPase activating protein, GAP, is a protein that stimulates GTPase activity of normal *ras* proteins without affecting oncogenic mutants.[3,23] GAP is predominantly a cytosolic protein. However, in

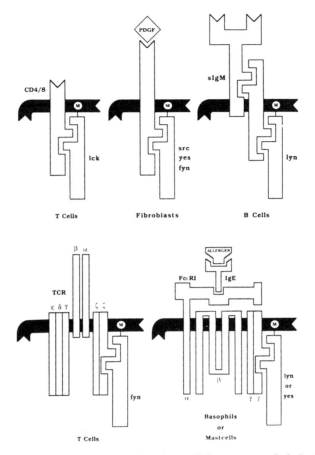

Figure 5. *Association of NRPTKs with various cellular receptors. Only in the case of lck and CD4/CD8 receptors have the domains of interaction been mapped and crucial amino acids involved in the association been identified. Cysteine residues are involved in the lck/CD4 complex. For other NRPTKs and receptors the interacting domains are not known. However, it seems likely that these interactions are mediated by SH2-phosphotyrosine binding and are therefore regulated by tyrosine phosphorylation. For simplicity, we assume here that the amino terminal regions of kinases are involved in the interaction with the receptor molecules. In many cases it is not known whether the interaction with the receptors is direct or through other components. This seems to be the case for the surface IgM receptor and the lyn kinase. Only three amino acids of the sIgM receptor are in the cytoplasm, therefore the direct association between these molecules is questionable. TCR, T cell receptor; PDGF, platelet-derived growth factor; sIgM, surface immunoglobulin M receptor; Fcepsilon RI, high-affinity immunoglobulin E (IgE) receptor.*[6,35,36]

response to stimulation of cells with PDGF, a substantial portion of the GAP population is found associated with membrane fractions. This membrane-bound form is enriched in phosphotyrosine residues. Recently, GAP protein was found to associate with the v-and c-*src* proteins.[3] This finding provides a biochemical link between the *src* kinase and GAP/*ras* signal-transduction pathways and could illuminate the possible crosstalk between NRPTKs and pathways of activated growth factor receptors. It would be interesting to determine whether the SH2 domains of *src* and GAP proteins are involved in these associations.

In sum, depending upon cell type, the same NRPTK can physically associate with different receptors, and the same receptors present in different types of cells can interact with different NRPTKs. In addition to receptors, other components of signal-transduction pathways interact with NRPTKs. With the exception of *lck*/CD4/8, interactions of NRPTKs with other molecules could be mediated by SH2-phosphotyrosine binding and therefore be regulated by tyrosine phosphorylation. It is apparent from these data that NRPTKs are involved in complex networks of transduction pathways.

NRPTKs and Human Cancers

Some oncogenes are known to be associated with different stages of human cancer, from initiation to progression and metastasis.[2] For NRPTKs, the best example is the chimeric *bcr-abl* oncogene expressed in human leukemias.[25,27] Virtually all patients with chronic myelogenous leukemia (CML) and approximately 15% with acute lymphoblastic leukemia (ALL) contain a chromosomal translocation, also called the Philadelphia chromosome, that juxtaposes *bcr* (breakpoint cluster region) and c-*abl* sequences that are normally found on chromosomes 22 and 9, respectively. The fusion proteins, p210[bcr-abl] (commonly associated with CML) and p190[bcr-abl] (commonly associated with ALL) (Fig. 4) have elevated tyrosine kinase activities. It is speculated that these chimeras confer growth advantages on target hematopoietic precursor cells. Although all the experimental evidence points to the *bcr-abl* oncogene as being associated with the initial or stable phase of the disease, the exact molecular events affected by this oncogene remain elusive.

It has been reported that overexpression, aberrant expression, and enzymatic activation of several members of the *src* family of proto-oncogenes occur in human colon carcinoma tissues and cell-lines as compared to normal mucosa adjacent to the tumor or to normal cells.[4] In one thorough study,[4] a high correlation was found between the relative increase in p60$^{c\text{-}src}$ activity and malignant potential in colonic polyps. Although the results of these studies provoke speculation and could be of potential diagnostic value, their contribution to the understanding of the molecular basis of the disease is unclear. A simple correlation cannot be considered as proof of causality. Activation of p60$^{c\text{-}src}$ and other NRPTKs is possibly one of many factors that contribute to malignant transformation of colonic epithelia.[4] It is important to emphasize here that proto-oncogenes have been selected or isolated by virtue of their involvement in important cellular processes controlling growth and differentiation. These genes encode proteins that participate in major cellular pathways that apparently cross each other and otherwise communicate. By affecting one of these gene products, we can apparently cause changes in the expression or behavior of others.

Recent Developments Concerning Nonreceptor Protein Tyrosine Kinases (NRPTKs)

Since the completion of this chapter, there have been several important developments further implicating the NRPTKs in various signaling pathways. For example, p56^{lck} was found to associate functionally with the interleukin-2 receptor (IL-2R).[13a] Contrary to the examples of CD4 and CD8, the IL-2R and p56^{lck} intermolecular association occurs at the kinase catalytic domain of p56^{lck}, not its amino-terminal region. In platelets, three kinases—*fyn*, *lyn*, and *yes*—were found in association with membrane glycoprotein IV (CD36).[13b] In B cells, in addition to *lyn*, two other kinases, *fyn* and *lck*, were shown to interact with the membrane immunoglobulin.[3a]

As expected, new NRPTKs were isolated. Among these new finds were *syk* and *csk* kinases which, because of their unique structures, constitute new subclasses of NRPTKs.[21b,33c] Csk was shown to be the sought-after kinase that phosphorylates the carboxy-terminal tyrosine of *src* and attenuates its enzymatic activity. There has been a change in the *src* family as well: *tkl* was shown to be the avian homolog of the mammalian *lck*.[4b] However, the number of *src* kinases did not change due to the recent characterization of *yrk* (*yes*-related kinase), which, like *fyn*, is highly expressed in neural and hematopoietic tissues.[33a]

Using the genetic complementation method and a mutant cell-line unresponsive to interferon, Laura Velazquez and colleagues have pointed to the *tyk2* kinase as a link between the interferon alpha/beta receptor and a cytoplasmic transcription factor, which mediates action of interferon-responsive genes.[35a] Seth Grant et al. from Eric Kandel's laboratory have shown that *fyn* kinase is involved in the long-term potentiation in the hippocampus and thus provided the first clue as to the function of *src* family NRPTKs expressed in neural tissues.[33b]

As to the SH2 and SH3 domains discussed in the chapter, the progress was quite impressive. By now more than 25 proteins have been identified that contain the SH2 domain. Some are protein-tyrosine phosphatases; others have features of transcription factors.[20a,21a] The *nck* protein was shown to transform mammalian fibroblasts in the absence of elevated phosphotyrosine levels.[4a] The crystal structure of the SH2 domain of v-*src* and the three-dimensional solution structure of the SH2 domain of *abl* were determined at high resolution, thus defining the amino acid residues involved in the specific recognition of phosphotyrosine.[21c,35b] A protein that interacts with the SH3 domain of *abl* was identified; it did not show any homology to a cytoskeletal protein. Instead, it contained stretches of sequence related to *bcr* and GAP-*rho*, implicating the SH3 domain, at least in *abl*, in signaling by *ras* related proteins.[4c]

Yes protein, normally found at elevated levels in keratinocytes, was found to be attenuated in human basal cell carcinomas.[17a]

The *src* receptor isolated by chemical crosslinking was shown to be an artifact. Rather than being the hypothesized protein anchor for myristoyl-*src*-protein, the 32 kd protein turned out to be a mitochondrial ADP/ATP carrier.[30a]

Concluding Remarks

In spite of intense research efforts from many laboratories, we are still left with major unanswered questions. The normal physiological functions of NRPTKs and the processes by which the activated forms of such kinases induce neoplastic transformation are unknown. It is anticipated that the number of answers to these questions will correlate with the number of tyrosine kinases described, and that complex networks of cellular pathways mediated by NRPTKs will be elucidated. Progress in the research on NRPTKs should have important ramifications for experimental biology and eventually for clinical medicine.

Acknowledgments: Special thanks are due to Rich Jove, Bruce Mayer, and Philippe Soriano for communicating unpublished results; and to Gerd Blobel, Melanie O'Brien, Hidesaburo Hanafusa, David Lehman, Bruce Mayer, and Jonathan Shannon for stimulating discussions and valuable comments on the manuscript. Space limitations make complete referencing impossible, and I ask the indulgence of my colleagues for numerous oversights. Supported by an NIH grant from the National Cancer Institute (CA45757) and by a Research Career Development Award (CA01605).

References

1. Anderson D, Koch AC, Grey L, et al. Binding of SH2 domains of phospholipase Cgamma1, GAP, and *src* to activated growth factor receptors. Science 1990; 250:979–982.
2. Bishop JM. The molecular genetics of cancer. Science 1987; 235:305–311.
3. Brott BK, Decker S, Shafer J, et al. GTPase-activating protein (GAP) interactions with viral and cellular *src* kinases. Proc Natl Acad Sci USA 1991; 88:755–759.
3a. Campbell MA, Sefton BM. Association between B-lymphocyte membrane immunoglobulin and multiple members of the *src* family of protein tyrosine kinases. Mol Cell Biol 1992; 12:2315-2321.
4. Cartwright CE, Meisler AI, Eckhart W. Activation of the pp60[c-src] protein kinase is an early event in colonic carcinogenesis. Proc Natl Acad Sci USA 1990; 87:558–562.
4a. Chou MM, Fajardo EJ, Hanafusa H. The SH2-and SH3-containing *nck* protein transforms mammalian fibroblasts in the absence of elevated phosphotyrosine levels. Mol Cell Biol 1992; 12:5834-5842.
4b. Chow LML, Ratcliffe MJH, Veillette A. *tkl* is the avian homolog of the mammalian *lck* tyrosine protein kinase gene. Mol Cell Biol 1992; 12:1226–1233.
4c. Cicchetti P, Mayer BJ, Theil G, et al. Identification of a protein that binds to the SH3 region of *abl* is similar to *bcr* and GAP-*rho*. Science 1992; 257:803–806.
5. Cooper JA. The *src*-family of protein-tyrosine kinases. In: Peptides and Protein Phosphorylation, Kemp B, ed. Boca Raton, CRC Press 1990; pp. 85–113.
6. Eiseman E, Bolen JB. *src*-related tyrosine protein kinases as signaling components in hematopoietic cells. Cancer Cells 1990; 2:303–310.
7. Fischman K, Edman JC, Shackleford GM, et al. A murine *fer* testis-specific transcript (*ferT*) encodes a truncated *fer* protein. Mol Cell Biol 1990; 10:146–153.
8. Frimbach-Kraft I, Byers M, Shows T, et al. *tyk2*, prototype of a novel class of non-receptor tyrosine kinase genes. Oncogene 1990; 5:1329–1336.
9. Golden A, Brugge JS. The *src* oncogene. In: The Oncogene Handbook, Reddy EP, Skalka AM, Curran T, eds. New York, Elsevier Science Publishers B.V. 1988; pp. 149–173.
10. Grandori C. Regulation of kinase activity. Nature (London) 1989; 338:467.

11. Gutkind SJ, Lacal PM, Robbins KC. Thrombin-dependent association of phosphatidylinositol-3 kinase with $p60^{c-src}$ and $p59^{fyn}$ in human platelets. Mol Cell Biol 1990; 10:3806–3809.

12. Hanafusa H. The *fps/fes* oncogene. In: The Oncogene Handbook, Reddy EP, Skalka AM, Curran T, eds. New York, Elsevier Science Publishers B.V. 1988; pp. 39–57.

13. Hanafusa H. Nonreceptor protein-tyrosine kinases and signal transduction. In: Proceedings of XXXIII Conference on Membrane Proteins: Targeting and Transduction. Houston, Texas 1989; pp. 237–245.

13a. Hatakeyama M, Kono T, Kobayashi N, et al. Interaction of the IL-2 receptor with *src*-family kinase $p56^{lck}$. Identification of novel intermolecular association. Science 1991; 252:1523–1528.

13b. Huang MM, Bolen JB, Barnwell JW, et al. Membrane glycoprotein IV (CD36) is physically associated with *fyn*, *lyn*, and *yes* protein-tyrosine kinases in human platelets. Proc Natl Acad Sci USA 1991; 88:7844–7848.

14. Jove R, Hanafusa H. Cell transformation by the viral *src* oncogene. Ann Rev Cell Biol 1987; 3:31–56.

15. Kanner SB, Reynolds AB, Vines RR, et al. Monoclonal antibodies to individual tyrosine-phosphorylated protein substrates of oncogene-encoded tyrosine kinases. Proc Natl Acad Sci USA 1990; 87:3328–3332.

16. Kaplan JM, Varmus HE, Bishop JM. The *src* protein contains multiple domains for specific attachment to membranes. Mol Cell Biol 1990; 10:1000–1009.

17. Kawakami T, Kawakami Y, Aaronson SA, et al. Acquisition of transforming properties by *fyn*, a normal *src*-related gene. Proc Natl Acad Sci USA 1988; 85:3870–3874.

17a. Krueger J, Zhao YH, Murphy D, et al. Differential expression of $p62^{c-yes}$ in normal, hyperplastic and neoplastic human epidermis. Oncogene 1991; 6:933–940.

18. Kruh GD, Perego R, Miki T, et al. The complete coding sequence of *arg* defines the Abelson subfamily of cytoplasmic tyrosine kinases. Proc Natl Acad Sci USA 1990; 87:5802–5806.

19. Lehmann JM, Riethmuller G, Johnson JP. Nck, a melanoma cDNA encoding a cytoplasmic protein consisting of the *src* homology units SH2 and SH3. Nucl Acid Res 1990; 18:1048.

20. Leto TL, Lomax KJ, Volpp BD, et al. Cloning of a 67-kd neutrophil oxidase factor with similarity to a noncatalytic region of $p60^{c-src}$. Science 1990; 248:727–730.

20a. Margolis B. Proteins with SH2 domains: Transducers in the tyrosine kinase signaling pathway. Cell Growth and Differentiation 1992; 3:73–80.

20b. Matsuda M, Mayer BJ, Fukui Y, et al. Binding of transforming protein, $P47^{gag-crk}$, to a broad range of phosphotyrosine-containing proteins. Science 1990; 248:1537-1539.

21. Mayer BJ, Hanafusa H. Association of the v-*crk* oncogene product with phosphotyrosine-containing proteins and protein kinase activity. Proc Natl Acad Sci USA 1990; 87:2638–2642.

21a. Mayer B, Baltimore D. Signaling through SH2 and SH3 domains. Trends in Cell Biol 1993; 3:8–13.

21b. Nada S, Okada M, MacAuley A, et al. Cloning of a complementary DNA for a protein-tyrosine kinase that specifically phosphorylates a negative regulatory site of p60$^{c\text{-}src}$. Nature 1991; 351:69–72.

21c. Overduin M, Rios CB, Mayer B, et al. Three-dimensional solution structure of the *src* homology domain of c-*abl*. Cell 1992; 70:697–704.

22. Parsons JT, Weber MJ. Genetics of *src*: Structure and functional organization of a protein tyrosine kinase. In: Current Topics in Microbiology and Immunology, Vogt PK, ed. Berlin, Springer-Verlag 1989; pp. 80–127.

23. Pawson T. Non-catalytic domains of cytoplasmic protein-tyrosine kinases: Regulatory elements in signal transduction. Oncogene 1988; 3:491–495.

24. Perlmutter RM, Marth JD, Ziegler SF, et al. Specialized protein tyrosine kinase proto-oncogenes in hematopoietic cells. Bioch Biophys Acta 1988; 948:245–262.

25. Ramakrishnan L, Rosenberg N. *abl* genes. Bioch Biophys Acta 1989; 989:209–224.

26. Resh MD, Ling H-P. Identification of a 32K plasma membrane protein that binds to the myristoylated amino-terminal sequence of p60$^{v\text{-}src}$. Nature (London) 1990; 346:84–86.

27. Risser R, Holland G. Structures and activities of *abl* oncogenes. In: Current Topics in Microbiology and Immunology, Vogt PK, ed. Berlin, Springer-Verlag, 1989; pp. 130–153.

28. Rodaway AR, Sternberg MJ, Bentley DL. Similarity in membrane proteins. Nature 1989; 342:624.

29. Sato K, Miki S, Tachibana H, et al. A synthetic peptide corresponding to residues 137 to 157 of p60$^{v\text{-}src}$ inhibits tyrosine-specific protein kinases. Bioch Biophys Res Comm 1990; 171:1152–1159.

30. Semba K, Kawai S, Matsuzawa, et al. Transformation of chicken embryo fibroblast cells by avian retroviruses containing the human *fyn* gene and its mutated genes. Mol Cell Biol 1990; 10:3095–3104.

30a. Sigal TC, Resh MD. The ADP/ATP carrier is the 32-kilodalton receptor for an NH$_2$-terminally myristylated *src* peptide but not for pp60*src* polypeptide. Mol Cell Biol 1993; 13:3084–3092.

31. Soriano P, Montgomery C, Geske R, et al. Targeted disruption of the c-*src* proto-oncogene leads to osteopetrosis in mice. Cell 1991; 64:693–702.

32. Sudol M. Expression of proto-oncogenes in neural tissues. Brain Res Rev 1988; 13:391–403.

33. Sudol M. Physiological functions of the *yes* proto-oncogene protein. Exp Med (Tokyo) 1990; 8:94–100.

33a. Sudol M, Greulich H, Newman L, et al. A novel *yes*-related kinase, *yrk*, is expressed in neural and hematopoietic tissues. Oncogene 1993; 8:823–831.

33b. Sudol M, Grant SGN, Maisonpierre PC. Proto-oncogenes and signaling processes in neural tissues. Neurochem International 1993; 4:369–384.

33c. Taniguchi T, Kobayashi T, Kondo J, et al. Molecular cloning of a porcine gene *syk* that encodes a 72-kDa protein-tyrosine kinase showing high susceptibility to proteolysis. J Biol Chem 1991; 266:15790–15796.

34. Ullrich A, Schlessiger J. Signal transduction by receptors with tyrosine kinase activity. Cell 1990; 61:203–212.

35. Veillette A, Bolen JB. src-related protein tyrosine kinases. In: Oncogenes, Benz C, Liu E, eds. Boston, Kluwer Academic Publishers 1989; pp. 121–142.

35a. Velazquez L, Fellous M, Stark GR, et al. A protein tyrosine kinase in the interferon alpha/beta signaling pathway. Cell 1992; 70:313–322.

35b. Waksman G, Kominos D, Robertson SC, et al. Crystal structure of the phosphotyrosine recognition domain SH2 of v-src complexed with tyrosine-phosphorylated peptides. Nature 1992; 358:646–653.

36. Yamanashi Y, Yamamoto T, Toyoshima K. Involvement of lck and lyn in signal-transduction pathways of lymphoid cells. Exp Med (Tokyo) 1990; 8:88–93.

37. Yee S-P, Mock D, Greer P, et al. Lymphoid and mesenchymal tumors in transgenic mice expressing the v-fps protein-tyrosine kinase. Mol Cell Biol 1989; 9:5491–5499.

Chapter 6

Growth Factor Receptors with Tyrosine Protein Kinase Activity

Diego Pulido

The response of a cell to an extracellular factor is mediated by the factor's binding to a cell surface receptor which then triggers a cascade of intracellular biochemical processes that result in a variety of biological responses of the cell. Growth factors and their receptors were recognized initially by their effects on cell proliferation; however, considerable evidence now exists implicating growth factors and their receptors on functional elements in developmental programs controlling different stages of embryogenesis and cell differentiation. Many of these growth factors mediate their actions by binding to activating cell surface receptors with intrinsic tyrosine protein kinase (TPK) activity. These receptors are the members of the TPK family of growth factor receptors.

Structural Characteristics and Classification

A large body of biochemical work in conjunction with the elucidation of the complete primary structures of several TPK receptors from cloned cDNAs suggest a common general architecture and membrane topology for this family of signal-transducing proteins. All possess an extracellular ligand-binding domain, designed to interact with a polypeptide ligand, a single hydrophobic transmembrane region, and a cytoplasmic domain that contains a tyrosine kinase

From *The Molecular Basis of Human Cancer:* edited by B. Neel, M.D., Ph.D., R. Kumar, Ph.D. © 1993, Futura Publishing Co. Inc., Mount Kisco, NY.

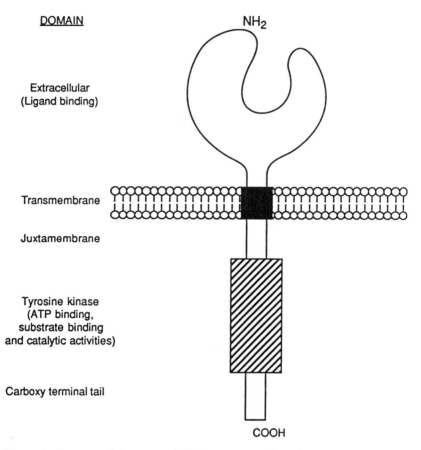

Figure 1. *Structure of the prototypic TPK receptors. Indicated are amino (NH₂) and carboxy (COOH) terminal ends of the receptor polypeptide chain.*

catalytic domain, capable of generating a signal that results in a pleiotropic cellular response (Fig. 1).[23,92,101] The combination of ligand-binding and catalytic functions within a single molecule represents a unique system for allosteric regulation within the context of the generation and control of biological signals.

Ligand-Binding Domain

Preceded by a typical cleavable signal sequence of 20 to 25 residues, a usually large extracellular domain of 500 to 800 amino acids comprises the ligand-binding domain of TPK receptors. As expected, most of the potential N-linked glycosylation sites are concentrated in this region, and biosynthetic studies have shown that these receptors are indeed glycosylated. Consistent with distinct ligand-binding specificities, this domain is characterized by a low degree of sequence conservation. Only those receptors which belong to a same subfamily share a significant level of homology between their sequences in the ligand-binding domain (e.g., *trk* and FGF family members).[2,15]

Transmembrane Domain

This domain comprises a short number of hydrophobic amino acids (22 to 30 residues) which are inserted in the plasma membrane. Besides its high degree of hydrophobicity and its conserved length, this region displays no primary structure conservation even between related TPK receptors.

Interestingly, the *neu* proto-oncogene (see below) can be activated as an oncogene when a single valine residue in its transmembrane region is substituted by a glutamic acid residue.[101] This mutation leads to the activation of the kinase catalytic domain which is essential for the transforming potential of the *neu* protein.[3] However, in spite of the involvement of the transmembrane domain in the activation of the *neu* proto-oncogene, different experiments suggest that the integrity of the transmembrane region is not directly involved in signal-transduction. Experiments with chimeric receptors consisting of combinations of the extracellular, intracellular, and transmembrane domains of several TPK receptors demonstrated that the origin of the transmembrane region had no influence on their signaling capacity.[44,92] Thus, the main function of the transmembrane domain would be to anchor the receptors in the plane of the plasma membrane, thereby connecting the extracellular environment with internal compartments of the cell.

The presence of a single transmembrane domain distinguishes the TPK receptors from another group of receptors that includes the β-adrenergic receptor,[100] rhodopsin,[60] and the muscarinic receptor,[66] each of which contain seven hydrophobic domains that are likely to span the membrane bilayer.

Juxtamembrane Domain

The transmembrane domain is separated from the cytoplasmic, catalytic TPK domain, by juxtamembrane sequences 40 to 60 amino acids in length. The primary structure of this domain has diverged among the different TPK receptors. However, remarkable conservation is apparent between the members of the same subclasses (see below). Different lines of evidence suggests that this domain is involved in modulation of receptor functions by heterologous stimuli, a process known as receptor transmodulation.[92] Activation of the protein kinase C (PKC) can trigger phosphorylation of the epidermal growth factor (EGF) receptor on serine and threonine residues. One of the PKC target residues is Thr654, which is located in the juxtamembrane region. This phosphorylation leads to the abolishment of the high affinity binding of the EGF to its receptors.[52,101] PKC may therefore act as a negative regulator of receptor activity.

On the other hand, the phorbol ester PMA is also able to modulate the binding affinity of EGF in a chimeric receptor composed of the extracellular domain of the EGF receptor fused to the transmembrane and cytoplasmic domains of the human *neu* receptor, suggesting that the binding affinity of the *neu* receptor for its as yet unidentified ligand is also controlled by PKC-mediated transmodulation.[45] Finally, the involvement of the juxtamembrane region in the regulation of the phosphorylation processes is emphasized by a mutant insulin receptor containing phenylalanine in place of a tyrosine located in the juxtamembrane region (Tyr960). This mutation abolishes the receptor's ability to phosphorylate a cellular substrate (p185) without affecting the ability of receptor autophosphorylation.[95]

Tyrosine Kinase Domain

The TPK catalytic domain is the most highly conserved region of all the TPK receptors (Fig. 1). This domain ranges from 250 to 300 amino acid residues. Fairly precise boundaries have been defined through an analysis of conserved sequences as well as by assay of truncated enzymes.[23] Hanks et al.[23] have defined 11 major conserved subdomains, separated by regions of lower conservation. The conserved subdomains must be important for catalytic function, either directly as components of the active site or indirectly by contributing to the formation of the active site through constraints imposed on secondary structure. The nonconserved regions, on the other hand, are likely to occur in loop structures, where folding allows the essential conserved regions to come together.

Among other highly conserved sequences, most of them of

unknown function, the tyrosine domain contains the denomined adenosine triphosphate-(ATP-) binding site. This site includes a conserved sequence, Gly-X-Gly-X-X-Gly-X (15 to 20) Lys, that function as part of the binding site for ATP. The lysine residue plays a key role in the binding activity, since replacement for other amino acids completely abolishes the kinase activity of these mutated TPK receptors, both in vitro and in living cells.[91,101]

Different types of receptor mutants have been generated to explore the role of the kinase domain. They include linker insertion mutants at the different positions of the catalytic regions, deletion mutants, and double mutants.[51] Those experiments indicated that while the kinase activity of those mutated receptors was dispensable for their expression and targeting to the cell surface, it was indispensable for signal-transduction and induction of cellular responses, including mitogenesis and transformation.[51]

Some of the members of the TPK receptor family contain the kinase domain divided into two halves, by insertion of up to 100 amino acid residues (subclass III, see below). The kinase insert of these receptors varies in length and shows minimal similarity. However, for a specific receptor, this insertion is conserved between different species, suggesting that it may play an important role in receptor function. Studies with deletion mutants in the kinase insert demonstrated that most of this insert region is dispensable for kinase activity and mitogenic signaling.[92] Finally, Kazlauskas and Cooper[35] reported that the platelet-derived growth factor (PDGF) receptor kinase insert contains an autophosphorylation site (tyr75l) that may regulate interaction with cellular substrates and effector proteins.

Carboxy-Terminal Tail

The carboxy-terminal tail corresponds to the most membrane distal, noncatalytic portion of the TPK receptors (Fig. 1). This region is among the most divergent (in sequence and length) between all known TPK receptors.[92,101] It is typically very hydrophilic and rich in small amino acids, which would impart a high degree of polypeptide chain flexibility. Several autophosphorylation sites have been mapped in this region of the EGF receptor, *neu* protein, and insulin receptor.[24,88]

Analysis of the EGF receptor mutants in which individual tyrosine autophosphorylation sites were replaced by phenylalamine residues, indicated that these mutant receptors had enzymatic and biological properties similar to wild type EGF receptor.[29] Several observations suggest that the carboxy-terminal tail of the EGF receptor may possess enough length and flexibility to interact with the substrate-binding sites of the protein tyrosine kinase region and thus modulate its capacity to interact with exogenous substrates[29,92] (see below).

TPK Receptor Subclasses

Comparison of the primary sequences of the different TPK receptors has led to the identification of both shared and unique structural subdomains which permit classification of the TPK receptor family in four distinct subclasses (Fig. 2 and Table 1).

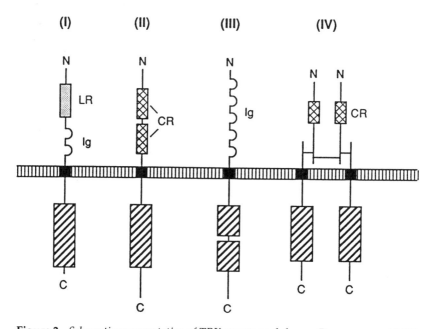

Figure 2. *Schematic representation of TPK receptor subclasses. Boxes represent LRG domain (LR) (shaded), cysteine-rich repeat (CR) region (cross-hatched), transmembrane region (black filled), and tyrosine kinase domain (hatched). Open circles indicated immunoglobulin-like (Ig) domains. N and C indicate amino and carboxy-terminal ends, respectively.*

TABLE 1.
Tyrosine Protein Kinase Receptors

Name	Protein (kDa)	Ligand	Subclass
Mammals			
EGF-R	170	EGF	II
IR	α: 135	Insulin	IV
	β: 95		
IGF1-R	α: 135	IGF-I	IV
	β: 90, 125		
PDGF-R (A)	180	PDGF	III
PDGF-R (B)	170	PDGF	III
CSF1-R	160	CSF1	III
FGF-Rs	125–135	aFGF, bFGF	III
kit	145	steel product	III
trk	140	NGF	I
trkB	145	BDNF	I
trkC	145	NT3	I
met	α: 50	HGF	IV
	β: 145		
neu (erbB2)	185	?	II
eph	130	?	II
elk	130	?	II
eck	130	?	II
ros	250	?	II
ret	135	?	II
sea	n.r.	?	II
Drosophila			
DER	*165*	?	*II*
DIR	*n.r.*	?	*II/IV*
sevenless	*280*	?	*IV*
torso	*n.r.*	?	*I*
DFGF-R	*n.r.*	?	*III*
Dtrk	*160*	*homophilic adh. molecule*	*III*

n.r.: not reported
?: unknown

1. Subclass I. This subclass is characterized by the presence in the extracellular region of three repeats of the denominated "leucine-rich glycoprotein" (LRG) domain, as well as two immunoglobulin-like (Ig-like) domains (Fig. 2).[2] Moreover, the kinase domain is not interrupted by insertions. Members of this subclass include the members of the mammalian *trk* family (*trk*, *trk*B, and *trk*C) of TPK receptors.[2,41,56]

2. Subclass II. This subclass is characterized by the presence of one or two cysteine-rich sequence repeat regions within the extracellular domain (Fig. 2). Two types of receptors can be grouped into this subclass depending on the conservation of cysteine residue, spacing and similarity of interspersed sequences in the cys-rich domain, as well as by the number of those domains. Members of the first group contain two cys-rich domains and include the EGF receptor[9] and the HER2/*neu*,[101] c-*erb*3, and x*mrk*[97] proteins (Fig. 2). Members of the second group contain only one cys-rich domain and include the *elk*, *eph*, and *eck* family of proteins,[49] and the *ros* protein[5] (Fig. 2).

3. Subclass III. Three distinct structural features define this subclass of TPK receptors: (i) the absence of cys-rich repeat clusters within their extracellular domains; (ii) the presence of several Ig-like domains in their ligand-binding domains; and (iii) the presence of hydrophilic insertion sequences in their catalytic kinase domains (Fig. 2). Members of this subclass are the PDGF-A and B receptors, the colony stimulating factor-1 (CSF-1) receptor, the steel receptor (c-*kit*), the members of the fibroblast (acidic and basic) growth factor (FGF) receptors (*flg*, *bek*, FGFR-3),[2,92,101] and the *flk* tyrosine kinase.[61]

4. Subclass IV. The members of this subclass of TPK receptors are thought to function as hetero-tetrameric structures, comprising two α and β subunits that are connected by disulfide bonds. The α subunits contribute to the formation of the ligand-binding domain, and are disulfide-linked to two β subunits which transverse the plasma membrane and carry the kinase domains (Fig. 2). In addition, one cys-rich repeated cluster is found in each of the α subunits. Members of this subclass are the insulin receptor and the insulin-like growth factor-I (IGF-I) receptors,[92,102] and recently it has been suggested that the *met* protein may also be included in this group of hetero-tetrameric receptors.[6,21,64]

TPK Receptors with Known Ligand

Epidermal Growth Factor Receptor

EGF is a well-characterized mitogen of 53 amino acids that stimulates the proliferation of numerous cell types in vitro and epithelial cells in vivo.[10] The EGF receptor is a 170 kDa single-chain transmembrane glycoprotein with intrinsic TPK activity.[9] The isolation, biochemical characterization, and cDNA cloning of the EGF receptor, has been greatly facilitated by the use of a cell-line (A431) derived from a human epidermoid carcinoma that overexpresses (20-to 50-fold) this receptor.[22]

The nucleotide sequence of the EGF receptor predicts an 1186 amino acid protein consisting of extra-and intracellular domains separated by a single hydrophobic transmembrane domain.[9] The extracellular EGF-binding domain is composed of 621 amino acids containing 12 putatives sites of N-linked glycosylation, as well as a high content of cysteine residue, that are clustered in two regions each 160 residues long. The 1:1 stoichiometry of EGF-binding predicts a single binding site in the extracellular domain of the EGF receptor.[9] The cytoplasmic domain of the EGF receptor contains the catalytic kinase domain. Analysis with mutant kinase-inactive EGF receptors indicated that the kinase-negative receptors are synthesized as cell-surface glycoproteins that bind EGF with expected affinity. However, although normal in its binding characteristics, these mutants were unable to stimulate calcium influx, inositol phosphate formation, Na$^+$/H$^+$ exchange, c-*fos* and c-*myc* expression, S6 ribosomal protein phosphorylation, and DNA synthesis and transformation.[92] After the kinase domain, the carboxy-terminal tail of the EGF receptor contains the major tyrosine sites of enzyme autophosphorylation, which occurs via an intermolecular mechanism.[89]

Until recently, no specific substrates for the EGF receptor were known, but two substrates have now been identified in living cells. They include the phosphatidylinositol-specific phospholipase C-γ (PLC-γ) and the GTPase activating protein (GAP), a protein which may be in the effector loop of the *ras* protein.[34,53,58,92] When cells are stimulated with either EGF or PDGF, these two proteins are rapidly phosphorylated on tyrosine residues both in vitro and in living cells. The tyrosine phosphorylation of PLC-γ has been found to be directly mediated by the EGF receptor and marks this enzyme as a direct substrate of the EGF receptor kinase.[53,61] These proteins are not only tyrosine phosphorylated, but also become physically associated with the EGF receptor in a stable noncovalent fashion. The association of GAP and PLC-γ mediated by regions known as SH2 and SH3 domains which are shared by GAP and PLC-γ.[42,53]

Insulin and Insulinlike Growth Factor I Receptors

Insulin was first discovered in the 1920s. Several physiological effects of insulin have been characterized, notably its ability to accelerate the transport of glucose into many types of cells.[48] The first step in the mechanism of action of insulin is the binding of the hormone to its cell surface receptor. The insulin receptor is a complex integral membrane glycoprotein present in extremely low abundance. Nucleotide sequence of the cDNA in combination with biochemical analysis indicated that the insulin receptor is a hetero-tetrameric structure composed of two α subunits of apparent molecular weight 120.000 and two β subunits of apparent molecular weight 90.000, held together by disulfide bridges.[48] The α and β subunits are cleavage products of a receptor precursor that is the product of a single gene.[47] Fifteen consensus sequences for N-linked glycosylation are distributed evenly over the 719-residue long α-subunit region, which is also characterized by a cluster of 37 cysteine residues between residues 155 and 312. The 620 amino acid-long β subunit contains only nine cysteine residues and can be divided in three domains: (i) an amino terminal 194 residue long domain contains four potential N-linked glycosylation sites and four cysteine residues; (ii) an adjacent stretch of 23 highly hydrophobic amino acids that represent the transmembrane domain; and (iii) a 403-residue long cytoplasmic domain containing the catalytic TPK domain. The insulin receptor kinase is activated by autophosphorylation, suggesting some functional significance for the sites of tyrosine phosphorylation of the β subunit.[48,91]

Blocking of signal-transduction has been observed when the insulin receptor kinase activity is abrogated by a mutation blocking the ability of the receptor to bind ATP.[47,88] This mutation not only results in the loss of insulin-stimulated tyrosine phosphorylation, but in reduced sensitivity to insulin-stimulated deoxyglucose uptake, activation by ribosomal protein S6 kinase, endogenous substrate phosphorylation, glycogen synthesis, and thymidine incorporation into DNA.[48,91] Riedel et al. (1986)[72] also demonstrated that the insulin receptor extracellular domain can efficiently couple hormone-binding to EGF receptor kinase activation by expressing a chimeric construct of the two receptor domains. However, it is not clear whether the insulin receptor/EGF receptor chimera could generate a biological response.[68]

IGF-I, a 70 amino acid polypeptide with extensive structural homology to insulin (49%) and IGF-II (61%), exerts its biological effects by binding to a specific receptor on the surface of target cells.[16] The IGF-I receptor is similar but distinct from the insulin receptor. Like the insulin receptor, the IGF-I receptor is a membrane glycoprotein of Mr 300,000 to 350,000 consisting of two α subunits (Mr~90.000) that are connected by disulfide bonds to form the functional β-α-α-β hetero-tetrameric receptor complex (Fig. 2).[70] In analogy with the insulin receptor, IGF-I receptor α and β subunits are encoded within a single 180.000 molecular weight receptor precursor that is glycosylated, dimerized, and proteolytically processed to yield the mature $\alpha_2\beta_2$ form of the receptor. Upon binding to the extracellular domain, IGF-I stimulates an intracellular, TPK activity which leads to β subunit autophosphorylation and phosphorylation of cytoplasmic components of an IGF-I specific signal transfer cascade.[91,92]

Although closely related to the insulin receptor, the IGF-I receptor gene maps to a distinct chromosome locus. The IGF-I receptor gene maps to 15g25→26, whereas the insulin receptor gene is localized on the chromosome 19 band p.13.3→13.2.[90]

Platelet-derived Growth Factor Receptors

PDGF is recognized as the major mitogen in serum for connective tissue and glial cells.[73] It has pleiotropic effects on cells and not only stimulates growth, but also elicits a mobility response including actin reorganization, membrane raffling, and chemotaxis.[25] PDGF was originally discovered as a product released by platelets. However, the finding that PDGF is produced by a number of normal and transformed cells indicated that PDGF may have an important role in growth, development, and tumorgenesis. Structurally, PDGF is a 30 kDa dimer of two disulphide-bonded polypeptide chains, denominated A and B. Homodimers (AA and BB) as well as the heterodimer (AB) have been identified and purified from natural sources and appear to participate in a number of processes in vivo, although the specific biological roles of the AB, AA, and BB dimeric forms have not been clarified.[25,96]

The PDGF receptor was first identified as a 180 to 190 kDa membrane glycoprotein by the covalent crosslinking of PDGF (AB heterodimeric form) to intact cells or to membrane preparations. Analysis of the binding of the various PDGF isoforms to cultured fibroblasts revealed two distinct PDGF receptor types, denoted type A and type B. The A-type receptor binds all three isoforms of PDGF, whereas the B-type receptor binds the BB isoform with high affinity, and AB with lower affinity, but does not appear to bind the AA isoform.[96]

The PDGF B-type receptor is a transmembrane glycoprotein of about 180 kDa with TPK activity. The deduced amino acid sequence of cDNA clones of this receptor reveals that it consists of 1074 amino acid residues after removal of the signal sequence, and that it has an extracellular ligand-binding domain, a single transmembrane, and a cytoplasmic region containing a TPK catalytic domain. The extracellular domain contains 11 potential acceptor sites for N-linked glycosylation and 10 cysteine residues regularly spaced which are organized in five Ig-like domains (Figs. 2, 3). The tyrosine kinase of the cytoplasmic domain of the PDGF B-type receptor contains an insert sequence of 104 amino acids which does not have homology to other kinases.[25,96] By deletion of the insert sequence of the B-type receptor, a receptor mutant was obtained that retained kinase activity and the ability to mediate a stimulatory effect on phosphatidylinositol turnover, but had lost its ability to transduce a mitogenic signal, suggesting that the insert sequence has an important role in signal-transduction.[96] Also, Kazlauskas and Cooper[35] have shown that the kinase insert of the PDGF B-type receptor contains a tyrosine residue that becomes phosphorylated and is able to regulate the interaction between the receptor and cellular substrates. The carboxy-terminal tail of this receptor is distinctive in sequence but has no easily predictable structure, and its function is unknown.[25,96]

The PDGF A-type receptor has been also characterized. It is synthesized as a 140 kDa precursor that matures to a 170 kDa product.[96] Purification and peptide mapping after partial proteolysis suggested that the A-and B-type PDGF receptors are structurally related. Analysis of PDGF A-type receptor cDNA clones revealed that this receptor is organized in a similar fashion to the B-type receptor,

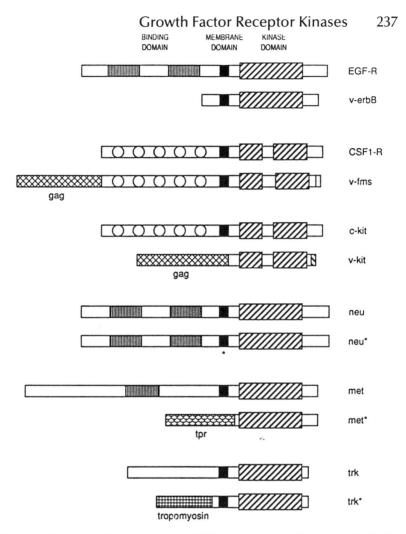

Figure 3. *Structure of some oncogenic TPK receptors and their normal cellular products. The protein kinase catalytic domain is indicated by a hatched box (thick box). This catalytic domain is interrupted in the case of the CSF receptor and c-*kit *protein. Where there are sequence differences between the cellular PTK receptor and its oncogenic derivative, these are indicated by a box with a different fill. An asterisk under the box indicates single amino acid differences that are essential for oncogenic activity. Cysteine-rich regions in the extracellular ligand-binding domains are indicated as vertically shaded bars, and the transmembrane domains are black filled boxes. Open circles indicate immunoglobulin-like domains. The identities of the new amino-termini for oncogenic derivatives are given under the relevant boxes. The oncogenic derivatives of* neu, met, *and* trk *are indicated with an asterisk.*

having five Ig-like domains and a split tyrosine kinase domain. The amino acid sequence similarity was found to be as high as 80% in the kinase domain and about 30% in the extracellular domain.[96]

How does the PDGF receptor transduce signals across the membrane? Several models have been proposed.[96] A possible mechanism of activation of the B-type PDGF receptor was suggested by the finding that the binding of the PDGF-BB to purify B-type receptor induced dimerization of the receptor in a concentration-dependent manner. This finding in conjunction with the dimeric structure of the ligand, indicates that each PDGF-BB molecule binds two receptor molecules. Dimerization was found to be closely associated with activation of the receptor kinase. It is thus likely that the ligand-induced dimerization allows an interaction between the tyrosine kinase domains of the cytoplasmic parts of the two receptors, leading to their activation.[25,92] This mechanism could be similar to that previously proposed for activation of the EGF receptor.[92]

The binding of the PDGF to its receptor rapidly stimulates a group of responses that occur in minutes. These include activation of the kinase domain, hydrolysis of phosphatidylinositol, alteration in cellular pH, increase in cytosolic calcium levels, dramatic changes in the cytoskeleton, elevation of cellular cyclic adenosine monophosphate, and internalization and degradation (downregulation) of the receptor.[96] In order to understand how these events occur and how these responses are interrelated, PDGF B-type receptors carrying different mutations in the transmembrane and tyrosine kinase domain, including the kinase insert, have been constructed and analyzed for their responses to PDGF.[25,96] Those experiments indicated that the transmembrane region of the PDGF receptor serves a specific role other than simply providing a membrane anchor for the molecule. When transmembrane regions of other receptors are substituted for the PDGF B-type receptor transmembrane sequences, the chimeric receptor fails to transduce signals.[25,96]

The tyrosine kinase activity of the receptor is important for most of the cellular responses to PDGF, including mitogenesis. However, tyrosine kinase activity is not required for ligand-induced receptor downregulation. The kinase insert domain is important for the specific mitogenic action of PDGF, and also may play a role in determining the substrate specificity of the receptor.[25,96] Finally, when the PDGF B-type receptor binds its ligand, the receptor physically associates with a phosphatidylinositol kinase that may be involved in the production of novel inositol phosphate second messengers.[25,35,96]

Colony-stimulating Factor-1 Receptor

The CSF-1, also called macrophage CSF, is a lineage-specific hematopoietin that stimulates proliferation and supports differentiation and survival of cells of the mononuclear phagocyte series.[84] The purified growth factor is a 70 to 90 kDa homodimeric glycoprotein synthesized primarily by fibroblasts, but its synthesis can be induced in endothelial cells and in monocytes and macrophages in response to other cytokines.[78,79] The CSF-1 exerts its pleiotropic effects by binding to a single class of high-affinity receptors expressed predominantly on mature mononuclear phagocytes and their immature bone marrow precursors.[78] The CSF-1 receptor is encoded by the c-*fms* proto-oncogene (see also below) and is a member of the family of growth factor receptors that exhibit ligand-induced tyrosine-specific protein kinase activity.[78]

The human CSF-1 receptor is an integral transmembrane glycoprotein of 972 amino acids. Including the signal peptide, it consists of a 512 amino acid extracellular-binding domain, a hydrophobic 25 amino acid transmembrane region, and a 435 amino acid intracellular domain that includes all the sequences necessary for tyrosine kinase activity.[79] Similar structures are predicted for the mouse and feline CSF-1 receptors. These show 75% and 84% overall homology to human CSF-1 receptor. The extracellular domain of the CSF-1 receptor is predicted to include five disulfide bonded loops, each representing five Ig-like domains. This extracellular domain is heavily glycosylated and contains 11 sites of N-linked glycosylation. The intracellular portion of the CSF-1 receptor includes the catalytic kinase domain. The kinase domain contains an insert sequence of 72 amino acids that are conserved among the human, mouse, and feline CSF-1 receptors, but are unrelated to analogous inserts of different lengths found in other TPK receptors, suggesting that they may function in specific substrate recognition.[79] Based on the analysis of conserved structural motifs as well as its genomic organization, the CSF-1 receptor is most closely related to the A and B isoforms of PDGF-receptor, the c-*kit* proto-oncogene product, and to the members of the fibroblast growth factor (FGF) family.

In absence of the ligand, the mature cell surface form of CSF-1 receptor is relatively stable (3 to 4 hours). However, ligand-receptor complexes are rapidly internalized, targeted to lysosome, and degraded ($\backsim$15 min), a process known as downregulation.[78] CSF-1-binding also upregulates TPK activity. The nature of this activation is poorly understood, but it has been suggested that, as in other systems, the receptors form dimers or higher order aggregates in response to ligand, thereby activating the receptor kinase through an intermolecular mechanism.[78,79] Three major sites of tyrosine phosphorylation within the kinase domain have been identified, two of them located within the kinase insert.[78]

In contrast to the ligand-induced phosphorylation of the EGF receptor which occurs at the multiple sites clustered within the receptor carboxy-terminal tail, the CSF-1 receptor carboxy-terminus contains only a single tyrosine residue which has not been shown to be phosphorylated either in the absence or presence of ligand.[78] Activation of CSF-1 receptor kinase activity leads to different and rapid effects including: phosphorylation of heterologous protein substrates, membrane ruffling and vacuolization, immediate cytoplasmic alkalinization through Na^+/H^+ exchange, increased hexose transport, and induction of a family of "immediate early response" genes, including the proto-oncogene c-*fos*.[78,79]

The human CSF-1 receptor gene (c-*fms* proto-oncogene) maps on chromosome 5 at band 5q33.3, close to other growth factor and receptor genes that play important roles in hematopoiesis.[78]

Fibroblast Growth Factor Receptor Family

The FGF family consists of seven related heparin-binding proteins, which include acidic (aFGF) and basic (bFGF) FGFs, the *int*-2 gene product, the *hst* gene product (Kaposi sarcoma-FGF), FGF-5, FGF-6, and the keratinocyte growth factor (KGF).[7,15,46] The members of the FGF family share 30% to 55% amino acid sequence identity, similar gene structure, and the ability to transform cultured cells when overexpressed in transfected cells. The response of cells to FGFs is mediated by binding and activation of specific cell surface receptors possessing intrinsic tyrosine kinase activity.[7,15,46] The existence of several related FGFs has raised the question as to whether all members of this family exert their effects through a common cell surface receptor or, alternatively, each factor might bind to a different receptor. Both aFGF and bFGF can be crosslinked to two receptor species of approximately 145 and 125 kDa. Competition studies suggest that the 145-kDa receptor species has a higher affinity for bFGF and the 125-kDa receptor species has a higher affinity for aFGF.[31]

Several genes coding for polypeptides with the ability to bind acidic and basic FGFs have been cloned from different species (human, mouse, and chicken) in different laboratories.[15,31,46] Two of them correspond to different genes denominated *flg* and *bek*.[15,76] Human *flg* and *bek* are similar yet distinct gene products, with structural features shared by the PDGF/CSF-1/c-*kit* family of receptor linked tyrosine kinases. Their coding sequences consist of a hydrophobic signal peptide sequence of 21 amino acids, an extracellular binding-domain of 355 (*flg*) and 356 (*bek*) amino acids, a transmembrane domain of 21 amino acids, and an intracellular region of 425 (*flg*) and 423 (*bek*) amino acids. The extracellular domains contain three Ig-like domains of similar size and location. The cytoplasmic domains of *flg* and *bek* consist of long juxtamembrane regions followed by conserved catalytic kinase domains which are split by 14 amino acid insertions. The kinase domains are followed by divergent carboxy-terminal tails. The overall identity between *flg* and *bek* is 71%, with the region of highest identity (88%) being the kinase domain. Reid et al.[71] and Johnson et al. (1990)[31] reported the isolation of cDNAs coding for truncated forms of *flg* and *bek* receptors. These truncated receptors include variants of *flg* and *bek* lacking the first Ig-like domain, a truncated version of *bek* encoding only a signal sequence, a single Ig-like domain and a stop codon, and a variant of *flg* encoding a signal sequence and two Ig-like domains. The last two clones may represent secreted forms of these receptors.[31,71]

Covalent crosslinking experiments with aFGFs or bFGFs to cells expressing either *flg* or *bek* indicate that both receptor proteins interact specifically with these factors. It is therefore concluded that *flg* and *bek* represent high affinity receptors for aFGF as well as bFGF.[15] Recently, Keegan et al.[36] reported the isolation of a human gene (FGFR-3) highly homologous to the previously described FGF receptors. They demonstrate that this gene encodes a biologically active FGF receptor by showing that human aFGF and bFGF activate this receptor as measured by Ca^{2+} efflux assays. The existence of several related FGFs that exhibit different biological effects suggests the existence of other FGF receptors.

White Spotting (W)/c-*kit* Protein

Mutations at the *white* spotting (W) locus in the mouse have pleiotropic effects on embryonic development and hematopoiesis. The characteristic phenotype of mutants at this locus, which include white coat color, sterility, and anemia, can be attributed to the failure of stem cell populations to migrate and/or proliferate effectively during development.[17,18] A major advance in the elucidation of the mechanism by which W mutations exert their pleiotropic effects came from the discovery that the c-*kit* proto-oncogene is the product of the W locus.[13,18]

The proto-oncogene c-*kit* is the cellular homolog of v-*kit*, the oncogene of an acute transforming feline retrovirus, which was isolated from a feline leukemia virus-associated fibrosarcoma (see below). The characterization of cDNAs of the proto-oncogene c-*kit* of mouse and human origin predicted that c-*kit* encodes a transmembrane kinase protein similar to PDGF and CSF-1 receptors.[99] The human c-*kit* gene encodes a 23 amino acid signal sequence, that precedes an amino terminal extracellular ligand-binding domain of 497 amino acid residues containing nine potential N-linked glycosylation sites. A transmembrane domain of 23 residues connects the extracellular domain with a cytoplasmic region of 933 amino acid residues containing the catalytic TPK domain. The c-*kit* protein shows a subdomain organization that is highly homologous to its closest relatives, the PDGF and CSF-1 receptors. Like these receptors, the extracellular domain of c-*kit* contains five Ig-like domains of similar size and location to those present in PDGF and CSF-1 receptors. In addition, the c-*kit* cytoplasmic kinase domain is bisected by a 77 amino acid insertion that, like the insertions present in the kinase domains of the PDGF and CSF-1 receptors, is composed of highly hydrophilic amino acid residues.[99] Molecular analysis of several of the W alleles indicated that alleles exhibiting severe phenotypes are due to large deletions within the c-*kit* gene, while more subtle phenotypes result from mutation within the kinase domain of the receptor.[98]

After the molecular identification of the W locus, a candidate for the c-*kit* ligand has been identified. Using quite different approaches, three groups have characterized a new hematopoietic growth factor with a broad range of biological activities that can bind to the c-*kit* receptor.[98] Different names have been assigned to this new molecule, including: stem cell factor (SCF), mast cell growth factor (MGF), *kit* ligand (KL) and *steel* factor (SLF). Physical characterization of this new growth factor shows that it is heavily glycosylated, and probably exists as a dimer. Finally, the *steel* locus has been identified as the gene coding for the c-*kit* ligand and, as expected, mutations in the mouse *steel* and W locus, have similar phenotype effects[98] (see below).

Hepatocyte Growth Factor Receptor/*met* Proto-oncogene

The *met* proto-oncogene codes for a protein of 1408 amino acids with features characteristic of the growth factor receptor TPK family. The predicted primary structure includes a putative 24 amino acid signal peptide and a candidate, hydrophobic, membrane-spanning segment of 23 amino acids which define an extracellular domain of 926 amino acids (ligand-binding domain), and a 435 amino acid cytoplasmic TPK catalytic domain.[64] The *met* protein is proteolytically processed to yield two subunits of 50 kDa (α) and 145 kDa (β) connected by disulfide bridges. In the fully processed *met* product, the α-subunit is extracellular, and the β-subunit has extracellular, transmembrane, and tyrosine kinase domains as well as sites for tyrosine phosphorylation.[20]

Recent data indicated that the *met* proto-oncogene product is the cell surface receptor for the hepatocyte growth factor (HGF).[6] HGF is a plasminogen-like protein thought to be a humoral mediator of liver regeneration.[59,74] HGF induces rapid tyrosine phosphorylation of proteins in intact target cells. One of these proteins, a 145 kDa tyrosylphosphoprotein was identified by immunoblot analysis as the β-subunit of the c-*met* proto-oncogene product. Covalent crosslinking of ^{125}I-labeled ligand to cellular proteins of appropriate size that were recognized by antibodies to c-*met* directly established the c-*met* proto-oncogene product as the cell surface receptor for HGF.[6]

The *trk* Family of Neurotrophin Receptors

The *trk* family of cell surface receptors comprise three mammalian genes denominated *trk*, *trk*B, and *trk*C, and a *Drosophila* gene denominated D*trk*, whose expression appears to be confined within defined structures of the mammalian and *Drosophila* nervous system.[2,37,39,43,69] They code for related TPKs, gp140[0trk], gp145[5trkB], gp14[trkC], and gp160[Dtrk], respectively. These observations indicated that the *trk* subfamily of receptors has evolved from a single ancestral gene that existed before the phylogenetic split between arthropods and chordates 800 million years ago (Fig. 4).[69]

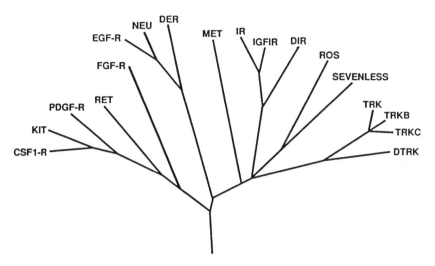

Figure 4. *Deduced phylogeny of TPK receptors according to their kinase catalytic domains. The phylogenetic tree is that proposed by Hanks et al. (1988)[23] with some additions.*

trk

The human *trk* locus was first identified by virtue of a somatic rearrangement that led to its malignant activation in a colon carcinoma patient.[2,55] This rearrangement generated a highly transforming gene that contained a subset of *trk* gene sequences fused to a nonmuscle tropomyosin gene (see below). Isolation and molecular characterization of this chimeric oncogene provided the necessary probes to identify and subsequently isolate cDNA clones encoding its normal allele, the *trk* proto-oncogene.[2,56]

The human *trk* proto-oncogene codes for a protein of 790 amino acid residues that has features characteristic of TPK receptors. They include a 32 amino acid signal peptide, a putative ligand-binding domain of 375 amino acid residues, rich in consensus N-linked glycosylation sites, a single transmembrane domain, a catalytic region of 266 amino acid residues highly related to that of known TPK, and a short carboxy-terminal tail of 15 amino acid residues.[56] Analysis of the deduced amino acid sequence of the *trk* proto-oncogene product indicates that this gene does not belong to any of the well characterized subfamilies of TPK receptors,[23] instead, in conjuntion with the related locus *trk*B and *trk*C, defines a new subclass of TPK receptors.

Biochemical analysis of NIH3T3 cells expressing *trk* proto-oncogene cDNA clones indicates that the primary translational product of this gene is a 110 kDa glycoprotein with a polypeptide backbone of 80 kDa. This 110 kDa glycoprotein becomes further glycosylated to yield a 140 kDa product. Both 110 and 140 kDa proteins exhibit in vitro kinase activity specific for tyrosine residues. Biochemical analysis indicated that only the 140 kDa glycoprotein is located on the cell surface, suggesting that this protein is the mature form of the human *trk* receptor.[2,56]

*trk*B

The mammalian *trk*B locus was identified by screening brain cDNA libraries using either a human *trk* proto-oncogene probe or a probe corresponding to a highly conserved region of kinase receptors.[2,41] Mouse *trk*B appears to be a large and complex locus with an intricate transcription pattern of at least six different transcripts, ranging in size from 2.0 kb to 9.0 kb. One of the products of the *trk*B gene is a 145 kDa glycoprotein (gp145[*trk*B]) with TPK activity.[41] gp145[*trk*B] is synthesized from two transcripts (9.0 kb and 5.5 kb in mouse and 9.0 kb and 4.8 kb in rat) likely to differ in their polyadenylation signals.[2,41] The deduced amino acid sequence of this glycoprotein indicates a polypeptidic backbone of 821 amino acid residues which exhibits all the characteristic features of tyrosine kinase cell surface receptors.[2,41] Comparison of the amino acid sequence of the *trk* and *trk*B proteins indicates a high degree of homology in both their extracellular domains (57% homology, 38% identity) and kinase catalytic regions (88% homology, 73% identity). In addition, both molecules exhibit a short carboxy-terminal tail (15 amino acids) characteristic of this gene family.[2,41] The mouse *trk*B locus also codes for a second class of molecules that lack a kinase catalytic domain.[37] Nucleotide sequence analysis of rat *trk*B cDNA clones suggest the existence of at least two noncatalytic *trk*B proteins which differ in their unique carboxy-termini.[2,37]

*trk*C

Recent studies have revealed the existence of *trk*C, a third member of the mammalian *trk* gene family of receptors.[2,43] Nucleotide sequence analysis of *trk*C cDNA clones have revealed a 825 amino acid

putative cell surface receptor with all the structural features characteristic of TPK receptors. The putative extracellular sequence of the *trk*C
gene product is 54% homologous (35% identical) to that of the *trk*
proto-oncogene and 52% homologous (39% identical) to the corresponding domain of the *trk*B protein. Much higher homologies were
observed between the catalytic TPK domains of these three genes
(86% homology with the human *trk* gene and 90% homology with the
mouse *trk*B). Thus, it appears that the *trk*C gene is equally related to
trk and *trk*B.[2,43]

Dtrk

Drosophila also contains a *trk*-related locus denominated D*trk*.
Molecular analysis of cDNA clones of the D*trk* locus revealed a
putative gene product of 1033 amino acid residues with structural
features characteristic of tyrosine kinase cell surface receptors.[2,69] The
overall homology between D*trk* and mammalian *trk* and *trk*-related
genes is 42% to 48% in the extracellular domain and 60% to 63% in the
catalytic kinase domain. The D*trk* protein exhibits some distinct
structural features including a stretch of 60 amino acid residues in the
cytoplasmic kinase region which creates a second putative ATP-
binding site. Moreover, the extracellular domain contains structural
motifs characteristic of the Ig superfamily of proteins, in particular
those found in neural adhesion molecules. In situ hybridization and
immunocytochemistry studies indicate that D*trk* is expressed during
Drosophila embryogenesis in several neurogenic areas of peripheral
and central nervous system (CNS).[69]

The product of the D*trk* gene is a 160 kDa glycoprotein (gp160^{Dtrk})
with TPK activity. When expressed in nonadhesive S2 *Drosophila* cells,
D*trk* protein-mediated adhesion of S2 cells in a homophilic, Ca^{2+}
independent manner. This adhesion process specifically activated the
TPK activity of D*trk* protein. These findings suggest that D*trk* encodes
a novel class of neural cell adhesion molecules with TPK activity.[69]

Mammalian *trk* Proteins: Functional Receptors for Neurotrophic Factors

Recent studies have revealed that these TPKs are receptors for a
family of neurotrophic factors which include nerve growth factor

(NGF), brain-derived neurotrophic factor (BDNF), and neurotrophin-3 (NT-3).[26,33,38,40,43,81,83,94]

The gp140[trk] kinase serves as a primary receptor for NGF,[12,26,32,33,38] a factor capable of inducing growth and differentiation of sensory and sympathetic neurons in the peripheral nervous system (PNS), as well as of certain cholinergic neurons of the forebrain.[26,38,67]

The gp145[trkB] kinase responds preferentially to BDNF,[40,81,83] a factor that plays a central role in the growth and survival of a wide spectrum of CNS neurons including cholinergic and dopaminergic neurons, as well as in certain sensory neurons of the PNS.[40,81,83] In addition, gp140[trk] and gp145[trkB] receptors can bind NT-3.[12,40,81,83]

The product of the trkC gene has been identified as a functional receptor for NT-3.[43] However, gp145[trkC] does not bind the highly related neurotrophic factors NGF or BDNF. In proliferating cells, the interaction between gp145[trkC] and NT-3 elicits a more efficient biological response than when NT-3 binds to its other receptors gp140[trk] and gp145[trkB] indicating that gp145[trkC] may play an important role in mediating the neurotrophic effects of NT-3.

The trk TPKs mediate signal-transduction initiated by these neurotrophic factors. Addition of either NGF, BDNF, and NT-3 to quiescent NIH3T3 cells ectopically expressing each of the trk family of receptors leads to their rapid phosphorylation in tyrosine residues.[32,38,40,43,81,83] Moreover, they induce c-fos expression and drive resting cells to enter the S-phase.[12,38,40] In addition, constitutive expression of any of these trk-related receptors with their respective cognate ligands results in cellular transformation.[12,40,43] These responses are not limited to proliferative cells, since BDNF and NT-3 can induce the neuronal differentiation of PC12 cells ectopically expressing gp145[trkB] receptors.[83]

TPK-Like Receptors with Unknown Ligand

The characterization of oncogenes from retroviruses and tumors in parallel with other genetic approaches, such as screening cDNA libraries with tyrosine kinase-derived oligonucleotides or antiphosphotyrosine antibodies has led to the discovery of new proteins. By comparing their primary amino acid sequences with the previously identified TPK receptors, they can be classified as putative TPK receptor proteins. In these proteins, the putative ligand(s) remain to be characterized, and thus their biological functions are unknown.

eph, elk, eck Receptor Family

The members of this family of putative growth factor receptors were isolated by different approaches. The *eph* gene was initially isolated from a human genomic library by cross-hybridization with a probe consisting of the kinase domain of the viral oncogene v-*fps*.[27] The *eph* gene is over-expressed in several human carcinomas, suggesting that this gene may be involved in the neoplastic process of some tumors.[27]

The *elk* gene was isolated from an expression library using antiphosphotyrosine antibodies as probes.[47] Among rat tissues, *elk* expression appears restricted to brain and testes, with the brain having higher levels of both *elk* RNA and protein.[47]

The *eck* gene was recently isolated by screening a human cell-line (HeLa) cDNA library with degenerate oligonucleotides that were designed to hybridize to regions that code for a highly conserved motif in the catalytic domains of TPK.[49] The *eck* gene is expressed in several cell-lines of epithelial origin and also in normal tissues that contain a high proportion of epithelial cells, e.g., skin, intestine, lung, and ovaries.[49]

In addition to having sequence homology, *eph*, *elk*, and *eck* proteins show similarities in domain topology. Seventeen cysteine residues in their external domains are conserved and clustered in a region that could be considered a cysteine-rich box, but the cysteine spacing is distinct from that in the EGF and insulin receptor boxes.[49]

Other Receptor-like Tyrosine Kinases

The HER2 gene, also denominated as *erb*B2 or *neu* proto-oncogene, also codes for a putative TPK receptor. The HER2 protein is highly related to the EGF receptor (80% homology in the kinase domain). This gene was initially isolated as the *neu* oncogene (see below) from a rat neuroglioblastoma.[101]

The *Xmrk* (*Xiphophorus* melanoma receptor kinase) gene was isolated from a malignant melanoma in the fish *Xiphophorus*. It also codes for a putative TPK cell surface receptor which shows significant similarity with the human EGF receptor.[92,97]

The *ros*-1 proto-oncogene was isolated and characterized from a glioblastoma cell-line. Analysis of the nucleotide sequence of cDNA clones revealed that it codes for a TPK receptor with a predicted molecular mass of 259 kDa.[5] The putative extracellular domain of the *ros*-1 shows some homology with the extracellular domain of the *sevenless* gene product from *Drosophila*.[5]

The *ret* proto-oncogene was isolated from a cDNA library of a THP-1 human monocytic leukemia cell-line. Analysis of the nucleotide sequence indicates that it encodes to a protein which is structurally related to transmembrane receptors with a cytoplasmic tyrosine kinase domain. However, unlike most growth factor receptors, it contains two hydrophobic regions which are potential transmembrane domains.[87] The *ret* proto-oncogene is frequently detected in an activated form in vivo in human thyroid papillary carcinomas (see below).

The *sea* proto-oncogene is also a member of the TPK receptor family. Sequence comparisons revealed that the *sea* protein is most closely related to the human *met* proto-oncogene product.[80]

Finally, the denominated "fetal liver kinase" or *flk*, is also a member of the TPK receptor family.[57] *flk* encodes a protein that is related to the W locus (c-*kit*) gene product, and appears to be expressed only in hematopoietic populations enriched in multipotential and self-renewing stem/progenitor cells.[57]

Oncogenic Protein Kinase Receptors: Mechanism of Activation

Growth factor receptor tyrosine kinases are key components of the biological control networks that govern cellular growth and differentiation. Because of their ability to generate a mitogenic signal, these molecules harbor a latent oncogenic potential which, when activated, results in subversion of normal signaling pathway controls.

The discovery that the v-*erb*B oncogene of avian erythroblastosis virus (AEV) was derived from the chicken EGF receptor gene was the first evidence that many oncogenes are derived from genes for growth factor receptors with protein tyrosine kinase activity.[101] Another example is the v-*fms* oncogene, which was derived from the gene for the receptor for the CSF-1.[78] There are several other oncogenes that appear to be growth factor receptor protein tyrosine kinase genes (Table 2).[101]

TABLE 2.
Oncogenic TPK Receptors

Oncogene	Species of Origin	Virus or Method of Detection	Oncogenic Product	Cellular Homolog Product	Human Chromosome Location
v-erbB	Avian	Erythroblastosis ES4 virus	gp70	gp170 (EGF-R)	7p11-p13
v-fms	Feline	McDonough sarcoma virus	gp180 (gag-fms)	gp160 (CSF1-R)	5q34
v-kit	Feline	Hardy-Zuckerman-4 sarcoma virus	p80 (gag-kit)	gp145	4q11-q21
v-ros	Avian	Rochester-2 sarcoma virus	p68 (gag-ros)	gp280	6q16-q22
v-sea	Avian	Erythroblastosis S13 virus	gp155 (env-sea)	n.r.	n.r.
neu (erbB2)	Rat	Transfection of mouse NIH3T3 cells with tumor DNA	gp185	gp185	17p11-q21
met	Human	Osteosarcoma cell line treated with carcino-gen	gp65 (tpr-met)	gp195 ($\alpha + \beta$)	7q21-q31
trk	Human	Transfection of mouse NIH3T3 cells with tumor DNA	p70 (trop-trk)	gp140	1q32-q41
ret	Human	Transfection of mouse NIH3T3 cells with tumor DNA	n.r. (rfp-ret)	gp135	10q11-q12

n.r.: not reported

How can a normal growth factor receptor protein kinase become a protein with oncogenic potential? In order to understand the possible mechanism of oncogenic activation it is necessary to understand the mechanism through which the binding of the ligand to the normal receptor stimulates its TPK activity. The most widely accepted model of signal-transduction by TPK receptors proposes that ligand-binding to the extracellular domain induces a conformational change that leads to dimerization of the receptor in the plane of the plasma membrane, followed by autophosphorylation reaction, which results in the phosphorylation of the cytoplasmic tyrosine kinase domains.[92,101] The phosphorylation of the tyrosine kinase domains "activates" this catalytic domain, resulting in an increase in protein kinase activity.

Two main levels of regulation of TPK receptors have been suggested, both of which ensure that the catalytic domain is normally in an inactive state. First, ligand-binding is needed as a positive signal. Second, negative regulation of the protein kinase domain has to be nullified by autophosphorylation. When we examine the different TPK receptor-derived oncogenes, it becomes clear that there are several mechanisms of oncogenic activation, rather a universal principle of activation. However, they can be grouped in two categories: qualitative, when the activated oncogene is a mutated version of the normal allele, and quantitative, when the simple overexpression of normal receptor is sufficient to induce the transformed phenotype.

Qualitative: Mutated Version of Normal Receptors

In all these cases, the oncogenic activation involves mutations causing structural changes in the receptor that result in deregulation of protein kinase activity. The most common change is the loss of all or part of the amino-terminal extracellular ligand-binding domain. This has occurred in the v-*erb*B, *trk*, *met*, *kit*, *ros*, *sea*, and *ret* genes.[8,56,87,101] In every case except the v-*erb*B protein, the amino-terminal truncation has taken place through recombination with another sequence, which results in a chimeric protein. In most cases, the foreign amino-terminus contains a signal peptide or a lipid attachment signal, and these oncoproteins are membrane-associated.

v-*erb*B Oncogene

v-*erb*B was identified in a retrovirus causing AEV and erythroleukemia. This avian retrovirus contained a cell-derived gene denominated *erb*B responsible for the transformed phenotype.[93] The v-*erb*B gene product represents a truncated version of the EGF receptor. It arose by insertion of viral DNA into the EGF-receptor gene, this resulted in expression of a protein that lacked the amino-terminal ligand-binding domain.[101] This finding was surprising in light of the fact that AEV selectively transforms erythroid cells, which are not known to express the EGF receptor.[8]

The fact that *erb*B retains the TPK domain of the EGF receptor implied that constitutive expression of this activity was the basis for its capacity as a transforming oncoprotein. Because viral isolates containing *erb*B lack most of the extracellular ligand-binding domain, it appears that this region inhibits activity of the intrinsic TPK domain. Genetic deletion of the ligand-binding domain from the EGF receptor is sufficient to create a transforming oncogene.[101] Moreover, mutations within the TPK domain of *erb*B abolish its transforming activity. *erb*B is thus transforming due to constitutively active protein tyrosine kinase resulting from deletion of the regulatory ligand-binding domain. Additional removal of carboxy-terminal regulatory sequences may enhance its transforming activity; however, they are not essential for the oncogenic activation.[101]

neu Oncogene

Rat neuroglioblastomas induced by exposure in vitro to ethylnitrosourea frequently carry an oncogene detectable upon transfection into NIH3T3 cells. This oncogene, called *neu*, was found to be more related to c-*erb*B than other members of the tyrosine kinase class of oncogenes.[8] The *neu* oncogene encodes a protein of 185 kDa, which is serologically related to the EGF receptor and is present on the surface of induced rat neuroblastomas. More than 50% of the amino acids coding for *neu* are shared with the EGF receptor, and there is 80% homology in the tyrosine kinase domain.[3,8] Structural comparison of the normal and transforming *neu* genes revealed no gross rearrangements, and comparable levels of the 185 kDa protein are expressed in nontransformed cell-lines. Sequence analysis revealed that the *neu* oncogene contains a single point mutation in its transmembrane domain (to change valine to glutamic acid) that renders the protein transforming.[3] The *neu* oncogene also can be activated by exposure of animals to another alkylating agent, methylnitrosourea. In this case the *neu* gene is activated by T to A transversions.[8]

The human *neu* gene, denominated c-*erb*B2, maps to chromosome 17p11-q21. This chromosome band is involved in a nonrandom reciprocal translocation in acute promyelocytic leukemia. The human c-*erb*B2 gene encodes a protein of 183 kDa with a transmembrane topology similar to that of the EGF receptor. Thus, it is likely that the gene encodes a growth factor tyrosine kinase receptor.[1] The fact that the ligand for c-*erb*B2/*neu* is still being sought, and that a single base change that alters the codon from valine to glutamine results in an increase in TPK activity, indicates that a normal cell surface receptor can be converted into a transforming protein, presumably by inducing a conformational change that mimics the change induced by ligand-binding.[8]

v-*fms* Oncogene

The v-*fms* gene is the transforming gene of the McDonough strain of feline sarcoma virus. This oncogene is derived from the proto-oncogene for the macrophage CSF-1 receptor.[8,101] Comparison of the amino acid sequences of the human CSF-1 receptor (c-*fms*) with feline v-*fms* reveals 84% amino acid homology. At least two mutations appear to be required for conversion to a transforming protein. First, deletion of 40 amino acids at the carboxy-terminus which have been replaced by 11 amino acids of the viral *env* protein. This deletion includes a tyrosine residue in position 969 of CSF-1 receptor. This tyrosine does not appear to be a major site for ligand-induced phosphorylation, but is suspected to have a negative regulating function for the catalytic activity.[78] Restoration of the normal carboxy-terminus reduces, but does not abolish, its transforming activity, suggesting that a second mutation is necessary for the complete transforming activity. This mutation appears to be a conversion of a leucine residue to serine at the position 301 of the extracellular ligand-binding domain, with a second enhancing mutation at residue 374. This mutation confers ligand-independent, constitutively active TPK activity, probably by inducing an active conformation of the receptor.[78] Finally, transfection of the nontransforming c-*fms* gene into cells that constitutively express CSF-1, results in cell transformation, indicating that chronic activation of the growth factor receptor can be induced by continuous binding to its ligand.[78]

v-*kit* Oncogene

The v-*kit* gene can be activated by transduction by the Hardy-Zuckerman-4 strain of feline sarcoma virus.[8] Mutants with extensive structural deletions at both ends of the gene, including the entire extracellular and transmembrane domains and part of the juxtamembrane domain have been described.[8] At the carboxy-terminus, 49 amino acids were replaced by five unrelated residues. In contrast to the protein products of v-*erb*B and v-*fms* oncogenes, which are inserted in the plasma membrane by hydrophobic segments, the v-*kit* oncogene product achieves membrane association by fusion with myristilated *gag* sequences.[101]

trk Oncogene

The *trk* oncogene was one of the first transforming genes identified in human malignancies. This oncogene was first detected during the course of gene transfer assays using DNA isolated from a colon carcinoma biopsy.[2,55] The molecular structure of this oncogene revealed a hybrid gene consisting of seven of the eight exons of a nonmuscle tropomyosin gene followed by sequences coding for the transmembrane and cytoplasmic tyrosine kinase domain of the *trk* proto-oncogene. Comparison of the deduced amino acid sequences of the *trk* oncogene and proto-oncogene products indicated that the transforming protein lacks the signal peptide and most of the normal *trk* receptor. No differences were observed within the *trk*-derived sequences, thus indicating that the fusion of tropomyosin sequences is sufficient to confer transforming properties to the *trk* tyrosine kinase.[2,58]

Although initially identified in a colon carcinoma, recent studies have indicated that the *trk* oncogenes are infrequently detected in this type of tumor. Instead, they appear to be activated frequently in thyroid papillary carcinomas.[2] These *trk* oncogenes exhibit an overall structure similar to the original colon carcinoma isolate, coding for hybrid molecules with an identical set of *trk* proto-oncogene-derived sequences. However, these oncogenes differ in the nature of the foreign sequences that replace the ligand-binding domain of the *trk* gene. To date, sequences derived from at least three different loci have been identified in the four thyroid carcinoma *trk* oncogenes that have been characterized so far, including: (i) the same nonmuscle tropomyosin locus that participated in the generation of the colon carcinoma oncogene; (ii) sequences derived from the *tpr* locus, a gene first identified as part of the *met* oncogene; and (iii) other sequences that remain to be identified but appear to be distinct from both tropomyosin and *tpr*.[2]

trk oncogenes can also be generated by in vitro recombinational events involving either genomic or cDNA sequences. In two cases, these oncogenes depict the same basic structure as those present in human tumors, including the same recombination region within the *trk* locus. However, these oncogenes possess different amino-terminal sequences which, in one case, have been identified as derived from the human ribosomal protein L7a.[2] In other cases, the structure of these in vitro-generated *trk* oncogenes indicated that they were generated either by rearrangements within the transfected *trk* sequences or by their recombination with the host genome. Finally, small mutations in the extracellular ligand-binding domain (replacement of a cysteine residue by serine) generated by in vitro site-directed mutagenesis also resulted in the generation of a *trk* transforming gene.[2]

met Oncogene

The *met* oncogene is another example of a transforming gene generated by fusion of two chromosomal loci. The oncogene originally was activated by treatment of a human osteosarcoma cell-line in vitro with N-methyl-N'-nitrosoguanidine and was isolated from *met*-transformed NIH3T3 cells.[8,14] Malignant activation of the *met* locus resulted from a DNA rearrangement joining two separate loci: *tpr* (mapping to chromosome 1) and c-*met* (mapping to chromosome 7q21–31) (Fig. 3). The normal c-*met* generates a 9 kb transcript found in human fibroblast and epithelial cell-lines. In contrast, the truncated, chimeric *met* oncogene is expressed as a 5 kb transcript consisting of 5' sequences derived from the *tpr* locus (which replaces most of the extracellular ligand-binding domain of the *met* locus) and 3' sequences of the *met* locus (containing the transmembane and tyrosine kinase domain).[63] The product of the *met* oncogene is a 65 kDa protein phosphorylated on tyrosine and serine residues and has tyrosine-specific autophosphorylation activity.[20,64]

ret Oncogene

The *ret* oncogene was activated by recombination between two unlinked segments of human DNA, during transfection of NIH3T3 cells with DNA of a human T-cell lymphoma.[87] The nucleotide sequence indicated that the active *ret* transforming gene encodes a fusion protein with an amino-terminal region corresponding to a human protein with zinc-finger structures, and a carboxy-terminal region which is 40% to 50% homologous to members of the tyrosine kinase gene family. This tyrosine kinase domain is preceded by a hydrophobic sequence characteristic of a transmembrane protein.[85,86] The *ret* proto-oncogene was found to be activated by rearrangement upon transfection of human colon carcinoma and human gastric carcinoma DNAs. These rearrangements occurred in vitro during the transfection assay, since no such rearrangements were detected in the DNAs of the original tumors.[21] In contrast, the *ret* proto-oncogene is frequently activated in vivo in human thyroid papillary carcinomas and in lymph node metastases.[21]

v-*ros* and v-*sea* Oncogenes

Additional cell surface receptors with intrinsic TPK activity have been identified in retroviral oncogenes, although the ligands for the proto-oncogene receptors have not been identified. Among these are the oncogenes v-*ros* and v-*sea*.

The v-*ros* oncogene was isolated by a transfection-tumorigenicity assay. The *ros* proto-oncogene was activated by a rearrangement in which all but eight amino acids of the *ros* proto-oncogene extracellular domain were replaced with sequences of unknown origin.[5]

The v-*sea* gene is the transforming gene of the AEV S13. The v-*sea* oncogene was found to be another member of the TPK gene family.[8] This oncogene was fused in frame with the retrovirus S13 envelope gene, thus generating a fusion protein with a structure resembling that of a growth factor receptor.[8] Sequence comparison revealed that the v-*sea* gene was most closely related to the insulin receptor family of protein tyrosine kinases, the greatest similarity being with the human *met* proto-oncogene.[8]

Quantitative: Activation by Overexpression

Activation by overexpression does not require any change in the structure of the receptor protein. Quantitative increases in either ligand or receptor are sufficient to perturb the equilibrium and result in transformation. For example, v-*sis*, the oncogene of the simian sarcoma virus, represents the B-chain of PDGF. Constitutive overexpression of c-*sis* to form B-chain homodimers of PDGF results in activation of the PDGF receptor.[8]

Overexpression of either the EGF receptor in the presence of EGF or the closely related normal *neu* protein in NIH3T3 cells leads to transformation.[30] In addition, there are human tumors where either the EGF receptor gene or the *neu* gene is found to be amplified between 10-and 50-fold. This amplification is accompanied by a large increase in protein expression.[30]

Amplification of the c-*erb*B2 gene was also found in three human adenocarcinomas: one of salivary origin, one mammary, and one gastric cancer cell-line.[8] Amplification of *erb*B2 in human breast carcinomas is correlated with more aggressive tumors and a worse prognosis. In addition, when normal *erb*B2/*neu* cDNA is placed under control of a strong viral transcription promoter, it behaves as a transforming protein in focus-forming, soft agar colony-forming, and thymic mice tumor-forming assay systems.[8] Similarly, the EGF and CSF-1 receptors are transforming when transcription of their respective genes is enhanced by strong viral promoters.[30] Finally, some human cancer cells have been found to overexpress the *eph* gene without gene amplification.[27]

Signal-Transduction Pathways

Signaling, initiated by activation of growth factor receptors, must be propagated and diffused throughout the cell to elicit complex cellular responses. Upon ligand-binding, a plethora of events are initiated, including stimulation of Na^+/H^+ exchange, Ca^{2+} influx, activation of PLC-γ, and stimulation of glucose and amino acid transport.[92,101]

What are the essential early substrates phosphorylated by activated TPK growth factor receptors? Using antiphosphotyrosine antibodies, many cellular proteins can be identified as putative target of receptor-specific phosphorylation. However, the problem is to sort out which of these phosphorylations are relevant and which are gratuitous. This difficulty is compounded by the fact that we know little about what processes are normally controlled by tyrosine phosphorylation.

Recently, several receptor tyrosine kinase substrates of potential biological importance have been identified (Fig. 5).[92] The different nature of these proteins that include a G protein (GAP), a proto-oncogene with threonine/serine protein kinase activity (c-*raf*), and two enzymes of phosphatidyl-inositol turnover (PLC-γ and PI3 kinase),

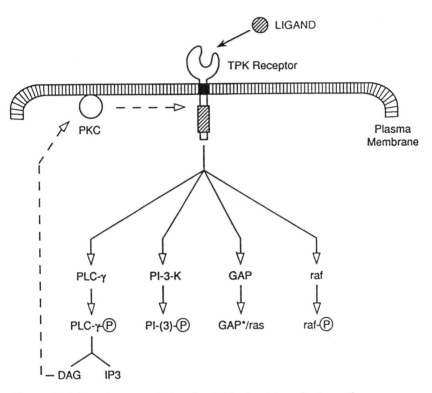

Figure 5. *Schematic representation of multiple signal-transduction pathways generated by TPK receptors. DAG: diacylglycerol; GAP: GTPase-activating protein; IP3: inositol 1,4,5-triphosphate; PI-3-K: phosphatidylinositol 3-kinase; PI-(3)-P: phosphatidylinositol 3-phosphate; PKC: protein kinase C; PLC-γ: phospholipase Cγ.*

revealed that multiple pathways are involved in the response triggered by TPK growth factor receptors.[92] Both PDGF and EGF can induce tyrosine phosphorylation of PLC-γ in vitro and in living cells. In addition, PLC-γ was observed to associate with the activated receptor kinases in a ligand-and kinase-dependent manner.[53,58,92] The stimulation of PLC-γ leads to the generation of phosphatidyl-inositol metabolites, such as inositol 1,4,5-triphosphate, which cause the release of Ca^{2+} from intracellular compartments and the generation of diacylglycerol, an activator of PKC.[92]

Several laboratories have also reported that the CSF-1 receptor associates with and activates phosphatidylinositol-3 kinase.[92] It has also been demonstrated that the *ras* GAP and the c-*raf* proto-oncogene product are direct substrates for some receptor tyrosine kinases. In some instances, this tyrosine has been shown to activate these proteins (e.g., PLC-γ).[92] The exact significance of the tyrosine phosphorylation of these proteins, however, remains to be determined.

TPK Receptors in Development

In the last few years, a growing body of genetic evidence implicates TPK receptors and their ligands as important elements in developmental programs controlling multiple stages of embryogenesis and cell differentiation. These studies indicate that TPK receptors play functional roles in a number of developmental processes, including oocyte maturation, embryonic cell proliferation and differentiation, pattern formation and morphogenesis in early embryos, and differentiation of continually renewing cell lineages.[28,65]

TPK Receptors in Mouse Development

Genetic analysis of mutations in several loci coding for TPK receptors (*white, Patch*) and growth factors (*Steel, Osteopetrotic*), in conjunction with detailed expression analysis (*trk, trkB*), have revealed specific developmental-linked functions.

white/Steel

The dominant W locus encodes the c-*kit* proto-oncogene. Mutations at the W locus result in pleiotropic developmental defects during both embryonic development and, in the blood-forming system, during adult life.[13,17,18] Severe W mutations produce homozygotes that are characterized by partial or complete lack of hair pigmentation, severe macrocytic anemia, mast cell deficiency, and sterility. W heterozygotes have varying degrees of hair pigmentation and occasionally anemia and reduced fertility. These cellular defects in W mutants reflect an inability of hematopoietic stem cells, melanoblasts and primordial germ cells to proliferate, migrate, and/or survive during embryogenesis. Analyses of chimeras have shown that the cellular defects in all three lineages are cell-autonomous, indicating that the W gene product is expressed and required by early stem cells within these three lineages.[13,18,65]

The *steel* locus codes for a new growth factor molecule and is a ligand for the c-*kit* proto-oncogene.[98] As expected, mutations in the *steel* locus, as in W mutations, also result in dominant W, severe macrocytic anemia, and sterility.[98] Unlike W mutations, however, the *steel* lesion does not result in an intrinsic, cell-autonomous defect but rather appears to perturb some aspect of the microenvironment that supports the growth and differentiation of these three lineages. Various studies have suggested that the function encoded by *steel* is not a long-range factor, such as a diffusible hormone, but rather appears to be mediated through local cell-cell interactions.[98]

trk, *trk*B, and *trk*C

As described previously, these genes are the mammalian members of the *trk* family of neurotrophin receptors. They encode closely related tyrosine kinases whose expression appears to be confined within defined structures of the mammalian nervous system.[2,38,39,41,84]

In situ hybridization analysis of 9.5-day-old mouse embryos indicated that the *trk* proto-oncogene is expressed in the condensing spinal ganglia.[54] During later stages of embryogenesis (13.5 and 14.5 days long), *trk* gene expression extends to other structures of the PNS, including dorsal root ganglia and visceral sensory ganglia. Analysis of late (17.5-day-old) embryos and adult mouse brain indicates that *trk* gene expression continues to be limited to visceral sensory ganglia of neural crest origin. No *trk* expression could be detected in other sensory ganglia of nonneural crest origin or in other cranial ganglia that are not strictly sensory.[54]

In situ hybridization studies indicate that in 9.5-day-old embryos, the *trk*B gene is expressed in a wide variety of structures of the developing CNS and PNS, including the forebrain, caudal midbrain, hind brain, spinal cord, the trigeminal ganglion, and differentiating neural crest cells, which will form the dorsal root ganglia. During late fetal development, the pattern of *trk*B expression appears to reflect the entire network of the developing CNS and PNS.[2,39] Unlike the *trk* proto-oncogene whose expression is confined to sensory neurons of neural crest origin, *trk*B transcripts are found in cells derived from both the neuroepithelium and the neural crest.[39]

Not all *trk*B transcripts are equally distributed throughout mouse neural tissues. Indeed, expression analysis revealed different and highly specialized patterns of expression for transcripts encoding the catalytic and noncatalytic *trk*B receptors. The specific expression of the noncatalytic form of *trk*B in the choroid plexus suggested that it may have a role in the active transport of a putative ligand within the brain as well as across the blood-brain barrier.[2,39,41]

In situ hybridization analysis of adult mouse brain, revealed *trk*C expression in several regions of the brain, including the pyramidal cell layer of the hippocampus, the dentate gyrus, and the cerebral cortex. In addition, expression is also detected in specific regions of the cerebellum such as the granular cell layer.

Patch

The *Patch* locus is another gene that appears to control coat color by controlling the behavior of melanoblasts in development.[65,75] Embryos homozygous for the *Patch* mutant allele die in utero with severe craniofacial abnormalities. Recent data suggested that the *Patch* locus codes for the PDGF receptor (α type).[65] Thus, indicating that mutations in a TPK receptor can lead to severe developmental defects.

Osteopetrotic

Mice homozygous for mutation at the *Osteopetrotic* locus have a marked deficiency in macrophages and osteoclasts. Similar to the *Steel* mutations, these defects cannot be reversed by transplantation of normal bone marrow stem cells, suggesting that the defect is in the microenvironment. Recent data suggested that this locus codes for the CSF-1, a growth factor for macrophages that is the ligand of the CSF-1 receptor.[102]

TPK Receptors in *Drosophila* Development

Several *Drosophila* genes coding for TPK receptors (see below) are prototypes for tyrosine kinases that convey positional and developmental information by interpreting cues provided by nearby cells. This type of local cellular interaction is likely to assume even greater significance in defining the developmental fate of cells during embryogenesis.

Drosophila EGF Receptor Homolog

The gene for the *Drosophila* EGF receptor homolog (DER) was cloned by cross-hybridization to the chicken oncogene v-*erb*B.[50] The DER protein is a transmembrane tyrosine kinase very similar in structure to the EGF receptor and *neu* proteins (37% and 55% similarity with the extracellular and cytoplasmic kinase domains, respectively), although it does not bind EGF or transforming growth factor, two agonists for the vertebrate EGF receptor.[28] So far, the ligand for the DER protein remains to be identified. A number of *Drosophila* developmental mutations, including the loss of function *faint-little-ball* (*flb*) and *torpedo* (*top*) alleles, and the gain-of-function *ellipse* (*elp*) allele, are allelic to the DER gene.[68,77] These mutations give rise to different phenotypes because some involve loss of function (*flb*, *top*), and some gain of function (*elp*), and some act in the embryo directly (*flb*), while others act in maternal cells (*torpedo*).[28,65] In embryos homozygous for severe *flb* alleles the anterior head structures deteriorate, the germ band does not retract, and the embryonic CNS fails to develop normally.[28] Recessive mutations in the maternal locus *torpedo* reveal that DER function is required in the female somatic follicle cells for proper egg formation. In contrast to these recessive mutations, dominant mutations in the DER gene have a rather specific effect on development of the *Drosophila* compound eye. In flies that are heterozygous for *ellipse* mutations, the regular spacing between the ommatidia is disrupted (each eye is composed of approximately 800 ommatidia), and in *ellipse* homozygotes few ommatidia develop.[26]

Drosophila FGF Receptor Homolog

The *Drosophila* homolog of the vertebrate FGF receptor (DFGF-R) was isolated by low-stringency hybridization.[19] In contrast to the diversity of this subclass of receptor tyrosine kinases in vertebrates, the *Drosophila* genome appears to encode only a single homolog. Nucleotide sequence analysis indicated that the DFGF receptor protein has a conserved sequence, size, and organization. The extracellular region encodes three Ig-like domains, and the cytoplasmic kinase domain exhibits a high degree of similarity (60%) to the vertebrate FGF receptors with the typical split kinase and comparably sized juxtamembrane and carboxy-terminal regions.[19] The DFGF receptor gene is expressed at all stages of development. Localization of the transcript and protein in embryos has shown that the gene is predominantly expressed in a restricted set of tissues: the developing tracheal system and the delaminating midline glial cells.[19] In embryos homozygous for a deletion of several genes including the DFGF receptor locus, the initial formation of the tracheal pits is not affected; however, the extension of tracheal cell processes leading to the formation of the elaborate tree structure is blocked.[19] The DFGF receptor protein may thus participate in receiving spatial cues that guide tracheal cell outgrowth.

sevenless

The *sevenless* gene encodes a transmembrane TPK receptor whose only known biological function is in a single photoreceptor of the ommatidial clusters that comprise the *Drosophila* compound eye.[4] The cells within each ommatidia apparently sense their position and adopt a specific fate as a consequence of short-range interactions with adjacent cells. Expression of the *sevenless* gene is required in the progenitor of the photoreceptor R7 for development of a neuronal phenotype. In the absence of *sevenless* function, this cell develops into a lens secreting cone cell.[4] Although expression of the *sevenless* gene is not normally restricted to R7, and can be widely induced in other cells, R7 is the only cell in which *sevenless* has a demonstrated biological effect in a wild type background. The *sevenless* ligand is probably expressed in a localized fashion by a neighboring cell, probably photoreceptor R8.

torso

The *torso* gene is a maternally encoded *Drosophila* gene that is required for the formation of embryos with normal anterior and posterior structures.[62,82] The *torso* gene product acts within the embryo to include the expression of zygotic genes required for the development of terminal structures. Loss of function *torso* mutations result in truncation of the anterior head skeleton, and failure to form any structures posterior to the seventh abdominal segment. Dominant *torso* gain-of-function mutations produce the opposite phenotype, elements of the termini are formed but the segmentation of the thorax and abdomen is suppressed.[62]

The *torso* gene codes for a TPK receptor which is ubiquitously expressed at the cell surface of the early *Drosophila* embryo, with no apparent localization to the terminal regions.[11] The distribution of the gene product of a *torso* gain-of-function mutant, is indistinguishable from wild type, indicating that simple overexpression of the wild type allele has no obvious phenotypic effect on anterior-posterior development; its kinase tyrosine activity is dependent on the binding of a ligand whose distribution is restricted to the terminal regions of the embryo.[11]

Dtrk

The *Drosophila* Dtrk gene was isolated by cross-hybridization to the human *trk* proto-oncogene and codes for a TPK receptor with cell-adhesion properties (see above).[2,69] Dtrk expression is developmentally regulated. High levels of a 5.7 kb transcript can be detected during medium-late embryogenesis. Expression of this transcript decreases during late embryogenesis to become almost undetectable in larvae. A second peak of expression is observed during late, third-instar larvae and adult flies.[69] In situ hybridization and antiDtrk antibody staining experiments indicate that Dtrk is expressed during *Drosophila* embryogenesis in several neurogenic areas of the PNS and CNS.[65] The Dtrk protein accumulates on the surface of neural cells including developing axons and cell bodies of neurons. During postembryonic development the Dtrk protein is localized in the optic lobes of the brain and in clusters of proliferating neuroblasts and mature neurons in the ventral ganglion.[2,69]

The pattern of expression of the Dtrk protein in the nervous system, and the discovery that Dtrk protein mediates cell-cell adhesion, indicate that Dtrk encodes a novel class of neural cell-adhesion molecules that may mediate cell-cell interaction and signal-transduction processes during the development of the *Drosophila* nervous system.[65]

Summary

TPK receptors are key components of the biological control network that govern cell growth and differentiation. Information received at the cell surface must be processed by activated TPK receptors through cytoplasmic intermediates to finally elicit different cellular responses. In the last few years, many new putative TPK receptors have been isolated; however, for many of them, their ligands remain to be identified. Despite these limitations, two new interesting concepts have been revealed: first, the implication of TPK receptors as important elements in developmental programs, in particular, during embryogenesis and in the development of the nervous system; and second, the confirmation that the pleiotropic cellular response initiated by TPK-activated receptors is mediated throughout multiple signal-transduction pathways. Activation of TPK receptors as oncogenes can result from a variety of different molecular alterations, with the common end result of increased unregulated catalytic activity. Although the physiological roles of many of the TPK receptors are still unknown, valuable information has emerged from the study of TPK receptor-derived oncogenes. First, the fact that some of these oncogenes are derived from receptors from known growth factors clearly indicates that their normal function is to transduce information across the plasma membrane, coupling growth factor-binding to an intracellular response. Moreover, transforming receptor tyrosine kinase derivatives serve as valuable model systems not only for studying the mechanism of oncogenesis but also for the analysis of structure-function relationships for these signal transmission molecules.

Acknowledgments: I wish to thank Ramesh Kumar for stimulating discussions, Peter Tapley and Joyce Shaffer for critically reading the manuscript, and Mariano Barbacid for support and facilities. I apologize to those whose references have had to be omitted, which was necessitated by space constraints.

References

1. Akiyama T, Sudo C, Ogawara, et al. The product of the human c-*erb*B gene: A 185-kilodalton glycoprotein with tyrosine kinase activity. Science 1986; 232:1644–1646.
2. Barbacid M, Lamballe F, Pulido D. The *trk* family of tyrosine protein kinase receptors. Biochem Biophys Acta 1991; 1072:115–127.
3. Bargmann C, Hung MC, Weinberg RA. Multiple independent activations of the *neu* oncogene by a point mutation altering the transmembrane domain of p185. Cell 1986; 45:649-654.
4. Basler K, Hafen E. *Sevenless* and *Drosophila* eye development: A tyrosine kinase control cell fate. Trends Genet 1988; 4:74–79.
5. Birchmeier C, O'Neill K, Riggs M, et al. Characterization of ROS1 cDNA

from a human glioblastoma cell line. Proc Natl Acad Sci USA 1990; 87:4799–4803.

6. Bottaro DP, Rubin JS, Faletto DL, et al. Identification of the hepatocyte growth factor receptor as the c-*met* proto-oncogene product. Science 1991; 251:802–804.

7. Burgess WH, Maciag T. The heparin-binding (fibroblast) growth factor family of proteins. Ann Rev Biochem 1989; 58:575–606.

8. Burk KB, Liu ET, Larrick JW. Oncogenes: An Introduction to the Concept of Cancer Genes. New York, Springer Verlag 1988; pp. 133-181.

9. Carpenter G. Receptors for epidermal growth factor and other polypeptides mitogens. Ann Rev Biochem 1987; 56:881–914.

10. Carpenter G, Cohen S. Epidermal growth factor. Ann Rev Biochem 1979; 48:193–216.

11. Casanova J, Struhl G. Localized surface activity of *torso*, a receptor tyrosine kinase, specifies terminal body pattern in *Drosophila*. Genes Dev 1989; 3:2025–2038.

12. Cordon-cardo C, Tapley P, Nandury V, et al. The *trk* tyrosine protein kinase mediates the mitogenic properties of nerve growth factor and neurotrophin-3. Cell 1991; 66:173–183.

13. Chabot B, Stephenson DA, Chapman VM, et al. The proto-oncogene c-*kit* encoding a transmembrane tyrosine kinase receptor maps to the mouse W locus. Nature 1988; 335:88–89.

14. Dean M, Park M, LeBeau MM, et al. The human *met* oncogene is related to the tyrosine kinase oncogenes. Nature 1985; 318:385–388.

15. Dionne CA, Crumley G, Bellot F, et al. Cloning and expression of two distinct high-affinity receptors cross-reacting with acidic and basic fibroblast growth factors. EMBO J 1990; 9:2685-2692.

16. Froesch ER, Schmid C, Schwander J, et al. Actions of insulin-like growth factors. Ann Rev Physiol 1985; 47:443–467.

17. Geissler EN, McFarland EC, Russell ES. Analysis of pleiotropism at the dominant spotting (W) mutations of the house mouse: A description of ten new W alleles. Genetics 1981; 97:337-361.

18. Geissler EN, Ryan MA, Housman DE. The dominant-white spotting (W) locus of the mouse encodes the c-*kit* proto-oncogene. Cell 1988; 55:185–192.

19. Glazer L, Shilo B-Z. The *Drosophila* FGF-R homolog is expressed in the embryonic tracheal system and appears to be required for directed tracheal cell extension. Genes Dev 1991; 5:697–705.

20. Gonzatti-Haces M, Seth A, Park M, et al. Characterization of the TPR-*met* oncogene p65 and the *met* proto-oncogene p140 protein-tyrosine kinases. Proc Natl Acad Sci USA 1988; 85:21–25.

21. Grieco M, Santoro MTB, Melillo RM, et al. PTC is a novel rearranged form of the *ret* proto-oncogene and is frequently detected in vivo in human thyroid papillary carcinomas. Cell 1990; 60:557–563.

22. Haigler H, Ash J, Singer SJ, et al. Visualization by fluorescence of the binding and internalization of epidermal growth factor in human carcinoma cells A431. Proc Natl Acad Sci USA 1978; 75:3317–3321.

23. Hanks SK, Quinn AM, Hunter T. The protein kinase family: Conserved features and deduced phylogeny of the catalytic domain. Science 1988; 241:42–52.

24. Hazan R, Margolis B, Dombalagian M, et al. Identification of auto-phosphorylation sites of HER2/*neu*. Cell Growth Differ 1990; 1:3–7.
25. Heldin CH, Westermark B. Platelet-derived growth factor: Three isoforms and two receptor types. Trends Genet 1989; 5:108-111.
26. Hempstead B, Martin-Zanca D, Kaplan DR, et al. High-affinity NGF binding requires co-expression of the *trk* proto-oncogene and the low-affinity NGF receptor. Nature 1991; 350:678-683.
27. Hirai H, Maru Y, Hagiwara K, et al. A novel tyrosine kinase receptor encoded by the *eph* gene. Science 1987; 238:1717-1720.
28. Hoffman FM. Roles of *Drosophila* proto-oncogene and growth factor homologs during development of the fly. Curr Top Microbiol Immunol 1989; 147:1–25.
29. Honenegger A, Dull TJ, Szapary D, et al. Kinetic parameters of protein tyrosine kinase activity of EGF-receptor mutants with individually altered autophosphorylation sites. EMBO J 1988; 7:3053–3060.
30. Hunter T. Oncogene products in the cytoplasm: The protein kinases. In: Oncogenes and the Molecular Origins of Cancer, Weinberg RA, ed. Cold Spring Harbor, Cold Spring Harbor Laboratory Press 1989; pp. 147–173.
31. Johnson DE, Lee PL, Williams LT. Diverse forms of a receptor for acidic and basic fibroblast growth factors. Mol Cell Biol 1990; 10:4728–4736.
32. Kaplan DR, Hempstead B, Martin-Zanca, D, et al. The *trk* proto-oncogene product: A signal transducing receptor for nerve growth factor. Science 1991; 252:554–558.
33. Kaplan DR, Martin-Zanca D, Parada LF. Tyrosine phosphorylation and tyrosine kinase activity of the *trk* proto-oncogene product induced by NGF. Nature 1991; 350:158-160.
34. Kaplan DR, Morrison DK, Wong G, et al. PDGF beta-receptor stimulates tyrosine phosphorylation of GAP and association of GAP with a signaling complex. Cell 1990; 61:121–133.
35. Kazlauskas A, Cooper J. Autophosphorylation of the PDGF receptor in the kinase insert region regulates interactions with cell proteins. Cell 1989; 58:1121–1132.
36. Keegan K, Johnson DE, Williams LT, et al. Isolation of and additional member of the fibroblast growth factor receptor family, FGFR-3. Proc Natl Acad Sci USA 1991; 88:1095–1099.
37. Klein R, Conway D, Parada LF, et al. The *trk*B tyrosine kinase gene codes for a second neurogenic receptor that lacks the catalytic kinase domain. Cell 1990; 61:647–656.
38. Klein R, Jing S, Nanduri V, et al. The *trk* proto-oncogene encodes a receptor for nerve growth factor. Cell 1991; 65:189–197.
39. Klein R, Martin-Zanca D, Barbacid M, et al. Expression of the tyrosine kinase receptor *trk*B is confined to the murine embryonic and adult nervous system. Development 1990; 109:845-850.
40. Klein R, Nanduri V, Jing S, et al. The *trk*B tyrosine protein kinase is a receptor for brain-derived neurotrophic factor and neurotrophin-3. Cell 1991; 66:395–403.
41. Klein R, Parada LF, Coulier F, et al. *trk*B, a novel tyrosine protein kinase receptor expressed during mouse neural development. EMBO J 1989; 8:3701–3709.

42. Kock CA, Anderson D, Moran MF, et al. SH2 and SH3 domains: Regulatory elements that control the interactions of signaling proteins. Science 1991; 252:668–674.

43. Lamballe F, Klein R, Barbacid M. *trk*C, a new member of the *trk* family of tyrosine protein kinases is a receptor for neurotrophin-3. Cell 1991; 66:1–20.

44. Lammers R, Gray A, Schlessinger J, et al. Differential signalling potential of insulin and IGF-1 receptor cytoplasmic domains. EMBO J 1989; 8:1369–1375.

45. Lee J, Dull T, Lax I, et al. HER2 cytoplasmic domain generates normal mitogenic and transforming signals in a chimeric receptor. EMBO J 1989; 8:167–173.

46. Lee P, Johnson D, Cousens L, et al. Purification and complementary DNA cloning of a receptor for basic fibroblast growth factor. Science 1989; 245:57–60.

47. Letwin K, Yee SP, Pawson T. Novel protein tyrosine kinase cDNAs related to *fps/fes* and *eph* cloned using anti-phosphotyrosine antibody. Oncogene 1988; 3:621–627.

48. Lewis RE, Czech MP. Molecular biology of the insulin receptor. In: Progress in Nucleic Acid Research. New York, Academic Press, 1988; pp. 157–172.

49. Lindberg RA, Hunter T. cDNA cloning and characterization of *eck*, and epithelial cell receptor protein-tyrosine kinase in the *eph/elk* family of protein kinases. Mol Cell Biol 1990; 10:6316–6324.

50. Livneh E, Glazer L, Segal D, et al. The *Drosophila* EGF receptor gene homolog: Conservation of both hormone binding and kinase domains. Cell 1985; 40:599–607.

51. Livneh E, Prywes R, Kashles O, et al. Reconstitution of human epidermal growth factor receptor and its deletion of mutants in cultured hamster cells. J Biol Chem 1986; 261:12490–12497.

52. Livneh E, Reiss N, Berent E, et al. An insertional mutant of epidermal growth factor receptors allows dissection of diverse receptor functions. EMBO J 1987; 6:2669–2676.

53. Margolis B, Li N, Koch A, et al. The tyrosine phosphorylated carboxy terminus of the EGF receptor is a binding site for GAP and PLC-γ. EMBO J 1990; 9:4375–4380.

54. Martin-Zanca D, Barbacid M, Parada LF. Expression of the *trk* proto-oncogene is restricted to the sensory cranial and spinal ganglia of neural crest origin in mouse development. Genes Dev 1990; 4:683–694.

55. Martin-Zanca D, Hughes S, Barbacid M. A human oncogene formed by the fusion of truncated tropomyosin and protein tyrosine kinase sequences. Nature 1986; 319:743–748.

56. Martin-Zanca D, Oskam R, Mitra G, et al. Molecular and biochemical characterization of the human *trk* proto-oncogene. Mol Cell Biol 1989; 9:24–33.

57. Matthews W, Jordan CT, Wilegand GH, et al. A receptor tyrosine kinase specific to hematopoietic stem and progenitor cell-enriched populations. Cell 1991; 65:1143–1152.

58. Molloy CJ, Bottaro DP, Fleming TP, et al. PDGF induction of tyrosine phosphorylation of GTPase activating protein. Nature 1989; 342:711–714.

59. Nakamura T. Molecular cloning and expression of human hepatocyte growth factor. Nature 1989; 342:440–442.
60. Nathans J, Hogness DS. Isolation, sequence analysis, and intron-exon arrangement of the gene encoding bovine rhodopsin. Cell 1983; 34:807–814.
61. Nishibe S, Wahl MI, Rhee SG, et al. Tyrosine phosphorylation of phospholipase C-II in vitro by the epidermal growth factor receptor. J Biol Chem 1989; 264:10335–10338.
62. Nüsslein-Volhard C, Frohnhofer HG, Lehmann R. Determination of auteroposterior polarity in *Drosophila*. Science 1987; 238:1675–1681.
63. Park M, Dean M, Cooper CS, et al. Mechanism of *met* oncogene activation. Cell 1986; 45:895–904.
64. Park M, Dean M, Kaul K, et al. Sequence of MET proto-oncogene cDNA has features characteristic of the tyrosine kinase family of growth factor receptors. Proc Natl Acad Sci USA 1987; 84:6379-6383.
65. Pawson T, Bernstein A. Receptor tyrosine kinases: Genetic evidence for their role in *Drosophila* and mouse development. Trends Genet 1990; 6:350–356.
66. Peralta EG, Winslow JW, Peterson GL, et al. Primary structure and biochemical properties of an M2 muscarinic receptor. Science 1987; 236:600–605.
67. Pintar JE. Structure and expression of the nerve growth factor gene. In: Oncogenes, Genes and Growth Factor, Guroff G, ed. New York, John Wiley and Sons 1987; pp. lO3–131.
68. Price JV, Clifford RJ, Schupbach T. The maternal ventralizing locus *torpedo* is allelic to *faint little ball*, an embryonic lethal, and encodes the *Drosophila* EGF receptor homolog. Cell 1989; 56:1085–1092.
69. Pulido D, Campuzano S, Koda T, et al. D*trk*, a *Drosophila* gene related to the *trk* family of neurotrophin receptors, encodes a novel class of neural cell adhesion molecule. EMBO J 1992; 11:391–404.
70. Rechler MM, Nissley SP. The nature and regulation of the receptors for insulin-like growth factors. Ann Rev Physiol 1985; 47:425–442.
71. Reid HH, Wildks AF, Bernard O. Two forms of the basic fibroblast growth factor receptor-like mRNA are expressed in the developing mouse brain. Proc Natl Acad Sci USA 1990; 87:1596-1600.
72. Riedel H, Dull TJ, Schlessinger J, et al. A chimaeric receptor allows insulin to stimulate tyrosine kinase activity of epidermal growth factor receptor. Nature 1986; 324:68–70.
73. Ross R, Raines EW, Bowen-Pope DF. The biology of platelet-derived growth factor. Cell 1986; 46:155–169.
74. Rubin JS, Cham AM, Bottaro DP, et al. A broad spectrum human lung fibroblast-drived mitogen is a variant of hepatocyte growth factor. Proc Natl Acad Sci USA 1991; 88:415–418.
75. Russell ES. Hereditary anemias of the mouse: A review for geneticists. Adv Genet 1979; 20:357–459.
76. Ruta M, Burgess W, Givol D, et al. Receptor for acidic fibroblast growth is related to the tyrosine kinase encoded by the *fms*-like gene (FLG). Proc Natl Acad Sci USA 1989; 86:8722–8726.
77. Schejter ED, Shilo BZ. The *Drosophila* EGF receptor homolog (DER) gene

is allelic to *faint little ball*, a locus essential for embryonic development. Cell 1989; 56:1093–1104.

78. Sherr CJ. Colony-stimulating factor-1 receptor. Blood 1990; 75:1–12.
79. Sherr CJ, Roussel MF, Rettenmier CW. Colony stimulating factor-1 receptor. J Cell Biochem 1988; 38:29–37.
80. Smith DR, Vogt PK, Hayman MJ. The v-*sea* oncogene of avian erythroblastosis retrovirus S13: Another member of the protein-tyrosine kinase gene family. Proc Natl Acad Sci USA 1989; 86:5291–5295.
81. Soppet D, Scandon E, Maragos J, et al. The neurotrophic factors brain-derived neurotrophic factor and neurotrophin-3 are ligands for the *trk*B tyrosine kinase receptor. Cell 1991; 65:895–903.
82. Sprenger F, Stevens LM, Nüsslein-Volhard C. The *Drosophila* gene *torso* encodes a putative receptor tyrosine kinase. Nature 1989; 338:478–483.
83. Squinto S, Stitt TN, Aldrich T, et al. *trk*B encodes a functional receptor for brain-derived neurotrophic factor and neurotrophin-3 but not nerve growth factor. Cell 1991; 65:885-893.
84. Stanley ER, Guilbert LJ, Tushinski RJ, et al. A mononuclear phagocyte lineage-specific hemopoietic growth factor. J Cell Biochem 1983; 21:151–156.
85. Takahashi M, Burma Y, Hiai H. Isolation of *ret* proto-oncogene cDNA with an amino-terminal signal sequence. Oncogene 1989; 4:805–806.
86. Takahashi M, Buma Y, Iwamoto T, et al. Cloning and expression of the *ret* proto-oncogene encoding a tyrosine kinase with two potential transmembrane domains. Oncogene 1988; 3:571–578.
87. Takahashi M, Ritz J, Cooper GM. Activation of a novel human transforming gene, *ret*, by DNA rearrangement. Cell 1985; 42:581–588.
88. Tornquist HE, Avruch J. Relationship of site-specific β subunit tyrosine kinase autophosphorylation to insulin activation of insulin receptor (tyrosine) protein kinase activity. J Biol Chem 1988; 263:4593–4601.
89. Ullrich AL, Coussens JS, Hayflick TJ, et al. Human epidermal growth factor receptor cDNA sequence and aberrant expression of the amplified gene in A431 epidermoid carcinoma cells. Nature 1984; 309:418–425.
90. Ullrich A, Gray A, Taru AW, et al. Insulin-like growth factor I receptor primary structure: Comparison with insulin receptor suggest structural determinants that define functional specificity. EMBO J 1986; 5:2503–2512.
91. Ullrich A, Ramachandran J. Insulin and type I insulin-like growth factor receptors. In: The Molecular Biology of Receptors, Stroberg AD, ed. Heidelberg, VCH Publishers 1977; pp. 35–48.
92. Ullrich A, Schlessinger J. Signal transduction by receptors with tyrosine kinase activity. Cell 1990; 61:203–212.
93. Vennstrom B, Bishop JM. Isolation and characterization of chicken DNA homologous to the two putative oncogenes of avian erythroblastosis virus. Cell 1982; 28:135–143.
94. Weskamp G, Reichardt LF. Evidence that biological activity of NGF is mediated through a novel subclass of high affinity receptors. Neuron 1991; 6:649–663.
95. White MF, Livingston JN, Backer JM, et al. Mutation of the insulin receptor at tyrosine 960 inhibits signal transmission but does not affect its tyrosine kinase activity. Cell 1988; 54:641-649.

96. Williams LT. Signal transduction by the platelet-derived growth factor receptor. Science 1989; 243:1564–1570.
97. Wittbrodt J, Adam D, Malitschek B, et al. Novel putative receptor tyrosine kinase encoded by the melanoma-inducing Tu locus in *Xiphophorus*. Nature 1989; 341:415–421.
98. Witte ON. *Steel* locus defines new multipotent growth factor. Cell 1990; 63:5–6.
99. Yarden Y, Kuang WJ, Yang-Feng T, et al. Human proto-oncogene c-*kit*: A novel cell surface receptor tyrosine kinase for an unidentified ligand. EMBO J 1987; 6:3341–3351.
100. Yarden Y, Rodriguez H, Wong SK, et al. The avian beta-adrenergic receptor: Primary structure and membrane topology. Proc Natl Acad Sci USA 1986; 83:6795–6799.
101. Yarden Y, Ullrich A. Growth factor receptor tyrosine kinase. Ann Rev Biochem 1988; 57:443–478.
102. Yoshida H, Hayashi S, Kunisada T, et al. The murine mutation *osteopetrosis* is in the coding region of the macrophage colony stimulating factor gene. Nature 1990; 345:442–443.

Chapter 7

Transforming Growth Factors

Anthony F. Purchio,
Greg D. Plowman

Sarcoma growth factor (SGF) was first described as an activity isolated from media conditioned by murine sarcoma virus-transformed rodent cells,[48] which promoted the growth of normal rat kidney (NRK) fibroblasts in soft agar. Subsequent analysis of SGF showed that it consists of two structurally unrelated proteins, named transforming growth factor (TGF)-α and TGF-β, which act synergistically to reversibly transform NRK cells.[7,8,240] Independently, both factors have quite different biological activities and act via separate and specific cell surface receptors.[35,36,150,151,240,251,256] However, in certain cell types, TGF-α and TGF-β show dramatic synergy. The precise mechanism of their cooperative interaction is not known, but it may in part result from the ability of TGF-β to alter the availability of cellular TGF-α-binding sites.

TGF-α and TGF-β are now recognized as representing two distinct families of molecules whose study has provided a basis for understanding the biochemical and molecular events involved in the control of both normal and malignant cell growth. The intent of this chapter is to summarize the structural and molecular biological characteristics of these molecules.

From *The Molecular Basis of Human Cancer:* edited by B. Neel, M.D., Ph.D., R. Kumar, Ph.D. © 1993, Futura Publishing Co. Inc., Mount Kisco, NY.

TGF-β

Protein Characterization

Biological activities

The component of SGF identified as TGF-β,[7,8,197,198] proved to represent a new class of growth factors capable of synergizing with epidermal growth factor (EGF). Although it was originally described for its ability to promote the growth of NRK fibroblasts in soft agar,[198] TGF-β isolated from media conditioned by a monkey cell-line (BSC-1) was also found to be a potent inhibitor of some cells in culture.[199,248] Further experiments showed that TGF-β possesses a multitude of biological activities that affect the growth and differentiation of a wide variety of cell types.[11,102,151,200,231,232] These included the inhibition of the growth of T and B lymphocytes,[100,101,258] mouse keratinocytes,[41,194] and several cancer cell-lines,[191,199] or the proliferation of early hematopoietic progenitor cells.[75] In addition, it increased the synthesis and secretion of collagen and fibronectin,[32,90] stimulated the differentiation of rat muscle mesenchymal cells and their subsequent production of cartilage-specific macromolecules,[218] and induced bone formation.[172] The specific effects of TGF-β are dependent on the presence of other growth factors as well as the physiological state of the cell.

TGF-β may also play an important role in wound healing. It was reported to accelerate the healing of incisional wounds in rats[166] and of surgical incisions in the rabbit gastrointestinal tract.[165] It reversed the glucocorticoid-induced and adriamycin-impaired wound healing in rats.[47,179] TGF-β also stimulated the formation of both periosteal bones in rat calvaria[172] as well as intramembranous bone formation upon injection into the subperiosteal region of newborn rat femurs.[97]

A second protein similar in function and structure to TGF-β has recently been described. Originally isolated from demineralized bone,[217] it has since been purified from human prostatic adenocarcinoma cells,[91] human glioblastoma cells,[267] and porcine platelets. This latter protein is now termed TGF-β2, while the protein described above is called TGF-β1. The complete amino acid sequence of TGF-β2 has been reported,[147] and it shares 71% homology with TGF-β1. Further analysis of cDNA clones encoding these proteins has indicated that TGF-β constitutes a family of highly related proteins that include TGF-β3,[55,94,237,238] TGF-β4,[93] and TGF-β5.[109] More distantly related proteins include Mullerian inhibitory substance[30] and the inhibins.[149]

This review will focus mainly on the molecular biology of the two original members of this family, TGF-β1 and TGF-β2; more extensive characterization of the biological activities of the TGF-β family can be found in the references.[11,102,151,171, 200,231,232]

Structure

TGF-β1 is a 24 kDa homodimer containing two identical 112 amino acid subunits which are held together by disulfide bonds.[9,54,68] TGF-β2 is also a disulfide-bonded homodimer (25.4 kDa) of two identical 112 amino acid monomers, displaying 71.4% homology with TGF-β1.[91,147] The mature dimers bind to specific receptors located in the cell membrane (see below) and are responsible for initiating the biological effects of TGF-β described above.

Latency

TGF-β1 and -β2, when isolated from most cell-lines and tissues under neutral conditions, are latent and require treatment such as heating in the presence of strong detergents, exposure to urea or extremes of pH, or treatment with certain proteolytic enzymes in order to become activated.[118,137,159,174,182,260] Latent TGF-β1 has been most extensively characterized from human platelets.[159,260] It fractionates as a large 210 to 230 kDa complex by nonreducing sodium dodecyl sulfate polyacrylamide gel electrophoresis (SDS-PAGE), which consists of mature TGF-β1, a 40 to 74 kDa pro-region-containing protein (see below) and a 130 to 160 kDa TGF-β1-binding protein. The human fibroblast TGF-β1-binding protein has been cloned[98]: cDNA sequence analysis indicates that the protein is made up of cysteine repeats, 16 of which are EGF-like. It was determined that the human-binding protein did not bind TGF-β1 directly, and it has been suggested that it might play a role in stabilization of the latent complex.[98]

Latent TGF-β1 from rat platelets is found associated with a 200 kDa complex called masking protein.[174] When analyzed by SDS-PAGE this complex consisted of a 110 kDa protein and a 78 kDa dimer composed of two pro-regions containing 39 kDa proteins. The complex had a molecular mass of 400 kDa when analyzed by gel filtration chromatography. Interestingly, the rat masking protein, unlike the human, was able to bind to and inhibit the activity of mature TGF-β1.[174] Sequence analysis of cDNA encoding the 110 kDa component of rat masking protein indicated that it is cleaved from a larger precursor and, like the human-binding protein, contains multiple EGF-like repeats.[243] Immunoblotting analysis of serum-free media conditioned by several cell-lines showed that TGF-β1 migrated as a 220 to 235 kDa complex after chemical crosslinking, and that this complex contained pro-region sequences.[260] Latent TGF-β2 has also been purified from BSC-40-(a monkey kidney cell-line) conditioned media[132] and chromatographs by gel filtration as a 130 and 400 kDa complex. These complexes contain mature TGF-β2 pro-region molecules as well as pro-TGF-β2 (see below for definition of these terms). Latent TGF-β purified from bone matrix chromatographs as a 400 to 600 kDa complex on an S400 column.[95]

It therefore appears that most cell-lines and tissues synthesize TGF-β1 and -β2 as part of a larger, latent protein complex. This implies that cells must have a mechanism of activating TGF-β such that active growth factor can become available when and where it is needed. Latent TGF-β has been reported to be activated by co-cultures of pericytes and smooth muscle cells as well as pericytes and endothelial cells.[5,209] Latent TGF-β can also be activated by activated osteoclasts,[177] by treatment with certain proteases,[137] or by enzymatic deglycosylation of the purified latent complex.[158] Further work into the various mechanisms of activation of latent TGF-β will certainly aid in our understanding of this multifunctional growth modulator.

TGF-β receptors

The various biological effects of TGF-β are thought to be mediated by its binding to specific cell surface receptors which are present on almost all cells examined[150,215,247]; however, receptor-deficient cell types have been noted.[106,196] Characterization of the β-receptor has relied mainly on the specific binding of [[125I]-labeled TGF-β to cell surfaces followed by chemical crosslinking and SDS-PAGE. These experiments revealed the presence of three major TGF-β-binding proteins having molecular weights of 250 to 350 kDa (type III receptor), 80 to 120 kDa (type II receptor), and 53 to 70 kDa (type I receptor).[21,35,36,37,116] The type III receptor is a proteoglycan[34,216] and binds TGF-β1 and -β2 with equal affinity[36]; type I and type II receptors are glycoproteins and have a higher affinity for TGF-β1 and TGF-β3 than for TGF-β.[36,116] The type I and II receptors have been implicated in signal-transduction,[21,116] while the type III receptor has been suggested to be an extracellular storage protein.[215]

Signal-transduction

Little is known about the various signal-transduction mechanisms involved after TGF-β-binding. Tyrosine kinase activity does not seem to be stimulated by TGF-β.[66,128] A report by Press et al.[187] showed that TGF-β1-induced c-*sis* mRNA in a human glioblastoma cell-line could be inhibited by the compound H7, suggesting serine and threonine phosphorylation may be involved in mediating some of the effects of TGF-β1. Early reports indicated that the TGF-β pathway was not linked to phosphoinositol (PI) turnover[128]; however, subsequent work showed that TGF-β1 treatment did lead to increased PI turnover in RAT-1 cells[162] and in canine kidney proximal tubular basolateral membranes.[202] Some of the effects of TGF-β may be coupled to G protein activation. Growth inhibition of CCL-64 cells by TGF-β was prevented by pertussis toxin,[87] while stimulation of c-*sis* and c-*myc* mRNA in AKR-2B fibroblasts was blocked by pertussis toxin and cholera toxin.[86] Increased incorporation of [^{3}H]-thymidine into DNA and [^{35}S]-GTP-binding to membranes in AKR-2B cells by TGF-β was also inhibited by pertussis toxin,[164] suggesting that GTP-binding proteins may be implicated in TGF-β-mediated signal-transduction.

Recent experiments have also suggested that the product of the retinoblastoma gene, pRB, may be involved in TGF-β1-mediated events.[115,181] pRB is a nuclear phosphoprotein of 110 kDa: loss of this gene has been associated not only with retinoblastoma but also with several carcinomas and sarcomas.[108,124–126] pRB undergoes cell cycle-dependent phosphorylation; it is unphosphorylated in G1 and phosphorylated in S and G2.[134] The growth suppressive activity[88] of pRB has led to its classification as an antioncogene, and the under-phosphorylated form is thought to be responsible for its growth suppressive ability.

TGF-β1 inhibits the growth of keratinocytes[40] and downregulates the expression of c-*myc*; keratinocyte proliferation requires the expression of c-*myc*.[180] Skin keratinocytes expressing proteins which bind unphosphorylated pRB (SV$_{40}$ TAg, Ad5 EIA protein) and presumably block pRB normal function, do not downregulate c-myc after TGF-β1 treatment and are resistant to the growth inhibition by TGF-β1.[181] In the case of mink lung epithelial cells where TGF-β1 is growth inhibitory and prevents phosphorylation of pRB, the expression of SV40 T-antigen, which binds underphosphorylated pRB in these cells, reduced the growth inhibitory effects of TGF-β1,[115] again suggesting a role for pRB in the signal pathway of TGF-β1.

Another way TGF-β may exert its effects on cell proliferation is by modulation of the synthesis of other growth factors and their receptors. Battegay et al.[15] have shown that, in smooth muscle cells, low concentrations of TGF-β induce the synthesis of platelet-derived growth factor (PDGF) and stimulate these cells to grow: higher concentrations of TGF-β are less stimulating and result in downregulation of the PDGF receptor α subunit suggesting that the PDGF-autocrine loop is involved in growth regulation of smooth muscle cells by TGF-β1.

Gene Regulation

cDNA cloning

Analysis of cDNA clones encoding human,[54,56] murine,[53] porcine,[110] bovine,[253] and simian[221] TGF-β1 have indicated that it is synthesized as a larger precursor (390 amino acids in the human, simian, and murine protein), the carboxy-terminal 112 residues of which constitutes the TGF-β1 monomer. There are nine cysteine residues in the mature region, allowing for the formation of one interchain disulfide bond and four intrachain disulfide bonds (H. Marquardt, personal communication). Sequence analysis of cDNA clones encoding TGF-β2 indicates that it too is cleaved from a larger precursor.[50,80,141] However, in the case of TGF-β2, alternative splicing produces transcripts predicted to encode a 442 [TGF-β2(442)] and a 414 [TGF-β2(414)] amino acid precursor protein,[262] due to a 28 amino acid insertion within the pro-region of TGF-β2(414). Although there is a 70% homology between mature TGF-β1 and -β2, there is only a 30% homology between the two molecules within the pro-region.[141] There are three cysteine residues in the TGF-β1 pro-region, five in the TGF-β2(414) pro-region, and eight in the TGF-β2(442) pro-region.

Analysis of the predicted amino acid sequences of cDNA clones encoding TGF-β3,[55,94,237] TGF-β4,[93] and TGF-β5[109] also show that the mature proteins are cleaved from larger precursors. All five proteins conserve the nine cysteine residues located within the mature region; interestingly, the TGF-β4 precursor, the cDNA sequence which was obtained from primary chick embryo chondrocytes,[93] does not contain a signal peptide. Further experiments are needed to determine whether or not this protein is secreted.

Transcriptional regulation

The major transcript of the TGF-β1 gene is a 2.5 kb polyadenyl-ated RNA species which has been detected in several cell-lines and tissues.[2,53,110,221] Transcription of this gene is developmentally regu-lated in the mouse fetus.[264]

The TGF-β2 gene is transcribed into three RNA species of 4.1, 5.1, and 6.5 kb,[50,141] which are produced both by alternative splicing and by differential polyadenylation.[262] Cell-lines vary with respect to expression of these three transcripts; the monkey kidney cell-line BSC-40 and human glioblastoma cells express mainly the 4.1 and 6.5 kb transcript,[50,141] while the human prostatic carcinoma cell-line PC-3 expresses all three messages equally.[141] The major TGF-β3 transcript is a 3.2 kb RNA species.[55,237]

TGF-β1 is capable of inducing its own message in several normal and transformed cell-lines.[254] Analysis of the human TGF-β1 promoter has uncovered two major transcriptional start sites, two regions responsible for autoinduction, and a site which inhibits transcrip-tion.[104,105] There were several SP1-binding sites and no "TATA" or "CAAT" boxes. In AKR-2B (mouse) fibroblasts, TGF-β1 treatment leads to a 25-fold induction in TGF-β1 mRNA after 6 to 12 hours.[13] TGF-β1 did not result in an increase in TGF-β2 or TGF-β3 mRNA in AKR-2B cells; however, TGF-β2 treatment of these cells resulted in increased expression of TGF-β1, TGF-β2, and TGF-β3,[13] each with different kinetics, suggesting that these genes are differently regu-lated.

The human TGF-β3 and TGF-β2 promoters have recently been characterized[114,143]; they differ greatly from the TGF-β1 promoter and from each other, supporting the notion of differential transcriptional regulation of these genes.

Expression of Recombinant TGF-β Proteins

Characterization of TGF-β1 proteins secreted by recombinant Chinese hamster ovary cells

Recombinant TGF-β1 (rTGF-β1) has been expressed to high levels in Chinese hamster ovary (CHO) cells.[74] These cells secreted TGF-β1 into serum-free media in a latent form, and acidification was required in order to detect optimal biological activity (Fig. 1), similar to TGF-β1 secreted by most cell-lines. Analysis of the TGF-β1-related proteins secreted by a clone of the recombinant CHO (rCHO) cells (clone 17) is shown in Figure 2. When analyzed by immunoblotting after SDS-PAGE under nonreducing conditions, the TGF-β1 proteins migrate as two components; a 90 to 110 kDa complex and a 24 kDa species (arrow in Fig. 2B, lane 1 and Fig. 2C, lane 1) which is the mature TGF-β1 dimer. Under reducing conditions, these proteins migrate as a 44 to 56

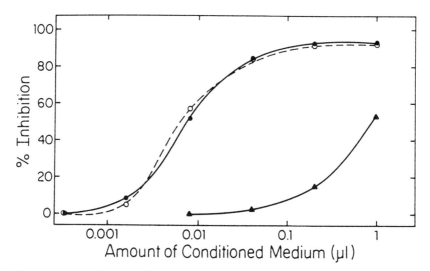

Figure 1. *Recombinant TGF-β secreted by CHO cells is latent. Serum-free media conditioned by a rCHO cell-line (TGF-β-3–2000) secreting TGF-β1 was dialyzed against 0.2 M acetic acid (●—●), 50 mM NH₄HCO₃, pH 7.0 (▲—▲) or 50 mM NH₄HCO₃, pH 7.0 followed by 0.2 M acetic acid (○- -○) and assayed for growth inhibitory activity on CCL-64 cells as described.*[74]

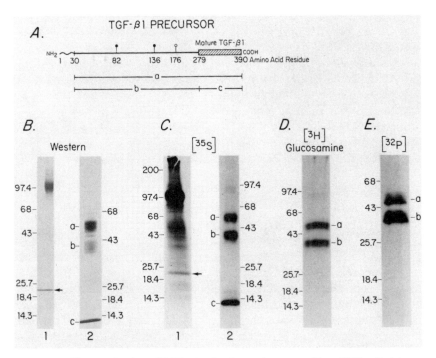

Figure 2. *Characterization of TGF-β1-related proteins secreted by rCHO cells (clone 17). A: Line diagram of TGF-β1 precursor.* ↑ *shows sites of glycosylation and* ↑ *shows sites of glycosylation containing mannose-6-phosphate. Line 'a' indicates pro-TGF-β1, line 'b' indicates the pro-region of TGF-β1, and line 'c' indicates TGF-β1 mature monomer. B: Serum-free media conditioned by clone 17 cells were analyzed by SDS-PAGE under nonreducing (lane 1) or reducing (lane 2) conditions followed by immunoblotting using mature and pro-region specific antipeptide antibodies.[74] Arrow points to mature TGF-β1 dimer. C: [35S]-cys and [35S]-met labeled serum-free media conditioned by clone 17 cells were fractionated by SDS-PAGE under nonreducing (lane 1) or reducing (lane 2) conditions. Bands were visualized by autoradiography. Arrow points to the mature TGF-β1 dimer. D: [3H]-glucosamine labeled serum-free media conditioned by clone 17 cells were fractionated by SDS-PAGE under reducing conditions: bands were visualized by fluorography followed by autoradiography. E: [32P]-orthophosphate labeled serum-free media conditioned by clone 17 cells were fractionated by SDS-PAGE under reducing conditions: bands were visualized by autoradiography.*

kDa species (band 'a', Fig. 2B, lane 2), a 30 to 42 kDa species (band 'b', Fig. 2B, lane 2) and a 12 kDa species (band 'c', Fig. 2B, lane 2). Band 'a' represents pro-TGF-β1, band 'b' represents the pro-domain (or pro-region) of TGF-β1, and band 'c' is the TGF-β1 monomer. The same proteins can be seen after fractionation of [^{35}S]-labeled proteins secreted by clone 17 cells, followed by SDS-PAGE and autoradiography (Fig. 2C). These proteins are diagramed in Figure 2A and have been identified both by immunoblotting with site-specific antipeptide antibodies and protein sequencing.[71,74] The 90 to 110 kDa complex consists of pro-TGF-β1, the pro-domain of TGF-β1, and mature TGF-β1 (see also Fig. 4). Similar proteins have been described in media conditioned by human 293S cells transfected with plasmids encoding TGF-β1.[259]

Secondary modifications of the pro-domain of TGF-β1

Figures 2D and 2E show that bands 'a' and 'b' can be labeled with [^{3}H]-glucosamine and [^{32}P]-orthophosphate.[26,188] The TGF-β1 cDNA sequence predicts three sites of N-glycosylation located at residues 82, 136, and 176,[221] and all three sites are glycosylated.[188] The phosphate is incorporated as mannose-6-phosphate (M-6-P) and is found primarily at the first two glycosylation sites. These M-6-P residues enable the pro-region-containing complex to specifically bind to the insulin-like growth factor II (IGF-II)/M-6-P-receptor (M-6-PR) and, in canine kidney proximal tubular basolateral membranes, activate phospholipase C.[111,202] The binding of the TGF-β1 pro-region-containing complex to the M-6-PR is a separate activity from the binding of mature TGF-β1 to its cell surface receptors, described previously.

Proteolytic cleavage of rTGF-β1 precursor can be inhibited by methylamine, ammonium chloride, monensin, and chloroquin,[139,219] agents which raise the pH of acidic vesicles and inhibit their acidic proteases.[58,157] The M-6-PR has been implicated in the transport of M-6-P-containing proteins to lysosomes or other intracellular acidic vesicles for proteolytic processing.[257] The above reagents may inhibit TGF-β1 processing either by direct inhibition of acidic proteases or by inhibiting the transport process itself. Further experiments are needed to clarify whether binding to the M-6-PR and subsequent transport to sites for proteolytic cleavage is involved in TGF-β1 processing.

Latency of recombinant TGF-β1

Characterization of latent recombinant TGF-β1 (LrTGF-β1) secreted by clone 17 cells shows that this complex fractionates as a 130 kDa species upon sizing chromatography under neutral conditions (Fig. 3A).[131] All bioactivity is found in this size region, and prior acidification of each fraction was required to detect optimal activity. Analysis of the TGF-β1-related proteins in this fraction by immunoblotting after nonreducing SDS-PAGE (Fig. 3B) identifies the 90 to 110 kDa species as well as the mature 24 kDa dimer (arrow in Fig. 3B). Acidification of this material, followed by chromatography under acidic conditions, separates the 24 kDa dimer from the 90 to 100 kDa species (Fig. 3D), and the bioactivity is now found in the same region as the 24 kDa mature dimer (Fig. 3C). This suggests that mature TGF-β1 is noncovalently associated with the 90 to 100 kDa pro-region-containing complex; acidification breaks this bond and frees the mature TGF-β1, which is now active. Chemical crosslinking experiments have also demonstrated that mature TGF-β1 is noncovalently associated with the 90 to 110 kDa species.[136] Mixing of the pro-region with mature TGF-β1 resulted in a loss of bioactivity, again suggesting a role for the pro-domain in conferring latency.[72]

There are three cysteines located within the TGF-β1 pro-region at positions 33, 223, and 225. Cysteine 33 has been shown to be disulfide bonded to one cysteine within the mature region.[71] Site-directed mutagenesis of Cys-33 to serine resulted in the production of increased amounts of active dimer when these DNAs were transfected into COS cells.[27] Cysteines 223 and 225 form interchain disulfide bonds.[27] Cells transfected with DNAs in which both Cys-223 and Cys-225 had been mutated to serine do not produce the 90 to 110 kDa complex; in addition, a significant proportion of the TGF-β1 secreted by these cells transfected with the double mutant is active.[27] This further supports the idea that the association of mature TGF-β1 with the 90 to 110 kDa complex is, in part, responsible for conferring latency.

Figure 4 shows a diagram of the structure of the LrTGF-β1 complex secreted by the rCHO cells which is consistent with all the experimental data accumulated to date. The model shows mature 24 kDa TGF-β1 noncovalently bound (indicated by three sets of three dots) to the 90 to 110 kDa complex; we suggest that this is the bond

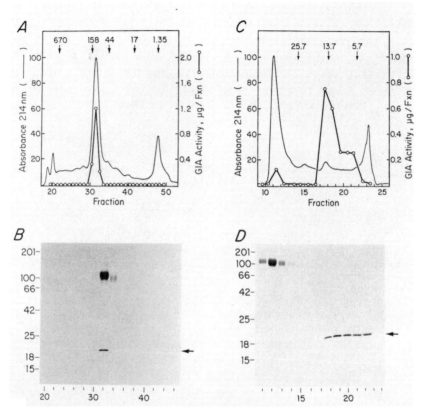

Figure 3. *Size fractionation of rTGF-β1 latent complex. A: Serum-free media conditioned by clone 17 cells were concentrated by ammonium sulfate precipitation and fractionated under neutral conditions on a Bio-Sil TSK 250 column (TSK) (Bio-Rad size exclusion chromatography). Individual fractions were then acidified and assayed for growth inhibitory activity GIA, ○—○) on CCL-64 cells as described.[131] B: Fractions from the neutral TSK column in panel A were analyzed by SDS-PAGE under nonreducing conditions followed by immunoblotting with mature and pro-region-specific antipeptide antibodies.[74] Arrow indicates the position of mature TGF-β1 dimer. C: Peak bioactive fractions from the neutral TSK column shown in panel A were pooled, acidified, and fractionated on a TSK column under acidic conditions. Individual fractions were assayed for growth inhibitory activity on CCL-64 cells (○—○) as described.[131] D: Fractions from the acidic TSK column shown in panel C were fractionated by SDS-PAGE under nonreducing conditions followed by immunoblotting with pro-and mature-region-specific antipeptide antibodies. Arrow indicates the position of mature TGF-β1 dimer.*

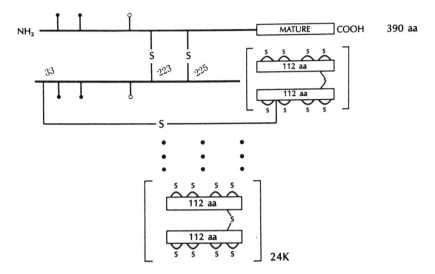

Figure 4. *Model of recombinant TGF-β1 latent complex. The figure shows a noncovalent bond (indicated by three sets of three dots) between mature TGF-β1 and the 90 to 110 kDa pro-region containing complex. This is the bond which is broken by acidification (see Fig. 3) and confers latency. Disulfide bonds are indicated by -S-. Cysteine residues located at position 223 and 225 form interchain disulfide bonds.[27] Cysteine 33 is disulfide bonded to one of the cysteine residues within a second mature TGF-β1 molecule.[71] Mutagenesis of this cysteine leads to the release of this additional, active TGF-β1.[27]*

which confers latency and is acid labile. The 90 to 110 kDa complex consists of pro-TGF-β1, the pro-domain of TGF-β1, and mature TGF-β1 dimer. Two cysteines located at residue 223 and 225 within the pro-region form interchain disulfide bonds (indicated by -S-) with a second pro-region-containing protein. Cys-33 within the pro-region forms a disulfide bond with a cysteine residue at various sites in a second mature TGF-β1 molecule; mutagenesis of this cysteine results in the release of this active protein in addition to what is released after acidification.[27] Also shown are the glycosylation sites ↑ and those sites containing M-6-P ↑ . It therefore appears that there are two ways of releasing active TGF-β1 from the LrTGF-complex: disruption of the noncovalent bond between mature TGF-β1 and the 90 to 110 kDa complex, and cleavage of the disulfide bond between Cys-33 and mature TGF-β1 within the 90 to 110 kDa complex.

Expression of Recombinant TGF-β2 and TGF-β3

TGF-β2(414) has also been expressed to high levels in CHO cells.[140] Analyses of the TGF-β2-related proteins secreted by the rCHO cells indicated that mature TGF-β2 was more efficiently cleaved from its precursor than was TGF-β1. The inhibition of proteolytic cleavage of TGF-β2 differed from that of TGF-β1 in that the cleavage of TGF-β2 precursor was inhibited by chloroquin and monensin but not by ammonium chloride and methylamine, as was the TGF-β1 precursor.[131]

Like rTGF-β1, rTGF-β2 is secreted in a latent form, noncovalently associated with a high molecular weight pro-region-containing complex.[131,140] However, the structure of the TGF-β2 latent complex differs from that of TGF-β1,[131] suggesting that different mechanisms of activating the two complexes may exist. Interestingly, the pro-domain of TGF-β1 can confer latency on mature TGF-β2, although only a 30% homology exists between the TGF-β1 and -β2 pro-regions.[138] Latent TGF-β2 has been partially purified from cell-free media conditioned by a nonrecombinant cell-line BSC-40.[132] These cells release TGF-β2 in a latent form as part of a high molecular weight complex which contains glycosylated pro-TGF-β2 and pro-domains of TGF-β2.[132]

Recently, rTGF-β3 has also been obtained.[77,237] Comparison of biological activities shows that TGF-β3 is similar to TGF-β1 and -β2; however, different potencies exist among the proteins depending on the exact assay and cell type used. Transient expression of TGF-β3 in COS cells led to the secretion of TGF-β3 in a latent form (L. Madisen, A.F. Purchio, unpublished observations).

Discussion and Future Directions

Purification and characterization of TGF-β1 and -β2 from various cell-lines and platelets has shown that these molecules are released as latent complexes. This implies that various cell types must have mechanisms for activating latent TGF-βs. The fact that LrTGF-β1 differs structurally from LrTGF-β2 suggests that different mechanisms for activating the two molecules may exist. This potential situation would give cells another level of control over where and when active growth factor is present.

Various systems have been described for activating latent TGF-β; these include co-cultures of endothelial cells and pericytes, endothelial cells and smooth muscle cells,[5,209] as well as activated osteoclasts.[177] Removal of carbohydrate from latent platelet TGF-β1 produced active growth factor,[158] and LrTGF-β1 can be activated by plasmin.[136] Since large quantities of LrTGF-β1 and -β2 are available, it is now possible to investigate and evaluate the potential of multiple cell types to activate the latent complexes. As recombinant proteins for other TGF-β family members become available, it will be important to characterize their latent complexes as well as their mechanisms of activation. The function of the platelet TGF-β1 masking protein will also require further clarification.

Further characterization of the TGF-β receptor is also needed, as well as the role of the cell surface proteoglycan-binding protein. Sequence analysis of cDNA clones encoding these proteins should provide valuable information with respect to secondary and tertiary structure of the molecule, ligand-binding sites, and interaction with other cellular effector proteins. Mechanisms of signal-transduction will also need to be investigated. Is PI turnover involved in all or just some cell types? Once antibodies to these receptor(s) are made, questions regarding secondary modifications (phosphorylation) of the receptor will be answered. These experiments will advance our understanding of how this multifunctional growth modulator exerts the multiplicity of its effects on cell growth and differentiation.

The availability of large amounts of recombinant proteins will now allow for the testing of any therapeutic potential of TGF-β. The ability of TGF-β to accelerate wound healing in an impaired animal model suggests that it might find use as a topical treatment for surgical wounds; its ability to promote collagen secretion suggests a use in decubitus ulcers. TGF-β, mixed with an appropriate slow-release vehicle, can also be tested for stimulation of bone formation in various clinical settings. Of particular interest is the recent finding that TGF-β can mediate cardioprotection.[83] Finally the inhibition of several tumor cell-lines by TGF-β suggests that it may be useful as an antitumor agent. Since TGF-β inhibits early hematopoietic stem cell division, it may be useful in myeloprotection in various chemotherapy and radiotherapy applications. Latent forms of TGF-β should also be tested. Testing the activity of the various TGF-βs in the above clinical settings will be an exciting new area in the study of these proteins.

TGF-α

Molecular Structure of TGF-α Family Members

Mammalian and viral homologs

TGF-α exists in several forms, including a secreted 6 kDa protein of 50 amino acids (aa), higher molecular weight (24 kDa, 40 kDa, 42 kDa) soluble forms, and 13 to 23 kDa transmembrane molecules.[22,23,73,145,236,266] The 50 aa form is structurally and functionally related to three other secreted mammalian growth regulatory molecules, specifically EGF,[210] amphiregulin (AR),[222,223] and a macrophage-derived heparin-binding molecule (HB-EGF).[83] These molecules exhibit 31% to 49% sequence homology in a region containing the conserved spacing of six cysteine residues that, for EGF, have been shown to form three disulfide bonds.[146] Functionally, TGF-α, EGF, AR, and HB-EGF all bind the 170 kDa EGF receptor and stimulate its intrinsic tyrosine kinase activity.[251,256] Recently another mammalian protein, gp30, has been partially characterized which may be capable of interacting with both EGF receptor and the related receptor HER2/*neu*.[135] Further purification and sequence analysis of gp30 is required for a more detailed comparison with this family of proteins. In addition, three pox virus proteins are structurally related to TGF-α and can also interact with the EGF receptor; they are vaccina growth factor (VGF),[25,249] myxoma growth factor (MGF),[252] and Shope fibroma growth factor (SFGF).[33]

TGF-α structure

Molecular cloning of TGF-α, EGF, AR, and HB-EGF revealed that each is a secreted protein which is first synthesized as a larger precursor molecule that contains two hydrophobic stretches, corresponding to a signal sequence and transmembrane domain.[57,76,83,123,184,214] The 4800 nucleotide human TGF-α mRNA contains a large 3' untranslated region preceded by a sequence that encodes a 159 aa or 160 aa precursor (the larger form results from the addition of Ala_{32} due to intron sliding at the 5' end of exon 3). The TGF-α precursor contains the following domains: a signal peptide; a 75 aa extracellular domain that includes the mature 50 aa growth factor; a

23 residue transmembrane domain; and a 39 aa cysteine-rich carboxy-terminal cytoplasmic domain.[57,123] Some larger forms of TGF-α have been shown to contain complex carbohydrates,[23,73,236] consistent with the presence of O-glycosylation sites in the precursor sequence. Membrane-bound TGF-α has been detected by immunohistochemical and biochemical methods in tumor cell-lines that express endogenous pro-TGF-α, but do not secrete soluble molecules.[22] The integral membrane form of TGF-α is biologically active, as demonstrated by characterization of cells transfected with noncleavable forms of the TGF-α precursor.[22,266] In this system, pro-TGF-α accumulates at the cell surface and is capable of binding the EGF receptor on adjacent cells, leading to increased cytosolic calcium levels and tyrosine autophosphorylation of the EGF receptor. Membrane associated TGF-α has been speculated to function in cell-cell adhesion and intercellular communication through contact-dependent mitogenic stimulation.[152] Adherant bone marrow-derived stromal cells that express pro-TGF-α can support the growth of a normally nonadherant hematopoietic cell-line that has been transfected with EGF receptors.[4] Association of the receptor-expressing cells with the ligand-expressing cells results in DNA replication and cell proliferation. In addition, the integral membrane form of TGF-α can induce transformation of NRK cells by autocrine stimulation of the EGF receptor.[19]

EGF structure

The EGF transcript is about the same size as that of TGF-α (4800 nucleotides), but encodes a considerably larger precursor of 1207 amino acids (Mr = 128 kDa). The mature 53 aa peptide is flanked by 970 amino-terminal residues and 184 residues on the carboxy-terminal side.[16,76,214] The flanking regions contain seven cysteine-rich EGF-like repeats, a domain with homology to the low-density lipoprotein receptor, a transmembrane sequence, and a 153 aa cytoplasmic domain. The EGF precursor appears to also exist as an unprocessed transmembrane molecule in certain kidney epithelial cells.[16,190]

Amphiregulin structure

The AR transcript is 1400 nucleotides and encodes a 252 residue precursor containing five structural domains[184]: a 19 aa signal sequence; an 81-residue serine-rich amino-terminal domain; an 84-

residue region encoding the mature soluble factor, the first half being composed of predominately hydrophilic amino acids followed by a 41-residue region bearing homology to EGF and TGF-α; a hydrophobic, 23-residue transmembrane domain; and a 31-residue carboxy-terminal cytoplasmic domain. The unglycosylated AR precursor minus the signal peptide has a predicted molecular weight of approximately 26 kDa. The major secreted forms of glycosylated AR (18 to 24 kDa) are composed of 78 or 84 amino acids (differing only in the presence or absence of six N-terminal residues) and are synthesized as the middle portion of a 252 aa transmembrane precursor.[184,223] Rat AR, isolated as a heparin-binding protein from a schwannoma cell-line, is larger (31 to 35 kDa) than the human protein presumably due to more extensive addition of N-linked oligosaccharides.[107]

Unlike other members of the TGF-α/EGF family, mature AR is a larger (18 to 35 kDa), glycosylated, heparin-binding protein. All of these unique features can be accounted for by the very basic 43 amino acid N-terminal region of the secreted protein. In addition, high molecular weight and transmembrane forms of AR have been identified, presumably the result of altered tissue-or temporal-specific proteolytic processing of the precursor (G. Plowman, unpublished). The N-terminal serine-rich domain of the AR precursor contains three potential tyrosine sulfation sites and multiple O-glycosylation and glycosaminoglycan attachment sites. Sulfation could serve to protect or stabilize the tyrosine residues in AR and thereby influence the activity or proteolytic processing of the precursor, whereas addition of complex carbohydrates might generate a latent form of the ligand by altering its binding affinity to the EGF receptor.

The transmembrane form of the AR precursor was established by immunostaining of the human breast carcinoma cell-line MCF-7, with an AR-specific monoclonal antibody (G. Plowman, unpublished). By light microscopy, the membrane bound precursor had a polarized distribution and was expressed predominantly on ruffled membranes of cells migrating into cell-free areas of the culture. The fibrillar staining pattern was explained by electron microscopy by which AR was localized to cell surface protrusions termed microspikes that have been associated with cell-substratum attachment, cell motility, and points of cell-cell contact. The appearance of microspikes often precedes the formation of membrane ruffles, one of the earliest observed morphological changes in cells responsive to EGF, TGF-α, or PDGF.[168] Expression of the transmembrane form of AR on the leading edge of the cell suggests AR may play a role in cell migration.

Recently, a heparin-binding EGF-like growth factor (HB-EGF) was identified from a human macrophage cell-line.[83] This molecule is most similar to AR, with 50% sequence homology in the region spanning the three disulfide loops, and exact conservation of a highly basic sequence, KRKKKG, in the N-terminal portion of the mature molecule which is believed to allow both AR and HB-EGF to bind to heparin. A transmembrane sequence is predicted by the HB-EGF cDNA, but further studies are required to assess if it is also expressed as an integral membrane protein.

The cytosplasmic domains of TGF-α, EGF, AR, and HB-EGF contain 39, 153, 31, and 24 residues, respectively. They share no obvious similarity between one another, but this region of TGF-α shows strict conservation between the rat and human molecules.[57,123] In addition, some of the cysteines in the cytoplasmic domain of TGF-α undergo covalent palmitate attachment, a feature proposed to affect its transit and processing in the Golgi apparatus.[23] In contrast, the cytoplasmic domains of EGF and AR show considerable divergence between rat and human sources (48% and 68% amino acid identity, respectively).

Structural studies of EGF-like motifs

What features define a functional EGF receptor-binding molecule? The primary sequence homology between these growth factors includes the conserved spacing of six cysteines which form three disulfide bonds and define their basic secondary structure. Only four additional residues are completely conserved between all other mammalian and viral proteins that can bind the EGF receptor (Gly_{18}, Tyr_{37}, Gly_{39}, and Arg_{41}; these amino acid positions are based on alignment with the mature human EGF sequence) (Fig. 5). Other highly conserved residues include Tyr_{13} or Phe_{13}, His_{16} (the exceptions are mouse and rat EGF, SFGF, and MGF which have Asn_{16}); Gly_{36} (the exceptions are SFGF and MGF which have Asn_{36}, and human AR which has Glu_{36}); and Leu_{47} (the only exception is mature AR which truncates prior to this residue). Two-dimensional nuclear magnetic resonance (NMR) studies of EGF[46] and TGF-α[160] suggest that the highly conserved spacing of cysteines and glycines may define the basic structure of the protein backbone while other conserved, or conservatively changed, residues may form the functional receptor-recognition site (residues 13, 16, 37, 39, and 47). Further support for

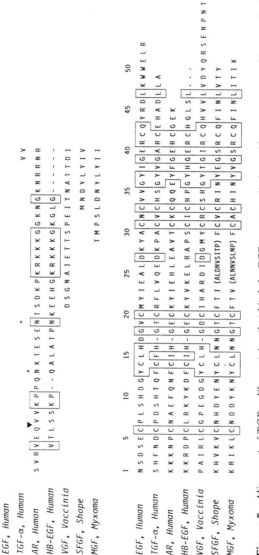

Figure 5. *Alignment of TGF-α-like proteins that bind the EGF receptor. Amino acids are represented by standard one letter symbols and are numbered in the cysteine-rich region based on alignment with the sequence of human EGF. Highly conserved residues are boxed and hyphens indicate a gap introduced to maximize homology. ★ , potential N-glycosylation site; ▼, beginning of the alternate 78 amino acid form of mature AR.*

their involvement in receptor-binding is provided by analyses that suggest these residues may all lie on the same face of the molecule.[28] Molecular and biochemical methods have been used to generate altered molecules for determining which residues are required for an active EGF-like molecule.[49,121] Some generalizations include the following: a) the six cysteines positioned in their disulfide loops and Arg_{41} are required for biological activity; b) an aromatic residue (Phe, Tyr) is required at position 13; c) a nonconservative change of Tyr_{37} results in loss of activity and/or dramatic loss in receptor-binding and autophosphorylation. In addition a nonconservative change or the elimination of Leu_{47} essentially inactivates these molecules, except in the case of AR which entirely lacks a residue at this position (Fig. 5). Possibly residues in the large N-terminal hydrophilic region of AR can fold back and fill in the "hole" in the receptor recognition site, created by its C-terminal truncation. AR provides a natural example of how functionally related molecules can apparently form a common three-dimensional receptor-binding site from regions with significant primary sequence differences.

Structural domains that are superficially similar to EGF are found in diverse proteins including: several of the blood coagulation factors; extracellular matrix proteins, tenascin and laminin; the invertebrate homeotic genes including *Notch*, *slit*, *Serrate*, *crumbs*, and *Delta* from *Drosophila*, and *lin-12* and *glp-1* from *Caenorhabditis elegans*; low-density lipoprotein (LDL) receptor and LDL receptor related protein (LRP); and members of a family of cell-adhesion proteins including the lymphocyte homing receptors and the endothelial leukocyte adhesion molecule, ELAM-1.[67,103,117,223,239,274] While structurally similar to EGF, none of these proteins maintain the precise spacing of all six cysteines and, likewise, none have been shown to interact with the EGF receptor. In addition, a gene termed Cripto, that was first isolated from a human teratocarcinoma cell-line, has intriguing primary sequence homology to EGF but, again, lacks verification of functional homology.[39]

In addition to the structural and functional similarities between TGF-α, EGF, and AR, they are also ancestrally related, according to an analysis of their exon organization.[16,20,184] The TGF-α and EGF genes are both > 100 kb and contain 6 and 24 exons, respectively. The AR gene is approximately 10 kb and is partitioned into six exons. The exon organization is conserved in the region encoding each mature active growth factor where an intron disrupts the coding sequence between the second and third disulfide loop of these proteins, and the adjacent exon of each contains the transmembrane domain.

Although TGF-α, EGF, and AR all arose from a common ancestral gene, they have since undergone considerable divergence, and each has a unique chromosomal location. Human TGF-α has been mapped to 2p13,[242] EGF to 4q25,[277] and AR to chromosome region 4q13 to 4q21.[184] Interestingly, the latter is near a site of the most common cytogenetic aberration in congenital acute lymphoblastic leukemia.[82] Determination of any link between AR and this malignancy requires a more detailed analysis of this translocation.

Tissue Distribution and Expression of TGF-α Family Members

Initially, TGFs were thought to be specifically associated with transformed cells, but subsequent studies have found significant levels of both TGF-α and TGF-β from a variety of normal sources. Northern analysis and immunohistochemical staining reveal the following generalizations regarding expression of TGF-α family members; EGF has a very limited pattern of expression, TGF-α is widely expressed in a variety of tumors and some fetal tissues, whereas AR has a much broader expression profile in normal adult tissues.

TGF-α

TGF-α expression has been demonstrated in a variety of tumors and retrovirally-transformed cells,[14,48,52,133,167] especially mammary and renal carinomas where it is often accompanied by high levels of EGF receptors (>100,000 receptors/cell). TGF-α expression has also been reported in early fetal development and preimplantation embryos.[122,192,263] In situ analysis revealed that the maternal rat deciduum is a major source of TGF-α during development.[79] TGF-α is expressed in these extraembryonic tissues from gestational day 7, until day 15, when the deciduum is resorbed. The TGF-α mRNA has also been detected in several murine fetal tissues, including the otic vesicle, oral cavity, pharyngeal pouch, developing kidneys, and the first and second branchial arches.[263]

Initial attempts to identify a normal adult tissue source of TGF-α expression were unsuccessful, due in part to low mRNA abundance and cell type specificity.[52] TGF-α has subsequently been shown to play a role in the growth of normal cells, since its mRNA has been detected in normal and psoriatic adult keratinocytes,[42,63] breast epithelial cells,[14] pituitary,[207] ovarian thecal cells,[112] seminiferous tubules,[225] several regions of the brain (dentate gyrus, caudate nucleus),[264] and activated alveolar macrophages.[142]

EGF

EGF is predominantly expressed in the male mouse submaxillary glands, the loop of Henle and distal convoluted tubules of the kidney, and lactating mammary gland, with lower levels in the pancreas, small intestine, and pituitary.[190,214] Humans do not produce detectable levels of submaxillary EGF. By Northern analysis, there is no detectable expression of EGF transcripts during fetal development, but in situ techniques reveal EGF mRNA in developing teeth and lungs and immunoreactive material has been described in the adult and fetal mouse brain (neuronal fibers and telencephalon) following the 14th day of gestation.[186] EGF first appears in the mouse kidney two weeks after birth and in the salivary gland after weaning. Immunoreactive material has also been identified in platelets.[173]

Amphiregulin

AR was first identified from a human breast cancer cell-line, MCF-7, following treatment with phorbol esters.[222] The protein has subsequently been isolated from human choriocarcinoma and colorectal carcinoma cell-lines, rat schwanoma cells,[107] and human keratinocytes (G. Plowman, unpublished). The AR transcripts and immunoreactive material have also been identified in several human breast carcinoma cells-lines and primary tumors, particularly those that are estrogen receptor-positive and contain low levels of EGF receptors.[184] Production of TGF-α also occurs in many human tumor cells and has been detected in 70% of primary breast tumors.[14] However, unlike AR, the expression of TGF-α correlated with overexpression of the EGF receptor.[52,60] The expression of AR is also found in several human carcinomas of colorectal, kidney, pancreatic, and ovarian origin, and most show an increase in AR transcripts following treatment with phorbol esters.[184]

Northern analysis revealed the 1.4 kb AR transcript was surprisingly abundant in RNA derived from human ovary, placenta, keratinocytes, and mammary epithelial cells, and was easily detected in RNA from normal human pancreas, cardiac muscle, testis, colon, breast, lung, spleen, brain, and kidney.[184] Little or no hybridization was seen in the adrenal, duodenum, epidermis, liver, parathyroid, prostate, or thymus, or mature hematopoietic cells.

The cellular sources of expression of TGF-α and AR are quite distinct from that of the much less prevalent EGF. Both TGF-α and AR are found in a variety of normal and malignant tissues including: normal keratinocytes, ovary, testis, brain, and breast, in addition to a variety of mammary, renal, and colorectal carcinomas. In addition, AR can be detected in placenta, lung, pancreas, colon, and spleen. In general, the AR transcripts are much more abundant in normal tissues than are those of TGF-α or EGF. The expression profiles of TGF-α, EGF, and AR suggest that all three factors may serve specific functional roles in the growth of normal tissues.

Biological Activities of TGF-α Family Members

In vitro activities

The name EGF reflects this protein's ability to stimulate epidermal maturation. The first activity recognized for EGF was the acceleration of eyelid opening and tooth eruption when injected into newborn mice.[44] Subsequently, EGF has been shown to be mitogenic for a wide range of mammalian cell types. Most mesenchymal and epithelial cells are stimulated by EGF and/or TGF-α, including fibroblasts,[8] keratinocytes,[12,42,213] endometrial stromal cells,[205] uterine epithelial cells,[241] gastrointestinal stem cells,[268] colonic epithelial cells,[144] embryonic palate mesenchymal cells,[43] rat calvaria cells,[6] fetal rat hepatocytes,[84] human fetal adrenal cells,[230] rat granulosa cells,[17] thyroid follicular cells,[280] mammary epithelial cells,[14] human proximal tubular kidney epithelial cells,[70] vascular smooth muscle,[83,279] and many neuronal cells including embryonic rat sympathetic ganglia,[61] glial cells, astrocytes, and Schwann cells.[3,107,161] The large number of EGF-responsive cell types reflects the finding that most tissues express EGF receptors. However, some exceptions are hematopoietic cells, parietal endoderm, and adult skeletal muscle, which are tissues that lack EGF receptors. In addition, human melanocytes[183] and pancreatic β-cells[224] are unresponsive to these growth factors. Alternatively, rapidly dividing cells, such as epidermal keratinocytes and the epithelial lining of the gut, are particularly responsive to EGF. Although hematopoietic cells also undergo rapid division and turnover, they appear to lack expression of ligands or receptors belonging to the EGF/TGF-α or EGF receptor family, with the exception of human macrophages which produced both TGF-α and HB-EGF.[83,142]

Role during development

The observation that embryonal carcinoma cells become responsive to EGF after being induced to differentiate, prompted early speculation that EGF/TGF-α may function during normal development.[193] Subsequently, EGF-binding activity was identified throughout gestation in the mouse.[1] Furthermore, in vivo administration of EGF accelerates the development of certain tissues, including tooth eruption and eyelid opening in newborn mice,[44] lung and liver maturation in fetal rabbits,[31,176] lung and skin development in fetal lambs,[234] and growth of rat gastric mucosa.[51] The identification of TGF-α mRNA in preimplantation embryos, the maternal decidua, and in several tissues during early gestation, further supports a role for these ligands in preparing the uterus for implantation and in early embryonic development.[79,192,263] However, recent studies involving overexpression of TGF-α in transgenic mice showed no marked effect on fetal development.[96,153,208] Conceivably the control of this proliferative response may be more at the level of the EGF receptor, rather than availability of ligand.

Role in adult physiology

The TGF-α and AR mRNAs are found in a variety of adult tissues, and their protein products appear to provide the mitogenic signals for many rapidly proliferating cells. Three in vivo approaches that suggest this ligand-receptor system may be important in adult physiology are the following: (1) mice made EGF-deficient by removal of the submandibular gland (sialoadenectomy), their major source of circulating EGF; (2) exogenous administration of EGF or TGF-α to animals or wounds and; (3) transgenic mice overexpressing TGF-α.

The EGF-deficient mice showed altered spermatogenesis, which was reversed on administration of EGF,[244] increased rate of abortion,[245] deficient mammary gland development with smaller size and decreased milk production,[175] decreased growth of the parotid gland and pancreas,[211] and diminished corneal wound healing with improved healing with topical application of EGF.[246]

Exogenous administration of EGF to adult animals can influence the growth of gastric mucosa,[51] the immature mammary glands,[45] and the female reproductive tract.[170] These factors may play a role in wound healing or tissue regeneration. Topical application of EGF or TGF-α accelerates healing of corneal grafts[64] and of partial thickness wounds of the skin due to enhanced epithelialization.[24] TGF-α also may be involved in regulation of liver regeneration.[156] One of the most extensive in vivo experiments with EGF involves administration of EGF to sheep to facilitate wool removal. EGF inhibits proliferation of hair follicle cells, resulting in thinning of the wool fiber, permitting easy removal of the wool several days after injection of EGF.[154,189] A depilatory dose of EGF in sheep also affected reproductive function by disrupting the hypothalamic pulse generator, resulting in decreased secretion of luteinizing hormone from the pituitary. In addition, EGF had a direct effect on the ovaries, diminishing their ability to respond to exogenous gonadotropin.[189] A similar inhibition of oocyte maturation was observed on administration of EGF to mice.[130]

Transgenic technology has provided another means for understanding the physiological role of TGF-α in whole animals. Three groups have recently reported the expression of TGF-α in transgenic mice.[96,153,208] They found that while overexpression of TGF-α had little effect on fetal development, it induced marked alterations in the growth and differentiation of several adult tissues. The pleiotropic effects included epithelial hyperplasia of the adult liver and gastrointestinal tract, interstitial fibroplasia and acinar cell hyperplasia of the pancreas, hyperplasia and dysplasia of the coagulation glands, and transformation of the breast and liver, which lead to postlactational mammary adenocarcinoma and hepatocellular carcinoma. These studies demonstrate that the gastrointestinal tract, liver, breast, and pancreas are predisposed to the effects of overproduction of TGF-α, and their responses range from epithelial proliferation to neoplastic transformation.

In addition to their mitogenic effects, EGF/TGF-α have been ascribed several other functions, including the stimulation of arachidonate metabolism,[127] the maintenance and stimulation of elongation of rodent neuronal cells,[161] the in vitro chemotaxis of vascular endothelial cells,[78] and the inhibition of gastric acid secretion.[195] Furthermore, TGF-α has been proposed as a candidate for initiation of morphogenesis in the embryonic kidney (metanephros) as a consequence of its being expressed in the developing mouse kidney and its ability to stimulate tubule formation of mouse kidney cells when cultured in a reconstituted basement membrane preparation.[235]

Differential activities of TGF-α family members

The mitogenic potency of EGF and TGF-α is similar on most mammalian mesenchymal and epithelial cells and both have the ability to stimulate epidermal cell migration and colony formation.[12] In vivo, EGF and TGF-α show similar induction of eyelid opening in newborn mice[229] and inhibition of gastric acid secretion in guinea pigs.[195] However, TGF-α is more potent on induction of neovascularization (angiogenesis) in vivo,[212] on induction of bone resorption and hypercalcemia in organ cultures,[89,233] and on constriction of vascular smooth muscle (especially renal glomerular mesangial cells).[18,69]

Amphiregulin has a mitogenic potency similar to EGF and TGF-α on keratinocytes and glial cells,[107,184] but is less active on fibroblasts and does not induce anchorage-independent growth of NRK cells in the presence of TGF-β.[184,222] In addition, AR also appears to abrogate the stimulatory effect of TGF-α on the growth of several aggressive epithelial carcinomas that overexpress EGFR.[184,222] All three factors specifically bind and activate the 170 kd EGF receptor tyrosine kinase,[223,240,251] but AR binds with lower affinity and can only partially compete with EGF.[223] These studies support the speculation that EGF, TGF-α, and AR may differ in their molecular interaction with the EGF receptor, that the internalized ligand-receptor complex may produce a temporally or qualitatively different signal, or that these ligands may recognize separate receptors in certain cell types.[119,185,265] Conceivably, multiple members of both the receptor and ligand families provide an organism with a greater repertoire to regulate homeostasis under various physiological and pathological conditions.

Cellular Transformation and Cancer

The subversion of the normal growth control mechanism transduced by the EGF receptor can lead to constitutive activation of its intrinsic tyrosine kinase, resulting in cell transformation. Constitutive activation of EGF receptor tyrosine kinase can occur by several mechanisms: truncation or point mutations; activation by viral proteins such as papillomavirus E5 or adenovirus E3 gene products; or autocrine activation by overproduction of both the normal receptor and ligand by tumor cells.

Activating mutations

Avian erythroblastosis virus (AEV) infection causes erythroleukemia and fibrosarcomas in chickens. The primary transforming gene contained in these retroviruses is the v-erbB oncogene, which was derived by transduction of the normal cellular EGF receptor.[62,120,269] v-erbB contains several activating mutations, the most important of which is truncation of the extracellular N-terminal ligand-binding domain.[256] The rat homolog of a related receptor c-erbB2/HER2/neu is activated by a single point mutation resulting in conversion of Val→Glu in the neu transmembrane domain.[10] This alteration results in constitutive receptor oligomerization in the absence of any ligand, and leads to transformation. Mutated versions of the EGF receptor have been identified in a few human tumors; for example, A431 epidermoid carcinoma cells overexpress a C-terminal truncated receptor,[250] and glioblastomas overexpress a receptor with specific deletions of certain extracellular domain exons.[129,270,271]

Activation by viral proteins

Papillomaviruses are the etiologic agents of certain benign and malignant epithelial tumors in humans, including warts and cervical carcinoma. The protein responsible for the transforming activity of these viruses is E5, a 44 aa protein that lacks homology with EGF/TGF-α. E5 appears to activate the EGF receptor in the absence of ligand by inhibition of receptor internalization.[148] The adenovirus E3 gene can induce EGF receptor internalization and degradation, presumably through an interaction with the cytoplasmic portion of the transmembrane domain.[29]

Autocrine activation

A common cellular lesion found in human cancers involves an autocrine interaction between a growth factor and its specific receptor that is overexpressed in the same cell. Increased expression of the EGF receptor (0.1 to 14 million receptors per cell) has been associated with more aggressive cancers of the breast, bladder, lung, and stomach,[169,204,255,272] and often occurs in tumors of the pancreas, brain, esophagus, and liver.[85,228,273] Frequently the overexpression has been determined to result from gene amplification. In breast and ovarian carcinoma, c-*erb*B-2/HER2/*neu* overexpression directly correlates with patient prognosis.[226,227] This EGF receptor-like tyrosine kinase appears to play an important role in tumor progression, but may also be involved in tumor initiation since transgenic expression results in single step induction of mammary carcinoma.[163] The HER2/*neu* protein is a substrate for the EGF receptor tryosine kinase and coexpression of the two proteins has a synergistic effect on cell transformation and correlates with a worse prognosis in breast cancer.[204,226]

Endogenous expression of TGF-α in the presence of high levels of EGF receptor can induce transformation through an autocrine mechanism. Originally detected in supernatants from retroviral or chemically-transformed cells, TGF-α is also abundantly expressed in cells transformed by *ras*, SV40, or polyoma virus,[99,178,206] and in a variety of human tumors where TGF-α expression often correlates with high levels of EGF receptor.[60,275,276,278] Specifically, many tumor cell-lines of mammary,[14,52,133] hepatic,[273] kidney,[167] or pancreatic[228] origin display elevated levels of TGF-α.

Initial evidence to suggest TGF-α might play a role in tumor formation came from the identification of TGF-α as one component of SGF. These studies demonstrate that TGF-α, together with TGF-β, can induce anchorage-independent growth of NRK fibroblasts. Three approaches have provided in vivo evidence of the tumor-inducing potential of TGF-α/EGF. First, exogenous or endogenous EGF increases the incidence of spontaneous mammary tumors in nude mice.[113] Second, TGF-α can cooperate with other factors to promote angiogenesis, an important component of tumor proliferation.[212] Third, transgenic mice that overexpress TGF-α exhibit a high incidence of adenocarcinoma of the breast and liver.[96,153,208] In vitro evidence of this oncogenic potential is demonstrated by reports where the transformation of either Rat-1 and NRK fibroblasts,[203,261] or NIH3T3 cells[81] occurs following high level expression of TGF-α, or EGF, respectively. These fibroblast cultured cell-lines contain only a moderate number of EGF receptors and exhibit a weakly transformed phenotype when maintained under normal growth conditions. For these cells to acquire a fully transformed phenotype requires expression of the EGF receptor to levels comparable to those reported in human epithelial tumors, and the exogenous addition of EGF or TGF-α to the culture medium.[59,81] Further studies suggest a threshold level of EGF receptors must be present as a prerequisite for efficient transformation through the autocrine mechanism of interaction between TGF-α and the EGF receptor.[60] When compared to fibroblast cultured cells (Rat-1, NIH3T3, NRK) mouse mammary epithelial cell-lines express more abundant levels of EGF receptor, and are more readily transformed by overexpression of TGF-α, in accordance with the autocrine loop mechanism.[155,220] Experiments using either blocking or neutralizing antibodies to the EGF receptor or TGF-α demonstrate that autocrine stimulation by TGF-α functions in a wide variety of target cell types. Anti-EGF receptor antibodies were shown to inhibit MDA-468 human breast carcinoma cells,[65] as well as a human colorectal carcinoma cell-line,[201] and a nontumorigenic colon adenoma cell-line.[144] Alternately, anti-TGF-α neutralizing antibodies inhibit the growth of both a human mammary epithelial cell-line either transformed by c-Ha-*ras* or infected with a retroviral vector containing TGF-α,[38] and two human lung adenocarcinoma cell-lines that express both TGF-α and its receptor.[92] These reports suggest that the TGF-α/EGF receptor autocrine loop may function to provide a growth advantage to tumor cells. Conceivably, interruption of this mitogenic signal by antibody-directed therapy or biological antagonists may provide a means by which to treat certain human malignancies.

Discussion and Future Directions

The TGF-α/EGF family of ligands has been implicated in both normal and malignant cell growth. These diverse roles are mediated in part by the interaction of these ligands with the widely expressed EGF receptor. While EGF and TGF-α behave almost identically in many in vitro assays, they have different potencies in models of angiogenesis, bone remodeling, and wound repair. The existence of a TGF-α-specific receptor has been proposed as one explanation for these findings. The recent discovery of two new members of this family of growth factors, AR and HB-EGF, increases the complexity of signaling possible through the EGF receptor. AR and HB-EGF are both heparin-binding molecules and exhibit striking differences from TGF-α and EGF in certain in vitro assays. The activity and availability of both these growth factors may be modulated by secreted, membrane-bound, or extracellular matrix-associated proteoglycans. In addition, HB-EGF is 15 to 40 times more potent as a mitogen for smooth muscle cells than EGF, suggesting its involvement in atherosclerotic hyperplasia.[83] Moreover, several functional assays distinguish AR from EGF and TGF-α and suggest AR may have potential as an anticancer agent.[184,222,223] AR does not induce anchorage-independent growth of NRK cells in the presence of TGF-β, an assay that was originally used to identify and characterize TGF-α. Biochemical studies show that AR only partially competes with TGF-α or EGF for binding the EGF receptor. Furthermore, the effect of AR on the growth of tumor cells differs from that of TGF-α. In vitro studies demonstrate that AR inhibits the growth of several human epithelial carcinoma cell-lines that overexpress both TGF-α and the EGF receptor.[184,222] At similar concentrations of ligand, these cells are stimulated by EGF and TGF-α. These cell-lines represent an aggressive tumor phenotype, yet AR inhibits their growth presumably by antagonizing the proliferative effects mediated through the TGF-α/EGF receptor autocrine loop. Conceivably this inhibition could be due to AR-binding the EGF receptor and failing to transduce a proliferative signal, or through its specific interaction with a distinct receptor that signals a growth inhibitory response. Further characterization of these differences in various animal models will be crucial.

Several groups have attempted to dissect the receptor-binding and mitogenic activities of TGF-α/EGF. It is hoped that this approach might generate a clinically useful superagonist or antagonist to the EGF receptor. Alternatively, one can look for naturally produced antagonists. Precedence for this approach include: IL-1ra, an interleukin-1 receptor antagonist; Krev-1, a protein that suppresses ras-induced transformation; and inhibin, a gonadal protein that opposes the biological effects of activin. In each case the antagonist is structurally related to the mitogen, suggesting that molecular approaches (such as low stringency hybridization or use of the polymerase chain reaction with degenerate primers) to search for natural homologs of TGF-α/EGF is a valid strategy for identification of a functional antagonist.

In lieu of a true receptor antagonist, other molecules can be used to inhibit proliferation through the EGF receptor. Monoclonal anti-EGF receptor antibodies that block ligand-binding and antibody-toxin conjugates are already being tested in in vivo models. In addition, specific tyrosine kinase inhibitors might be useful for blocking this autocrine loop.

Since related ligands often bind structurally similar receptors, it has been speculated that TGF-α, EGF, AR, or HB-EGF may differentially interact with a homolog of the EGF receptor. Two additional members of the EGF receptor family have been identified, HER2/*neu* and HER3/ERBB3. These homologs of the EGF receptor remain orphan receptors since, to date, their ligands appear elusive. It seems likely that additional ligands and receptors related to these molecules remain to be discovered, but the search is complicated by the almost ubiquitous expression of the EGF receptor. However, characterization of cell types where differential effects are seen by these growth factors may lead to the identification of additional receptors, specific for certain members of the TGF-α/EGF family. In addition, high molecular weight and trans-membrane forms of these growth factors should be examined for their ability to interact with these EGF receptor homologs.

EGF receptor-induced cell proliferation is important in normal as well as tumorigenic cells. Potential clinical applications which take advantage of the effect of TGF-α/EGF molecules on stimulation of normal cell growth include healing of partial or full thickness wounds, treatment of oral mucositis, and treatment of gastrointestinal ulcers. Availability of large quantities of recombinant protein, and improved formulation and delivery systems may make such studies clinically feasible. The challenge of in vivo models arises from their complexity. For example, wound healing involves the contribution of several components: epithelization, angiogenesis, synthesis and deposition of connective tissue, fibroplasia, inflammation, and contraction. To date several growth factors have shown some efficacy at these targets including TGF-α/EGF, PDGF, fibroblast growth factor (FGF), and insulin-like growth factor-1 (IGF-1). However, each has its own strength and weakness. EGF stimulates re-epithelialization but fails to induce formation of granulation tissue. FGF and PDGF are potent angiogenic agents, but tend to stimulate fibroblasts more than ker-atinocytes leading to increased scarring. Conceivably, other mole-cules, or combination of molecules, may provide a better balance of these features, leading to optimal wound repair.

Acknowledgment: We thank Cynthia Hagen for excellent assistance in prepa-ration of this manuscript.

References

1. Adamson ED, Deller MJ, Warshaw JB. Functional EGF receptors are present on mouse embryo tissues. Nature 1981; 291:656–659.
2. Akhurst RJ, Fee F, Balmain A. Localized production of TGF-β mRNA in tumor promoter-stimulated mouse epidermis. Nature 1988; 331:363–367.

3. Almazan G, Honegger P, Matthieu JM, et al. Epidermal growth factor and bovine growth hormone stimulate differentiation and myelination of brain cell aggregates in culture. Brain Res 1985; 353:257–264.
4. Anklesaria P, Teixidó J, Laiho M, et al. Cell-cell adhesion mediated by binding of membrane-anchored transforming growth factor alpha to epidermal growth factor receptors promotes cell proliferation. Proc Natl Acad Sci USA 1990; 87:3289–3293.
5. Antonelli-Orlidge A, Saunders KB, Smith SR, et al. An activated form of transforming growth factor β is produced by cocultures of endothelial cells and pericytes. Proc Natl Acad Sci USA 1989; 86:4544–4548.
6. Antosz ME, Bellows CG, Aubin JE. Effects of transforming growth factor beta and epidermal growth factor on cell proliferation and the formation of bone nodules in isolated fetal rat calvaria cells. J Cell Physiol 1989; 140:386–395.
7. Anzano MA, Roberts AB, Meyers CA, et al. Synergistic interaction of two classes of transforming growth factors from murine sarcoma cells. Cancer Res 1982; 42:4776–4778.
8. Anzano MA, Roberts AB, Smith JM, et al. Sarcoma growth factor from conditioned medium of virally transformed cells is composed of both type alpha and type beta transforming growth factors. Proc Natl Acad Sci USA 1983; 80:6264–6268.
9. Assoian RK, Komoriya A, Meyers CA, et al. Transforming growth factor beta in human platelets—identification of a major storage site, purification, and characterization. J Biol Chem 1983; 258:7155–7160.
10. Bargmann CI, Hung MC, Weinberg RA. The _neu_ oncogene encodes an epidermal growth factor receptor-related protein. Nature 1986; 319:226–230.
11. Barnard JA, Lyons RM, Moses HL. The cell biology of transforming growth factor β. Biochim Biophys Acta 1990; 1032:79–87.
12. Barrandon Y, Green H. Cell migration is essential for sustained growth of keratinocyte colonies: The roles of transforming growth factor-alpha and epidermal growth factor. Cell 1987; 50:1131–1137.
13. Bascom C, Wolfshohl JR, Coffey RJ, et al. Complex regulation of transforming growth factor β1, β2, and β3 mRNA expression in mouse fibroblasts and keratinocytes by transforming growth factors β1 and β2. Mol Cell Biol 1989; 9:5508–5515.
14. Bates SE, Davidson NE, Valverius EM, et al. Expression of transforming growth factor alpha and its messenger ribonucleic acid in human breast cancer: Its regulation by estrogen and its possible functional significance. Mol Endocrinol 1988; 2:543–555.
15. Battegay EJ, Raines EW, Seifert RA, et al. TGF-β induces bimodal proliferation of connective tissue cells via complex control of an autocrine PDGF loop. Cell 1990; 63:515–525.
16. Bell GI, Fong NM, Stempien MM, et al. Human epidermal growth factor precursor: cDNA sequence, expression in vitro and gene organization. Nucleic Acids Res 1986; 14:8427–8446.
17. Bendell JJ, Dorrington JH. Epidermal growth factor influences growth and differentiation of rat granulosa cells. Endocrinology 1990; 127:533–540.

18. Berk BC, Brock TA, Webb RC, et al. Epidermal growth factor, a vascular smooth muscle mitogen, induces rat aortic contraction. J Clin Invest 1985; 75:1083–1086.
19. Blasband AJ, Gilligan DM, Winchell LF, et al. Expression of the TGF alpha integral membrane precursor induces transformation of NRK cells. Oncogene 1990; 5:1213–1221.
20. Blasband AJ, Rogers KT, Chen XR, et al. Characterization of the rat transforming growth factor alpha gene and identification of promoter sequences. Mol Cell Biol 1990; 10:2111–2121.
21. Boyd FT, Massagué J. Transforming growth factor-β inhibition of epithelial cell proliferation linked to the expression of a 53-kDa membrane receptor. J Biol Chem 1989; 264:2272–2278.
22. Brachmann R, Lindquist PB, Nagashima M, et al. Transmembrane TGF-alpha precursors activate EGF/TGF-alpha receptors. Cell 1989; 56:691–700.
23. Bringman TS, Lindquist PB, Derynck R. Different transforming growth factor-alpha species are derived from a glycosylated and palmitoylated transmembrane precursor. Cell 1987; 48:429–440.
24. Brown GL, Nanney LB, Griffen J, et al. Enhancement of wound healing by topical treatment with epidermal growth factor. N Engl J Med 1989; 321:76–79.
25. Brown JP, Twardzik DR, Marquardt H, et al. Vaccinia virus encodes a polypeptide homologous to epidermal growth factor and transforming growth factor. Nature 1985; 313:491–492.
26. Brunner AM, Gentry LE, Cooper JA, et al. Recombinant type 1 transforming growth factor β precursor produced in Chinese hamster ovary cells is glycosylated and phosphorylated. Mol Cell Biol 1988; 8:2229–2232.
27. Brunner AM, Marquardt H, Malacko AR, et al. Site-directed mutagenesis of cysteine residues in the pro region of the transforming growth factor β1 precursor. J Biol Chem 1989; 264:13660–13664.
28. Campbell ID, Baron M, Cooke RM, et al. Structure-function relationships in epidermal growth factor (EGF) and transforming growth factor-alpha (TGF-alpha). Biochem Pharmacol 1990; 40:35-40.
29. Carlin CR, Tollefson AE, Brady HA, et al. Epidermal growth factor receptor is down-regulated by a 10,400 MW protein encoded by the E3 region of adenovirus. Cell 1989; 57:135–144.
30. Cate RL, Mattaliano RJ, Hession C, et al. Isolation of the bovine and human genes for Mullerian inhibiting substance and expression of the human gene in animal cells. Cell 1986; 45:685-698.
31. Catterton WZ, Escobedo MB, Sexson WR, et al. Effect of epidermal growth factor on lung maturation in fetal rabbits. Pediatr Res 1979; 13:104–108.
32. Centrella M, McCarthy TL, Canalis E. Transforming growth factor β is a bifunctional regulator of replication and collagen synthesis in osteoblast-enriched cell cultures from fetal rat bone. J Biol Chem 1987; 262:2869–2874.
33. Chang W, Upton C, Hu SL, et al. The genome of Shope fibroma virus, a tumorigenic poxvirus, contains a growth factor gene with sequence similarity to those encoding epidermal growth factor and transforming growth factor alpha. Mol Cell Biol 1987; 7:535-540.

34. Cheifetz S, Andres JL, Massague J. The transforming growth factor-β receptor type III is a membrane proteoglycan. J Biol Chem 1988; 263:16984–16991.

35. Cheifetz S, Bassols A, Stanley K, et al. Heterodimeric transforming growth factor-β. Biological properties and interaction with three types of cell surface receptors. J Biol Chem 1988; 263:10783–10789.

36. Cheifetz S, Hernandez H, Laiho M, et al. Distinct transforming growth factor-β (TGF-β) receptor subsets as determinants of cellular responsiveness to three TGF-β isoforms. J Biol Chem 1990; 265:20533–20538.

37. Cheifetz S, Like B, Massagué J. Cellular distribution of type I and type II receptors for transforming growth factor-β. J Biol Chem 1986; 261:9972–9978.

38. Ciardiello F, McGeady ML, Kim N, et al. Transforming growth factor alpha expression is enhanced in human mammary epithelial cells transformed by an activated c-Ha-ras protooncogene but not by the c-neu protooncogene, and overexpression of the transforming growth factor alpha complementary DNA leads to transformation. Cell Growth Diff 1990; 1:407–420.

39. Ciccodicola A, Dono R, Obici S, et al. Molecular characterization of a gene of the 'EGF family' expressed in undifferentiated human NTERA2 teratocarcinoma cells. EMBO J 1989; 8:1987–1991.

40. Coffey R, Bascom CC, Sipes NJ, et al. Selective inhibition of growth-related gene expression in murine keratinocytes by transforming growth factor beta. Mol Cell Biol 1988; 8:3088–3093.

41. Coffey RJ Jr, Sipes NJ, Bascom CC, et al. Growth modulation of mouse keratinocytes by transforming growth factor. Cancer Res 1988; 48:1596–1602.

42. Coffey RJ Jr, Derynck R, Wilcox JN, et al. Production and auto-induction of transforming growth factor-alpha in human keratinocytes. Nature 1987; 328:817–820.

43. Coffin-Collins PA, Hall BK. Chondrogenesis of mandibular mesenchyme from the embryonic chick is inhibited by mandibular epithelium and by epidermal growth factor. Int J Dev Biol 1989; 332:297–311.

44. Cohen S. Isolation of a mouse submaxillary gland protein accelerating incisor eruption and eyelid opening in the new born animal. J Biol Chem 1962; 237:1555–1562.

45. Coleman S, Silberstein GB, Daniel CW. Ductal morphogenesis in the mouse mammary gland: Evidence supporting a role for epidermal growth factor. Dev Biol 1988; 127:304–315.

46. Cooke RM, Wilkinson AJ, Baron M, et al. The solution structure of human epidermal growth factor. Nature 1987; 327:339–341.

47. Curtsinger LJ, Pietsch JD, Brown GL, et al. Reversal of adriamycin-impaired wound healing by transforming growth factor-beta. Surg Gynecol Obstet 1989; 168:517–522.

48. De Larco JE, Todaro GJ. Growth factors from murine sarcoma virus-transformed cells. Proc Natl Acad Sci USA 1978; 75:4001-4005.

49. Defeo-Jones D, Tai JY, Wegrzyn RJ, et al. Structure-function analysis of synthetic and recombinant derivatives of transforming growth factor alpha. Mol Cell Biol 1988; 8:2999–3007.

50. DeMartin R, Haendler B, Hoefer-Warbinek R, et al. Complementary DNA for human glioblastoma-derived T cell suppressor factor, a novel member of the transforming growth factor-β gene family. EMBO J 1987; 6:3673–3677.

51. Dembinski AB, Johnson LR. Effect of epidermal growth factor on the development of rat gastric mucosa. Endocrinology 1985; 116:90–94.

52. Derynck R, Goeddel DV, Ullrich A, et al. Synthesis of messenger RNAs for transforming growth factors alpha and beta and the epidermal growth factor receptor by human tumors. Cancer Res 1987; 47:707–712.

53. Derynck R, Jarret JA, Chen EY, et al. The murine transforming growth factor-beta precursor. J Biol Chem 1986; 261:4377–4379.

54. Derynck R, Jarrett JA, Chen EY, et al. Human transforming growth factor-beta complementary DNA sequence and expression in normal and transformed cells. Nature 1985; 316:701–705.

55. Derynck R, Lindquist PB, Lee A, et al. A new type of transforming growth factor-β, TGF-β3. EMBO J 1988; 7:3737-3743.

56. Derynck R, Rhee L, Chen EY, et al. Intron-exon structure of the human transforming growth factor-β precursor gene. Nucleic Acids Res 1987; 15:3188–3189.

57. Derynck R, Roberts AB, Winkler ME, et al. Human transforming growth factor-alpha: precursor structure and expression in E. coli. Cell 1984; 38:287–297.

58. Devault A, Zollinger M, Crine P, et al. Effects of the monovalent ionophore monensin on the intracellular transport and processing of pro-opiomelanocortin in cultured intermediate lobe cells of the rat pituitary. J Biol Chem 1984; 259:5146–5151.

59. Di Fiore PP, Pierce JH, Fleming TP, et al. Overexpression of the human EGF receptor confers an EGF-dependent transformed phenotype to NIH 3T3 cells. Cell 1987; 51:1063–1070.

60. Di Marco E, Pierce JH, Fleming TP, et al. Autocrine interaction between TGF alpha and the EGF-receptor: Quantitative requirements for induction of the malignant phenotype. Oncogene 1989; 4:831–838.

61. DiCicco-Bloom E, Townes-Anderson E, Black IB. Neuroblast mitosis in dissociated culture: Regulation and relationship to differentiation. J Cell Biol 1990; 110:2073–2086.

62. Downward J, Yarden Y, Mayes E, et al. Close similarity of epidermal growth factor receptor and v-erb-B oncogene protein sequences. Nature 1984; 307:521–527.

63. Elder JT, Fisher GJ, Lindquist PB, et al. Overexpression of transforming growth factor alpha in psoriatic epidermis. Science 1989; 243:811–814.

64. Elliott JH. Epidermal growth factor: In vivo ocular studies. Trans Am Ophthalmol Soc 1980; 78:629–656.

65. Ennis BW, Valverius EM, Bates SE, et al. Anti-epidermal growth factor receptor antibodies inhibit the autocrine-stimulated growth of MDA-468 human breast cancer cells. Mol Endocrinol 1989; 3:1830–1838.

66. Fanger BO, Wakefield LM, Sporn MB. Structure and properties of the cellular receptor for transforming growth factor type beta. Biochemistry 1986; 25:3083–3091.

67. Fleming RJ, Scottgale TN, Diederich RJ, et al. The gene Serrate encodes a putative EGF-like transmembrane protein essential for proper ectodermal development in *Drosophila* melanogaster. Genes Dev 1990; 4:2188–2201.
68. Frolik CA, Dart LL, Meyers CA, et al. Purification and initial characterization of a type beta transforming growth factor from human placenta. Proc Natl Acad Sci USA 1983; 80:3676-3680.
69. Gan BS, Hollenberg MD, MacCannell KL, et al. Distinct vascular actions of epidermal growth factor-urogastrone and transforming growth factor-alpha. J Pharmacol Exp Ther 1987; 242:331–337.
70. Gansler T, Hsu WC, Gramling TS, et al. Growth factor binding and bioactivity in human kidney epithelial cell cultures. In Vitro Cell Dev Biol 1990; 26:285–299.
71. Gentry LE, Lioubin M, Purchio AF, et al. Molecular events in the processing of recombinant type 1 pre-pro-transforming growth factor beta to the mature polypeptide. Mol Cell Biol 1988; 8:4162–4168.
72. Gentry LE, Nash BW. The pro domain of pre-pro-transforming growth factor β1 when independently expressed is a functional binding protein for the mature growth factor. Biochemistry 1990; 29:6851–6857.
73. Gentry LE, Twardzik DR, Lim GJ, et al. Expression and characterization of transforming growth factor alpha precursor protein in transfected mammalian cells. Mol Cell Biol 1987; 7:1585–1591.
74. Gentry LE, Webb NR, Lim GJ, et al. Type 1 transforming growth factor-beta: Amplified expression and secretion of mature and precursor polypeptides in Chinese hamster ovary cells. Mol Cell Biol 1987; 7:3418–3427.
75. Goey H, Keller JR, Back T, et al. Inhibition of early murine hemopoietic progenitor cell proliferation after in vivo locoregional administration of transforming growth factor-β1. J Immunol 1989; 143:877–880.
76. Gray A, Dull TJ, Ullrich A. Nucleotide sequence of epidermal growth factor cDNA predicts a 128,000-molecular weight protein precursor. Nature 1983; 303:722–725.
77. Graycar JL, Miller DA, Arrick BA, et al. Human transforming growth factor-β3: Recombinant expression, purification, and biological activities in comparison with transforming growth factors-β1 and -β2. Mol Endo 1989; 3:1977–1989.
78. Grotendorst GR, Soma Y, Takehara K, et al. EGF and TGF-alpha are potent chemoattractants for endothelial cells and EGF-like peptides are present at sites of tissue regeneration. J Cell Physiol 1989; 139:617–623.
79. Han VK, D'Ercole AJ, Lee DC. Expression of transforming growth factor alpha during development. Can J Physiol Pharmacol 1988; 66:1113–1121.
80. Hanks SK, Armour R, Baldwin JH, et al. Amino acid sequence of BSC-1 cell growth inhibitor (Polyergin) deduced from the nucleotide sequence of the cDNA. Proc Natl Acad Sci USA 1988; 85:79–82.
81. Heidaran MA, Fleming TP, Bottaro DP, et al. Transformation of NIH3T3 fibroblasts by an expression vector for the human epidermal growth factor precursor. Oncogene 1990; 5:1265–1270.
82. Heim S, Békassy AN, Garwicz S, et al. New structural chromosomal rearrangements in congenital leukemia. Leukemia 1987; 1:16–23.

83. Higashiyama S, Abraham JA, Miller J, et al. A heparin-binding growth factor secreted by macrophage-like cells that is related to EGF. Science 1991; 251:936–939.

84. Hoffmann B, Piasecki A, Paul D. Proliferation of fetal rat hepatocytes in response to growth factors and hormones in primary culture. J Cell Physiol 1989; 139:654–662.

85. Hollstein MC, Smits AM, Galiana C, et al. Amplification of epidermal growth factor receptor gene but no evidence of ras mutations in primary human esophageal cancers. Cancer Res 1988; 48:5119–5123.

86. Howe PH, Cunningham MR, Leof EB. Distinct pathways regulate transforming growth factor β1-stimulated proto-oncogene and extracellular matrix gene expression. J Cell Physiol 1990; 142:39–45.

87. Howe PH, Cunningham MR, Leof EB. Inhibition of mink lung epithelial cell proliferation by transforming growth factor-β is coupled through a pertussis-toxin-sensitive substrate. Biochem J 1990; 266:537–543.

88. Huang H-JS, Yee J-K, Shew J-Y, et al. Suppression of the neoplastic phenotype by replacement of the RB gene in human cancer cells. Science 1988; 242:1563–1566.

89. Ibbotson KJ, Twardzik DR, D'Souza SM, et al. Stimulation of bone resorption in vitro by synthetic transforming growth factor-alpha. Science 1985; 228:1007–1009.

90. Ignotz RA, Massague J. Transforming growth factor-β stimulates the expression of fibronectin and collagen and their incorporation into the extracellular matrix. J Biol Chem 1986; 261:4337–4345.

91. Ikeda T, Lioubin MN, Marquardt H. Human transforming growth factor type β2: Production by a prostatic adenocarcinoma cell line, purification, and initial characterization. Biochemistry 1987; 26:2406–2410.

92. Imanishi K, Yamaguchi K, Kuranami M, et al. Inhibition of growth of human lung adenocarcinoma cell lines by anti-transforming growth factor-alpha monoclonal antibody. J Natl Cancer Inst 1989; 81:220–223.

93. Jakowlew SB, Dillard PJ, Kondaiah J, et al. Complementary deoxyribonucleic acid cloning of a messenger ribonucleic acid encoding transforming growth factor beta 4 from chicken embryo chondrocytes. Mol Endocrinol 1988; 2:1064–1069.

94. Jakowlew SB, Dillard PJ, Kondaiah P, et al. Complementary deoxyribonucleic acid cloning of a novel transforming growth factor-beta messenger ribonucleic acid from chick embryo chondrocytes. Mol Endocrinol 1988; 2:747–755.

95. Jennings JC, Mohan S. Heterogeneity of latent transforming growth factor-β isolated from bone matrix proteins. Endocrinol 1990; 126:1014–1021.

96. Jhappan C, Stahle C, Harkins RN, et al. TGF alpha overexpression in transgenic mice induces liver neoplasia and abnormal development of the mammary gland and pancreas. Cell 1990; 61:1137–1146.

97. Joyce ME, Roberts AB, Sporn MB, et al. Transforming growth factor-β and the initiation of chondrogenesis and osteogenesis in the rat femur. J Cell Biol 1990; 110:2195–2207.

98. Kanzaki T, Olofsson A, Moren A, et al. TGF-β1 binding protein: A component of the large latent complex of TGF-β1 with multiple repeat sequences. Cell 1990; 61:1051–1061.

99. Kaplan PL, Topp WC, Ozanne B. Simian virus 40 induces the production of a polypeptide transforming factor(s). Virology 1981; 108:484–490.
100. Kasid A, Bell GI, Director EP. Effects of transforming growth factor-beta on human lymphokine-activated killer cell precursors. Autocrine inhibition of cellular proliferation and differentiation of immune killer cells. J Immunol 1988; 141:690-698.
101. Kehrl JH, Roberts AB, Wakefield LM, et al. Transforming growth factor β is an important immunomodulatory protein for human B-lymphocytes. J Immunol 1987; 137:3855–3860.
102. Keski-Oja J, Postlethwaite AE, Moses HL. Transforming growth factors in the regulation of malignant cell growth and invasion. Cancer Invest 1988; 6:705–724.
103. Kidd S, Kelley MR, Young MW. Sequence of the notch locus of *Drosophila* melanogaster: Relationship of the encoded protein to mammalian clotting and growth factors. Mol Cell Biol 1986; 6:3094–3108.
104. Kim S-J, Glick A, Sporn MB, et al. Characterization of the promoter region of the human transforming growth factor-β1 gene. J Biol Chem 1989; 264:402–408.
105. Kim S-J, Jeang K-T, Glick A, et al. Promoter sequences of the human transforming growth factor-β1 gene responsive to transforming growth factor-β1 autoinduction. J Biol Chem 1989; 264:7041–7045.
106. Kimchi A, Wang X-F, Weinberg RA, et al. Absence of TGF-β receptors and growth inhibitory responses in retinoblastoma cells. Science 1988; 240:196–199.
107. Kimura H, Fischer WH, Schubert D. Structure, expression and function of a schwannoma-derived growth factor. Nature 1990; 348:257–260.
108. Knudson AG Jr. Mutation and cancer: statistical study of retinoblastoma. Proc Natl Acad Sci USA 1971; 68:820–823.
109. Kondaiah P, Sands MJ, Smith JM, et al. Identification of a novel transforming growth factor-β (TGF-β5) mRNA in xenopus laevis. J Biol Chem 1990; 265:1089–1093.
110. Kondaiah P, Van Obberghen-Schilling E, Ludwig RL, et al. cDNA cloning of porcine transforming growth factor-β mRNAs. Evidence for alternate splicing and polyadenylation. J Biol Chem 1988; 263:18313–18317.
111. Kovacina KS, Steele-Perkins G, Purchio AF, et al. Interactions of recombinant and platelet transforming growth factor-β1 precursor with the insulin-like growth factor II/mannose-6-phosphate receptor. Biochem Biophys Res Commun 1989; 160:393–403.
112. Kudlow JE, Kobrin MS, Purchio AF, et al. Ovarian transforming growth factor-alpha gene expression: Immunohistochemical localization to the theca-interstitial cells. Endocrinology 1987; 121:1577–1579.
113. Kurachi H, Okamoto S, Oka T. Evidence for the involvement of the submandibular gland epidermal growth factor in mouse mammary tumorigenesis. Proc Natl Acad Sci USA 1985; 82:5940–5943.
114. Lafyatis R, Lechleider R, Kim S-J, et al. Structural and functional characterization of the transforming growth factor β3 promoter. J Biol Chem 1990; 265:19128–19131.
115. Laiho M, DeCaprio JA, Ludlow JW, et al. Growth inhibition by TGF-β

linked to suppression of retinoblastoma protein phosphorylation. Cell 1990; 62:175–185.

116. Laiho M, Weis FMB, Massagué J. Concomitant loss of transforming growth factor (TGF)-β receptor types I and II in TGF-β-resistant cell mutants implicates both receptor types in signal transduction. J Biol Chem 1990; 265:18518–18524.

117. Lasky LA, Singer MS, Yednock TA, et al. Cloning of a lymphocyte homing receptor reveals a lectin domain. Cell 1989; 56:1045–1055.

118. Lawrence DA, Pircher R, Jullien P. Conversion of a high molecular weight latent TGF-β from chicken embryo fibroblasts into a low molecular weight active TGF-β under acidic conditions. Biochem Biophys Res Commun 1985; 133:1026–1034.

119. Lax I, Burgess WH, Bellot F, et al. Localization of a major receptor-binding domain for epidermal growth factor by affinity labeling. Mol Cell Biol 1988; 8:1831–1834.

120. Lax I, Johnson A, Howk R, et al. Chicken epidermal growth factor (EGF) receptor: cDNA cloning, expression in mouse cells, and differential binding of EGF and transforming growth factor alpha. Mol Cell Biol 1988; 8:1970–1978.

121. Lazar E, Watanabe S, Dalton S, et al. Transforming growth factor alpha: Mutation of aspartic acid 47 and leucine 48 results in different biological activities. Mol Cell Biol 1988; 8:1247-1252.

122. Lee DC, Rochford R, Todaro GJ, et al. Developmental expression of rat transforming growth factor-alpha mRNA. Mol Cell Biol 1985; 5:3644–3646.

123. Lee DC, Rose TM, Webb NR, et al. Cloning and sequence analysis of a cDNA for rat transforming growth factor-alpha. Nature 1985; 313:489–491.

124. Lee EY-HP, To H, Shew J-Y, et al. Inactivation of the retinoblastoma susceptibility gene in human breast cancers. Science 1988; 241:218–221.

125. Lee W-H, Bookstein R, Lee EY-HP. Molecular biology of a human retinoblastoma gene. In: Immunology Series 51: Tumor Suppressor Genes, Klein G, ed. New York, Dekker, 1990; pp. 169-200.

126. Lee W-H, Shew J-Y, Hong FD, et al. Human retinoblastoma susceptibility gene: Cloning, identification, and sequence. Science 1987; 235:1394–1399.

127. Levine L, Hassid A. Epidermal growth factor stimulates prostaglandin biosynthesis by canine kidney (MDCK) cells. Biochem Biophys Res Commun 1977; 76:1181–1187.

128. Libby J, Martinez R, Weber MJ. Tyrosine phosphorylation in cells treated with transforming growth factor-β. J Cell Physiol 1986; 129:159–166.

129. Libermann TA, Nusbaum HR, Razon N, et al. Amplification, enhanced expression and possible rearrangement of EGF receptor gene in primary human brain tumours of glial origin. Nature 1985; 313:144–147.

130. Lintern-Moore S, Moore GP, Panaretto BA, et al. Follicular development in the neonatal mouse ovary; effect of epidermal growth factor. Acta Endocrinol (Copenh) 1981; 96:123–126.

131. Lioubin MN, Madisen L, Marquardt H, et al. Characterization of latent recombinant TGF-β2 produced by Chinese hamster ovary cells. J Cell Biochem 1991; 45:112–121.

132. Lioubin MN, Madisen L, Roth R, et al. Characterization of latent TGF-β2 from monkey kidney cells. Endocrinol 1991; 128:2291–2296.

133. Liu SC, Sanfilippo B, Perroteau I, et al. Expression of transforming growth factor alpha (TGF alpha) in differentiated rat mammary tumors: Estrogen induction of TGF alpha production. Mol Endocrinol 1987; 1:683–692.

134. Ludlow JW, Shon J, Pipas JM, et al. The retinoblastoma susceptibility gene product undergoes cell cycle-dependent dephosphorylation and binding to and release from SV40 large T. Cell 1990; 60:387–396.

135. Lupu R, Colomer R, Zugmaier G, et al. Direct interaction of a ligand for the *erb*B2 oncogene product with the EGF receptor and p185*erb*B2. Science 1990; 249:1552–1555.

136. Lyons RM, Gentry LE, Purchio AF, et al. Mechanism of activation of latent recombinant transforming growth factor β1 by plasmin. J Cell Biol 1990; 110:1361–1367.

137. Lyons RM, Keski-Oja J, Moses HL. Proteolytic activation of latent transforming growth factor-β from fibroblast-conditioned medium. J Cell Biol 1988; 106:1659–1665.

138. Madisen L, Farrand AL, Lioubin MN, et al. Expression and characterizaton of recombinant TGF-β2 proteins produced in mammalian cells. DNA 1989; 8:205–212.

139. Madisen L, Lioubin MN, Farrand AL, et al. Analysis of proteolytic cleavage of recombinant TGF-β1: Production of hybrid molecules with increased processing efficiency. *Transforming Growth Factor-βs* Chemistry, Biology, and Therapeutics. Ann NY Acad Sci 1990; 593:7–24.

140. Madisen L, Lioubin MN, Marquardt H, et al. High-level expression of TGF-β2 and the TGF-β2(414) precursor in Chinese hamster ovary cells. Growth Factors 1990; 3:129–138.

141. Madisen L, Webb NR, Rose TM, et al. Transforming growth factor-β2: cDNA cloning and sequence analysis. DNA 1988; 7:1-8.

142. Madtes DK, Raines EW, Sakariassen KS, et al. Induction of transforming growth factor-alpha in activated human alveolar macrophages. Cell 1988; 53:285–293.

143. Malipiero U, Höller M, Werner U, et al. Sequence analysis of the promoter region of the glioblastoma derived T cell suppressor factor/transforming growth (TGF)-β2 gene reveals striking differences to the TGF-β1 and -β3 genes. Biochem Biophys Res Commun 1990; 171:1145–1151.

144. Markowitz SD, Molkentin K, Gerbic C, et al. Growth stimulation by coexpression of transforming growth factor-alpha and epidermal growth factor-receptor in normal and adenomatous human colon epithelium. J Clin Invest 1990; 86:356–362.

145. Marquardt H, Hunkapiller MW, Hood LE, et al. Transforming growth factors produced by retrovirus-transformed rodent fibroblasts and human melanoma cells: Amino acid sequence homology with epidermal growth factor. Proc Natl Acad Sci USA 1983; 80:4684–4688.

146. Marquardt H, Hunkapiller MW, Hood LE, et al. Rat transforming growth factor type 1: Structure and relation to epidermal growth factor. Science 1984; 223:1079–1082.

147. Marquardt H, Lioubin MN, Ikeda T. Complete amino acid sequence of human transforming growth factor type β2. J Biol Chem 1987; 262:12127–12131.
148. Martin P, Vass WC, Schiller JT, et al. The bovine papillomavirus E5 transforming protein can stimulate the transforming activity of EGF and CSF-1 receptors. Cell 1989; 59:21–32.
149. Mason AJ, Hayflick JS, Ling N, et al. Complementary DNA sequences of ovarian follicular fluid inhibin show precursor structure and homology with transforming growth factor-beta. Nature 1985; 318:659–663.
150. Massagué J, Like B. Cellular receptors for type beta transforming growth factor. J Biol Chem 1985; 260:2636–2645.
151. Massagué J. The transforming growth factor-β family. Annu Rev Cell Biol 1990; 6:597–641.
152. Massagué J. Transforming growth factor alpha. A model for membrane anchored growth factors. J Biol Chem 1990; 265:21393-21396.
153. Matsui Y, Halter SA, Holt JT, et al. Development of mammary hyperplasia and neoplasia in MMTV-TGF alpha transgenic mice. Cell 1990; 61:1147–1155.
154. McDonald BJ, Waters MJ, Richards MD, et al. Effect of epidermal growth factor on wool fibre morphology and skin histology. Res Vet Sci 1983; 35:91–99.
155. McGeady ML, Kerby S, Shankar V, et al. Infection with a TGF-alpha retroviral vector transforms normal mouse mammary epithelial cells but not normal rat fibroblasts. Oncogene 1989; 4:1375–1382.
156. Mead JE, Fausto N. Transforming growth factor alpha may be a physiological regulator of liver regeneration by means of an autocrine mechanism. Proc Natl Acad Sci USA 1989; 86:1558-1562.
157. Mellman I, Fuchs R, Helenius A. Acidification of the endocytic and exocytic pathways. Annu Rev Biochem 1986; 55:663-700.
158. Miyazono K, Heldin C-H. Role for carbohydrate structures in TGF-β1 latency. Nature 1989; 338:158–160.
159. Miyazono K, Hellman U, Wernstedt C, et al. Latent high molecular weight complex of transforming growth factor β1. J Biol Chem 1988; 263:6407–6415.
160. Montelione GT, Winkler ME, Burton LE, et al. Sequence-specific 'H-NMR assignments and identification of two small antiparallel beta-sheets in the solution structure of recombinant human transforming growth factor alpha. Proc Natl Acad Sci USA 1989; 86:1519–1523.
161. Morrison RS, Kornblum HI, Leslie FM, et al. Trophic stimulation of cultured neurons from neonatal rat brain by epidermal growth factor. Science 1987; 238:72–75.
162. Muldoon LL, Rodland KD, Magun BE. Transforming growth factor β modulates epidermal growth factor-induced phosphoinositide metabolism and intracellular calcium levels. J Biol Chem 1988; 263:5030–5033.
163. Muller WJ, Sinn E, Pattengale PK, et al. Single-step induction of mammary adenocarcinoma in transgenic mice bearing the activated c-neu oncogene. Cell 1988; 54:105–115.
164. Murthy US, Anzano MA, Stadel JM, et al. Coupling of TGF-β-induced

mitogenesis to G-protein activation in AKR-2B cells. Biochem Biophys Res Commun 1988; 152:1228–1235.

165. Mustoe TA, Landes A, Cromack DT, et al. Differential acceleration of healing of surface incisions in the rabbit gastrointestinal tract by platelet-derived growth factor and transforming growth factor, type beta. Surgery 1990; 108:324-330.

166. Mustoe TA, Pierce GF, Thomason A, et al. Accelerated healing of incisional wounds in rats induced by transforming growth factor-β. Science 1987; 237:1333–1335.

167. Mydlo JH, Michaeli J, Cordon-Cardo C, et al. Expression of transforming growth factor alpha and epidermal growth factor receptor messenger RNA in neoplastic and nonneoplastic human kidney tissue. Cancer Res 1989; 49:3407–3411.

168. Myrdal SE, Auersperg N. An agent or agents produced by virus-transformed cells cause unregulated ruffling in untransformed cells. J Cell Biol 1986; 102:1224–1229.

169. Neal DE, Sharples L, Smith K, et al. The epidermal growth factor receptor and the prognosis of bladder cancer. Cancer 1990; 65:1619–1625.

170. Nelson KG, Takahashi T, Bossert NL, et al. Epidermal growth factor replaces estrogen in the stimulation of female genital-tract growth and differentiation. Proc Natl Acad Sci USA 1991; 88:21–25.

171. Nilsen-Hamilton M. Transforming growth factor-β and its actions on cellular growth and differentiation. Curr Top Dev Biol 1990; 24:95–136.

172. Noda M, Camilliere JJ. In vivo stimulation of bone formation by transforming growth factor-β. Endocrinology 1989; 124:2991-2995.

173. Oka Y, Orth DN. Human plasma epidermal growth factor/beta-urogastrone is associated with blood platelets. J Clin Invest 1983; 72:249–259.

174. Okada F, Yamaguchi K, Ichihara A, et al. Purification and structural analysis of a latent form of transforming growth factor-β from rat platelets. J Biochem 1989; 106:304–310.

175. Okamoto S, Oka T. Evidence for physiological function of epidermal growth factor: Pregestational sialoadenectomy of mice decreases milk production and increases offspring mortality during lactation period. Proc Natl Acad Sci USA 1984; 81:6059-6063.

176. Opleta K, O'Loughlin EV, Shaffer EA, et al. Effect of epidermal growth factor on growth and postnatal development of the rabbit liver. Am J Physiol 1987; 253:G622-G626.

177. Oreffo ROC, Mundy GR, Seyedin SM, et al. Activation of the bone-derived latent TGF beta complex by isolated osteoclasts. Biochem Biophys Res Commun 1989; 158:817–823.

178. Ozanne B, Fulton RJ, Kaplan PL. Kirsten murine sarcoma virus trans-formed cell lines and a spontaneously transformed rat cell-line produce transforming factors. J Cell Physiol 1980; 105:163-180.

179. Pierce GF, Mustoe TA, Lingelbach J, et al. Transforming growth factor β reverses the glucocorticoid-induced wound healing deficit in rats: Possible regulation in macrophages by platelet-derived growth factor. Proc Natl Acad Sci USA 1989; 86:2229–2233.

180. Pietenpol JA, Holt JT, Stein RW, et al. TGFβ1 suppression of c-*myc* gene transcription: Role in inhibition of keratinocyte proliferation. Proc Natl Acad Sci USA 1990; 87:3758-3763.

181. Pietenpol JA, Stein RW, Moran E, et al. TGF-β1 inhibition of c-*myc* transcription and growth in keratinocytes is abrogated by viral transforming proteins with pRB binding domains. Cell 1990; 61:777-785.

182. Pircher R, Lawrence DA, Jullien P. Latent β-transforming growth factor in nontransformed and Kirsten sarcoma virus-transformed normal rat kidney cells, clone 49F. Cancer Res 1984; 44:5538-5543.

183. Pittelkow MR, Shipley GD. Serum-free culture of normal human melanocytes: Growth kinetics and growth factor requirements. J Cell Physiol 1989; 140:565-576.

184. Plowman GD, Green JM, McDonald VL, et al. The amphiregulin gene encodes a novel epidermal growth factor-related protein with tumor-inhibitory activity. Mol Cell Biol 1990; 10:1969-1981.

185. Plowman GD, Whitney GS, Neubauer MG, et al. Molecular cloning and expression of an additional epidermal growth factor receptor-related gene. Proc Natl Acad Sci USA 1990; 87:4905-4909.

186. Popliker M, Shatz A, Avivi A, et al. Onset of endogenous synthesis of epidermal growth factor in neonatal mice. Dev Biol 1987; 119:38-44.

187. Press RD, Misra A, Gillaspy G, et al. Control of the expression of c-*sis* mRNA in human glioblastoma cells by phorbol ester and transforming growth factorβ1. Cancer Res 1989; 49:2914-2920.

188. Purchio AF, Cooper JA, Brunner AM, et al. Identification of mannose-6-phosphate in two asparagine-linked sugar chains of recombinant transforming growth factor-β1 precursor. J Biol Chem 1988; 263:14211-14215.

189. Radford HM, Avenell JA, Panaretto BA. Some effects of epidermal growth factor on reproductive function in Merino sheep. J Reprod Fertil 1987; 80:113-118.

190. Rall LB, Scott J, Bell GI, et al. Mouse prepro-epidermal growth factor synthesis by the kidney and other tissues. Nature 1985; 313:228-231.

191. Ranchalis JE, Gentry L, Agawa Y, et al. Bone-derived recombinant transforming growth factor βs are potent inhibitors of tumor cell growth. Biochem Biophys Res Commun 1987; 148:783-789.

192. Rappolee DA, Brenner CA, Schultz R, et al. Developmental expression of PDGF, TGF-alpha, and TGF-beta genes in preimplantation mouse embryos. Science 1988; 241:1823-1825.

193. Rees AR, Adamson ED, Graham CF. Epidermal growth factor receptors increase during the differentiation of embryonal carcinoma cells. Nature 1979; 281:309-311.

194. Reiss M, Dibble CL. Reinitiation of DNA synthesis in quiescent mouse keratinocytes; regulation by polypeptide hormones, cholera toxin, dexamethasone and retinoic acid. In Vitro Cell Dev Biol 1988; 24:537-544.

195. Rhodes JA, Tam JP, Finke U, et al. Transforming growth factor alpha inhibits secretion of gastric acid. Proc Natl Acad Sci USA 1986; 83:3844-3846.

196. Rizzino A. Appearance of high affinity receptors for type β transforming growth factor during differentiation of murine embryonal carcinoma cells. Cancer Res 1987; 47:4386-4390.

197. Roberts AB, Anzano MA, Lamb LC, et al. Isolation from murine sarcoma cells of novel transforming growth factors potentiated by EGF. Nature 1982; 295:417–419.

198. Roberts AB, Anzano MA, Lamb LC, et al. New class of transforming growth factors potentiated by epidermal growth factor: Isolation from non-neoplastic tissues. Proc Natl Acad Sci USA 1981; 78:5339–5343.

199. Roberts AB, Anzano MA, Wakefield LM, et al. Type beta transforming growth factor: A bifunctional regulator of cellular growth. Proc Natl Acad Sci USA 1985; 82:119–123.

200. Roberts AB, Sporn MB. The transforming growth factor-βs. In: Peptide Growth Factors and Their Receptors I, Sporn MB, Roberts AB, eds. Berlin, Springer-Verlag, 1990; pp. 417–472.

201. Rodeck U, Herlyn M, Herlyn D, et al. Tumor growth modulation by a monoclonal antibody to the epidermal growth factor receptor: Immunologically mediated and effector cell-independent effects. Cancer Res 1987; 47:3692–3696.

202. Rogers SA, Purchio AF, Hammerman MR. Mannose 6-phosphate-containing peptides activate phospholipase C in proximal tubular basolateral membranes from canine kidney. J Biol Chem 1990; 265:9722–9727.

203. Rosenthal A, Lindquist PB, Bringman TS, et al. Expression in rat fibroblasts of a human transforming growth factor-alpha cDNA results in transformation. Cell 1986; 46:301–309.

204. Sainsbury JR, Farndon JR, Needham GK, et al. Epidermal-growth-factor receptor status as predictor of early recurrence of and death from breast cancer. Lancet 1987; 1:1398–1402.

205. Saji M, Taga M, Minaguchi H. Epidermal growth factor stimulates cell proliferation and inhibits prolactin secretion of the human decidual cells in culture. Endocrinol Jpn 1990; 37:177-182.

206. Salomon DS, Perroteau I, Kidwell WR, et al. Loss of growth responsiveness to epidermal growth factor and enhanced production of alpha-transforming growth factors in ras-transformed mouse mammary epithelial cells. J Cell Physiol 1987; 130:397-409.

207. Samsoondar J, Kobrin MS, Kudlow JE. Alpha-transforming growth factor secreted by untransformed bovine anterior pituitary cells in culture. I. Purification from conditioned medium. J Biol Chem 1986; 261:14408–14413.

208. Sandgren EP, Luetteke NC, Palmiter RD, et al. Overexpression of TGF alpha in transgenic mice: Induction of epithelial hyperplasia, pancreatic metaplasia, and carcinoma of the breast. Cell 1990; 61:1121–1135.

209. Sato Y, Tsuboi R, Lyons R, et al. Characterization of the activation of latent TGF-β by co-cultures of endothelial cells and pericytes or smooth muscle cells: A self-regulating system. J Cell Biol 1990; 111:757–763.

210. Savage CR Jr, Inagami T, Cohen S. The primary structure of epidermal growth factor. J Biol Chem 1972; 247:7612–7621.

211. Schneyer CA, Humphreys-Beher M. Effects of epidermal growth factor and nerve growth factor on isoproterenol-induced DNA synthesis in rat parotid and pancreas following removal of submandibular-sublingual glands. J Oral Pathol 1988; 17:250-256.

212. Schreiber AB, Winkler ME, Derynck R. Transforming growth factor-

alpha: a more potent angiogenic mediator than epidermal growth factor. Science 1986; 232:1250–1253.

213. Schultz GS, White M, Mitchell R, et al. Epithelial wound healing enhanced by transforming growth factor-alpha and vaccinia growth factor. Science 1987; 235:350–352.

214. Scott J, Urdea M, Quiroga M, et al. Structure of a mouse submaxillary messenger RNA encoding epidermal growth factor and seven related proteins. Science 1983; 221:236–240.

215. Segarini PR, Rosen DM, Seyedin SM. Binding of TGF-β to cell surface proteins varies with cell type. Mol Endocrinol 1989; 3:261–272.

216. Segarini PR, Seyedin SM. The high molecular weight receptor to transforming growth factor-β contains glycosaminoglycan chains. J Biol Chem 1988; 263:8366–8730.

217. Seyedin SM, Segarini PR, Rosen DM, et al. Cartilage inducing factor-β is a unique protein structurally and functionally related to transforming growth factor-beta. J Biol Chem 1987; 262:1946–1949.

218. Seyedin SM, Thompason AY, Bentz H, et al. Cartilage-inducing factor-A: Apparent identity to transforming growth factor-beta. J Biol Chem 1986; 261:5693–5695.

219. Sha X, Brunner AM, Purchio AF, et al. Transforming growth factor β1: Importance of glycosylation and acidic proteases for processing and secretion. Mol Endo 1989; 3:1090–1098.

220. Shankar V, Ciardiello F, Kim N, et al. Transformation of an established mouse mammary epithelial cell line following transfection with a human transforming growth factor alpha cDNA. Mol Carcinog 1989; 2:1–11.

221. Sharples K, Plowman GD, Rose TM, et al. Cloning and sequence analysis of simian transforming growth factor-beta cDNA. DNA 1987; 6:239–244.

222. Shoyab M, McDonald VL, Bradley JG, et al. Amphiregulin: A bifunctional growth-modulating glycoprotein produced by the phorbol 12-myristate 13-acetate-treated human breast adenocarcinoma cell line MCF-7. Proc Natl Acad Sci USA 1988; 85:6528–6532.

223. Shoyab M, Plowman GD, McDonald VL, et al. Structure and function of human amphiregulin: A member of the epidermal growth factor family. Science 1989; 243:1074–1076.

224. Sjvholm A, Welsh N, Sandler S, et al. Role of polyamines in mitogenic and secretory responses of pancreatic beta-cells to growth factors. Am J Physiol 1990; 259:C828-C833.

225. Skinner MK, Takacs K, Coffey RJ. Transforming growth factor-alpha gene expression and action in the seminiferous tubule: Peritubular cell-Sertoli cell interactions. Endocrinology 1989; 124:845–854.

226. Slamon DJ, Clark GM, Wong SG, et al. Human breast cancer: Correlation of relapse and survival with amplification of the HER-2/*neu* oncogene. Science 1987; 235:177–182.

227. Slamon DJ, Godolphin W, Jones LA, et al. Studies of the HER-2/*neu* proto-oncogene in human breast and ovarian cancer. Science 1989; 244:707–712.

228. Smith JJ, Derynck R, Korc M. Production of transforming growth factor alpha in human pancreatic cancer cells: Evidence for a superagonist autocrine cycle. Proc Natl Acad Sci USA 1987; 84:7567–7570.

229. Smith JM, Sporn MB, Roberts AB, et al. Human transforming growth factor-alpha causes precocious eyelid opening in newborn mice. Nature 1985; 315:515–516.

230. Spencer SJ, Rabinovici J, Jaffe RB. Human recombinant activin-A inhibits proliferation of human fetal adrenal cells in vitro. J Clin Endocrinol Metab 1990; 71:1678–1680.

231. Sporn MB, Roberts AB, Wakefield LM, et al. Transforming growth factor-β: Biological function and chemical structure. Science 1986; 233:532–534.

232. Sporn MB, Roberts AB. Transforming growth factor-β: Multiple actions and potential clinical applications. JAMA 1989; 262:938–941.

233. Stern PH, Krieger NS, Nissenson RA, et al. Human transforming growth factor-alpha stimulates bone resorption in vitro. J Clin Invest 1985; 76:2016–2019.

234. Sundell HW, Gray ME, Serenius FS, et al. Effects of epidermal growth factor on lung maturation in fetal lambs. Am J Pathol 1980; 100:707–725.

235. Taub M, Wang Y, Szczesny TM, et al. Epidermal growth factor or transforming growth factor alpha is required for kidney tubulogenesis in matrigel cultures in serum-free medium. Proc Natl Acad Sci USA 1990; 87:4002–4006.

236. Teixidó J, Gilmore R, Lee DC, et al. Integral membrane glycoprotein properties of the prohormone pro-transforming growth factor-alpha. Nature 1987; 326:883–885.

237. Ten Dijke P, Iwata KK, Goddard C, et al. Recombinant transforming growth factor type β3: Biological activities and receptor-binding properties in isolated bone cells. Mol Cell Biol 1990; 10:4473–4481.

238. Ten-Dijke P, Hansen P, Iwata KK, et al. Identification of another member of the transforming growth factor type β gene family. Proc Natl Acad Sci USA 1988; 85:4715–4719.

239. Tepass U, Theres C, Knust E. Crumbs encodes an EGF-like protein expressed on apical membranes of *Drosophila* epithelial cells and required for organization of epithelia. Cell 1990; 61:787–799.

240. Todaro GJ, Fryling C, De Larco JE. Transforming growth factors produced by certain human tumor cells: Polypeptides that interact with epidermal growth factor receptors. Proc Natl Acad Sci USA 1980;77:5258–5262.

241. Tomooka Y, DiAugustine RP, McLachlan JA. Proliferation of mouse uterine epithelial cells in vitro. Endocrinology 1986; 118:1011–1018.

242. Tricoli JV, Nakai H, Byers MG, et al. The gene for human transforming growth factor alpha is on the short arm of chromosome 2. Cytogenet Cell Genet 1986; 42:94–98.

243. Tsuji T, Okada F, Yamaguchi K, et al. Molecular cloning of the large subunit of transforming growth factor type β masking protein and expression of the mRNA in various rat tissues. Proc Natl Acad Sci USA 1990; 87:8835–8839.

244. Tsutsumi O, Kurachi H, Oka T. A physiological role of epidermal growth factor in male reproductive function. Science 1986; 233:975–977.

245. Tsutsumi O, Oka T. Epidermal growth factor deficiency during pregnancy causes abortion in mice. Am J Obstet Gynecol 1987; 156:241–244.

246. Tsutsumi O, Tsutsumi A, Oka T. Epidermal growth factor-like, corneal

wound healing substance in mouse tears. J Clin Invest 1988; 81:1067–1071.

247. Tucker RF, Branum EL, Shipley GD, et al. Specific binding to cultured cells of ^{125}I-labeled type β transforming growth factor from human platelets. Proc Natl Acad Sci USA 1984; 81:6757–6761.

248. Tucker RF, Shipley GD, Moses HL, et al. Growth inhibitor from BSC-1 cells closely related to platelet type beta transforming growth factor. Science 1984; 226:705–707.

249. Twardzik DR, Brown JP, Ranchalis JE, et al. Vaccinia virus-infected cells release a novel polypeptide functionally related to transforming and epidermal growth factors. Proc Natl Acad Sci USA 1985; 82:5300–5304.

250. Ullrich A, Coussens L, Hayflick JS, et al. Human epidermal growth factor receptor cDNA sequence and aberrant expression of the amplified gene in A431 epidermoid carcinoma cells. Nature 1984; 309:418–425.

251. Ullrich A, Schlessinger J. Signal transduction by receptors with tyrosine kinase activity. Cell 1990; 61:203–212.

252. Upton C, Macen JL, McFadden G. Mapping and sequencing of a gene from myxoma virus that is related to those encoding epidermal growth factor and transforming growth factor alpha. J Virol 1987; 61:1271–1275.

253. Van Obberghen-Schilling E, Kondaiah P, Ludwig RL, et al. Complementary deoxyribonucleic acid cloning of bovine transforming growth factor-β1. Mol Endocrinol 1987; 1:693-699.

254. Van Obberghen-Schilling E, Roche NS, Flanders KC, et al. Transforming growth factor β1 positively regulates its own expression in normal and transformed cells. J Biol Chem 1988; 263:496–539.

255. Veale D, Ashcroft T, Marsh C, et al. Epidermal growth factor receptors in non-small cell lung cancer. Br J Cancer 1987; 55:513–516.

256. Velu TJ. Structure, function and transforming potential of the epidermal growth factor receptor. Mol Cell Endocrinol 1990; 70:205–216.

257. vonFigura K, Hasilik A. Lysosomal enzymes and their receptors. Ann Rev Biochem 1986; 55:167–193.

258. Wahl SM, Hunt DA, Wong HL, et al. Transforming growth factor-β is a potent immunosuppressive agent that inhibits IL-1-dependent lymphocyte proliferation. J Immunol 1988; 140:3026-3032.

259. Wakefield LM, Smith DM, Broz S, et al. Recombinant TGF-β1 is synthesized as a two-component latent complex that shares some structural features with the native platelet latent TGF-β1 complex. Growth Factors 1989; 1:203–218.

260. Wakefield LM, Smith DM, Flanders KC, et al. Latent transforming growth factor-β from human platelets. J Biol Chem 1988; 263:7646–7654.

261. Watanabe S, Lazar E, Sporn MB. Transformation of normal rat kidney (NRK) cells by an infectious retrovirus carrying a synthetic rat type alpha transforming growth factor gene. Proc Natl Acad Sci USA 1987; 84:1258–1262.

262. Webb NR, Madisen L, Rose TM, et al. Structural and sequence analysis of TGF-β2 cDNA clones predicts two different precursor proteins produced by alternative mRNA splicing. DNA 1988; 7:493-497.

263. Wilcox JN, Derynck R. Developmental expression of transforming

growth factors alpha and beta in mouse fetus. Mol Cell Biol 1988; 8:3415–3422.

264. Wilcox JN, Derynck R. Localization of cells synthesizing transforming growth factor-alpha mRNA in the mouse brain. J Neurosci 1988; 8:1901–1904.

265. Winkler ME, O'Connor L, Winget M, et al. Epidermal growth factor and transforming growth factor alpha bind differently to the epidermal growth factor receptor. Biochemistry 1989; 28:6373-6378.

266. Wong ST, Winchell LF, McCune BK, et al. The TGF-alpha precursor expressed on the cell surface binds to the EGF receptor on adjacent cells, leading to signal transduction. Cell 1989; 56:495–506.

267. Wrann M, Bodmer S, DeMartin R, et al. T cell suppressor factor from human glioblastoma cells is a 12.5-kd protein closely related to transforming growth factor-beta. EMBO J 1987; 6:1633-1636.

268. Wright NA, Pike C, Elia G. Induction of a novel epidermal growth factor-secreting cell lineage by mucosal ulceration in human gastrointestinal stem cells. Nature 1990; 343:82–85.

269. Yamamoto T, Hihara H, Nishida T, et al. A new avian erythroblastosis virus, AEV-H, carries erbB gene responsible for the induction of both erythroblastosis and sarcomas. Cell 1983; 34:225–232.

270. Yamazaki H, Fukui Y, Ueyama Y, et al. Amplification of the structurally and functionally altered epidermal growth factor receptor gene (c-erbB) in human brain tumors. Mol Cell Biol 1988; 8:1816–1820.

271. Yamazaki H, Ohba Y, Tamaoki N, et al. A deletion mutation within the ligand binding domain is responsible for activation of epidermal growth factor receptor gene in human brain tumors. Jpn J Cancer Res 1990; 81:773–779.

272. Yasui W, Hata J, Yokozaki H, et al. Interaction between epidermal growth factor and its receptor in progression of human gastric carcinoma. Int J Cancer 1988; 41:211–217.

273. Yeh YC, Tsai JF, Chuang LY, et al. Elevation of transforming growth factor alpha and its relationship to the epidermal growth factor and alpha-fetoprotein levels in patients with hepatocellular carcinoma. Cancer Res 1987; 47:896–901.

274. Yochem J, Greenwald I. glp-1 and lin-12, genes implicated in distinct cell-cell interactions in C. elegans, encode similar transmembrane proteins. Cell 1989; 58:553–563.

275. Yoshida K, Kyo E, Tsuda T, et al. EGF and TGF-alpha, the ligands of hyperproduced EGFR in human esophageal carcinoma cells, act as autocrine growth factors. Int J Cancer 1990; 45:131–135.

276. Yoshida K, Tsujino T, Yasui W, et al. Induction of growth factor-receptor and metalloproteinase genes by epidermal growth factor and/or transforming growth factor-alpha in human gastric carcinoma cell line MKN-28. Jpn J Cancer Res 1990; 81:793–798.

277. Zabel BU, Eddy RL, Lalley PA, et al. Chromosomal locations of the human and mouse genes for precursors of epidermal growth factor and the beta subunit of nerve growth factor. Proc Natl Acad Sci USA 1985; 82:469–473.

278. Zajchowski D, Band V, Pauzie N, et al. Expression of growth factors and oncogenes in normal and tumor-derived human mammary epithelial cells. Cancer Res 1988; 48:7041–7047.
279. Zaragoza R, Battle-Tracy KM, Owen NE. Heparin inhibits Na(+)-H+ exchange in vascular smooth muscle cells. Am J Physiol 1990; 258:46–53.
280. Zerek-Meen G, Lewinski A, Szkudlinski M. Influence of somatostatin and epidermal growth factor (EGF) on the proliferation of thyroid follicular cells in organ culture. Regul Pept 1990; 28:293–300.

Chapter 8

Transcription Factors

Pramod Sutrave

In recent years transcription factors have gained a wide interest in the field of molecular biology. This is because of the unusual characteristics of these factors which are essentially proteins of a wide variety of types ranging from oncogene products to determinants of tissue-specific regulation of gene expression.[41,67,71,121] This chapter is intended to provide a general overview and to explain the basic concepts in the ever-growing field of transcription factors.

In simple terms, transcription can be defined as the process of synthesis of RNA from a DNA template. Several different elements are involved in transcription and its regulation, ranging from enzymes and other specific proteins that bind to discrete DNA segments. Three different DNA dependent RNA polymerases are involved in the eukaryotic transcription: RNA polymerase I (pol I, pol A), II (pol II, pol B), and III (pol III). RNA pol I transcribes the ribosomal pre-RNA, while pol III transcribes the small RNA molecules or transfer RNA (tRNA). RNA pol II, on the other hand, is the enzyme that is involved in synthesis of divergent mRNAs after the formation of specific complexes with a variety of proteins termed transcription factors. Transcription is initiated by the formation of a preinitiation complex. This complex involves the interaction of RNA pol II and several different proteins. There are multiple proteins that interact with RNA pol II and the TATA box to form a preinitiation complex.[59,76,91,101] This complex also controls the basal transcription of a gene. These proteins include TFIIA, TFIIB,

The contents of this chapter do not necessarily reflect the views or policies of the Department of Health and Human Services, nor does mention of trade names, commercial products, or organizations imply endorsement by the U.S. Government.

From *The Molecular Basis of Human Cancer:* edited by B. Neel, M.D., Ph.D., R. Kumar, Ph.D. © 1993, Futura Publishing Co. Inc., Mount Kisco, NY.

TFIID, TFIIE, TFIIF, TFIIG, and TFIIH. Some of these have been purified and used for in vitro experiments aimed at the definition of their roles and possible functions.[33,76,101] The intricacies of the preinitiation complex at the transcription start site will not be discussed here. The role of TFIID, a protein that has been shown to interact with specific transcription factors, will be described briefly.[32] These transcriptional factors have unique structural and functional requirements. In addition to the transcription initiation site, there are regions of short conserved sequences with which specific transcriptional factors interact, resulting in the up- or down-regulation of gene expression. These unique sequences are described in the literature as enhancers or activators and are located upstream, downstream, or in the intronic sequences of a gene.[80]

Structure of Transcription Factors

Most known transcription factors can be classified into one of the structural categories described below.[35,104] The three-dimensional shape of the proteins which constitute the transcriptional activation or inactivation domain is extremely important in determining the function of a protein. Any alteration in these domains—either by mutation, deletion, or truncation—has a significant effect on the function of the protein. It is for this reason that these domains have been very well conserved in the course of evolution from prokaryotes to higher eukaryotes. These structural motifs may either directly interact with DNA sequences or may indirectly influence DNA protein interaction. X-ray crystallographic studies and mutational analyses of some of these proteins have contributed significantly to elucidating these structures in detail.

Zinc Fingers

The first eukaryotic transcription factor that was purified to homogeneity from *Xenopus* oocytes was TFIIIA. This protein is one of the transcription components for the expression of the ribosomal 5S RNA gene, and it also serves as a storage protein for the newly synthesized 5S RNA. This abundant protein was easily purified to homogeneity and its biochemical properties were readily analyzed. The specific interaction of this protein with DNA depends on the presence of zinc ions. During subsequent characterization of the protein through the isolation of cDNAs, a part of the protein identified as the zinc finger domains common to many different transcription factors. In this domain, a systematic arrangement of cysteines and histidines is observed; the spacing of Cys and His residues is such that the Cys-His pairs serve as a tetrahedral coordination site for a single zinc ion and the amino acids located between the Cys-His project out as fingers. This general motif was described as a zinc finger, having Cys-X4-Cys-X12-His-X3/4-His, where X is any amino acid (Fig. 1A).

A large number of proteins have been discovered from diverse species that have zinc finger motifs.[23,52] However, the structure of the zinc finger in different proteins can vary, and variations in both the spacing of the amino acids as well as in the Cys-His combinations in the motif have been observed (Fig. 1B). The most commonly observed change was in the receptors for the steroid hormones. Instead of the Cys-His combination, the receptors had four Cys residues that coordinated the zinc ion. The DNA-binding domains of the steroid hormone receptors contain two putative zinc fingers where the spacing of the amino acids between the Cys is not conserved and, also, the two fingers were not identical. However, the four amino acids interacting with zinc are either Cys or His. A further variant was discovered with the characterization of Gal 4 protein, a transcriptional activator from yeast. Gal 4 protein has a DNA-binding domain in the amino terminus where the Cys residues are spaced at regular intervals. Several proteins that interact with zinc and have no structural similarity to the canonical zinc finger proteins are termed zinc cluster proteins.[114] These include a number of other proteins that have Cys and His spaced at specific intervals. A Cys-x2-Cys-x17–19-His-x2-Cys-x2-Cys-x2-Cys-x1–7-11-Cys-x8-Cys motif is found in homeodomain proteins,[29,50] while a Cys-x1–4-Cys-x11–30-Cys-x-His-FIL-Cys-x2-Cys-ILM-x10–18-Cys-P-x-Cys domain has been found in a wide variety of proteins.[28] Another novel Cys-rich region is found in the *ski/sno* oncogene products identified from chicken and human sources. These proteins, which have a distinct array of Cys-His, have not yet been shown to bind zinc, nor has their DNA-binding activity been proven to be dependent on zinc ions, as has been shown for the Gal 4 protein of yeast. However, mutational and domain-swapping analyses of most of the zinc finger proteins have demonstrated that some of the zinc fingers may not directly interact with the target sequences but can cause structural changes that will disrupt the subsequent interaction of the active domain.[46,87,88] For example, specific amino acid changes in finger 1 will change the specificity from GRE to ERE.[46] A chimeric receptor having finger 1 of GRE and finger 2 of TRE loses the spacer requirement characteristic of TRE. GRE binds

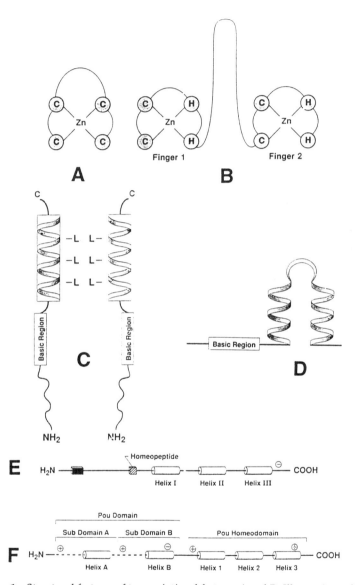

Figure 1. *Structural features of transcriptional factors. A and B: Illustrations of zinc finger domains of transcription factors TFIIIa and steroid hormone receptors. C: Leucine zipper containing factors showing the helical regions for dimerization followed by the basic region (DNA-binding). D: A simplistic structure of bHLH proteins showing the helix loop helix region and the basic region. E and F: Homeodomain and Pou/homeodomain factors showing various regions of the protein.*

to its target sequence as a dimer which is lost in the chimeric receptor, suggesting that finger 2 is essential for protein-protein interaction.[88]

Leucine Zippers

Although the sequence and the amino acid composition of the *fos*, *jun*, and *myc* proto-oncogene products were well known, it was only recently when the sequence of the transcriptional factor CAAT enhancer-binding protein (C/EBP) was described that a new domain in these proteins was identified.[13,53,68] C/EBP is a liver-specific transcriptional activator and has a region of structural homology with the *fos* and *jun* transforming proteins. In the newly discovered domain, the leucine zipper, leucine is repeated at every seventh position in a stretch of 35 to 40 amino acids. Just preceding the leucines is a cluster of basic amino acids. In the original model proposed by McKnight's group, the heptad stretch of leucines form an α-helical structure and could form stable dimers through what is now recognized as the leucine zippers (Fig. 1C). It was originally thought that the two α helices associate in an antiparallel fashion so that the basic domain that is known to interact with the DNA is on the opposite side of the leucine zipper. A scissor-grip model,[115] which is not very different from the coiled coil model proposed by O'Shea et al.,[82] is now widely accepted.[1] In the coiled coil model, the zipper regions associate in parallel in a fashion similar to that described for the fibrous proteins, keratin, lamins, and myosins. While the structure of the leucine zippers was being described, the mutational analyses of the specific regions confirmed the function of the two defined regions in this class of proteins. Mutations in the leucines of the zipper region prevented dimerization, suggesting that it is essential for protein-protein interaction. Modification in the basic domain prevents DNA-binding but does not interfere with dimerization. Further analyses have shown that the most conserved amino acids (Arg-Lys) in the basic domain are the DNA contact residues. Domain-swapping experiments in the basic region or the leucine zipper region suggested that the specificity of the DNA recognition or the homo- or heterodimerization capability of a particular protein can be altered. For example, *fos* proteins do not form homodimers, while GCN 4 protein, a transcriptional activator from yeast, readily forms homodimers. Exchanging the leucine zipper domain of *fos* with that of GCN 4 led to the formation of *fos* homodimers, suggesting that the leucine zippers do direct the homo-

or heterodimerization potential of a protein.[5] However, it is not known how, within a cell where there are a number of proteins that have leucine zippers, a particular protein forms a functional hetero-dimer with its active partner. It is possible that there are regions in each leucine zipper protein that determine this specific interaction. Most leucine zipper proteins are called basic-zipper (bZIP) proteins and are found in prokaryotes and eukaryotes.[110]

Helix Turn Helix

Most prokaryotic transcriptional regulatory proteins belong to the helix turn helix (HTH) group. The prokaryotic system provided the first and best characterized motif for the DNA-binding, the HTH.[10] Structural and X-ray crystallographic analyses of the cro and cI proteins of bacteriophage lambda and the catabolite activator protein of E coli defined a unique structure for the above proteins. These proteins have an α helix, then a β turn, and finally an α helix as the structural motif. Of the two helices, the second helix in the HTH has been considered the recognition helix. The region occupies the major groove and makes contacts with specific DNA sequences. The amino acids, numbers 1, 2, and 5, of this helix are important for sequence recognition. Mutations in these amino acids abolishes or decreases the transcriptional activation function of the protein. Further, most prokaryotic HTH proteins bind to palindromic DNA sequences as dimers, as opposed to similar HTH motifs found in homeodomain proteins (see below).

Helix Loop Helix

Helix loop helix (bHLH) is a major group of transcriptional proteins that have been discovered recently, and the family is rapidly expanding. Structurally, these proteins have two amphipathic helices separated by a variable region of 9 to 20 bases.[77] Unlike the HTH proteins, the bHLH proteins use the helical domain for dimerization and interact with DNA through a basic amino acid region which usually is located just upstream of the first helix and are commonly referred to as bHLH proteins (Fig. 1D).[42,77] They have gained a wide interest in the field of developmental biology since similar structural motifs were found in the muscle regulatory proteins (MyoD, myogenin, *myf5* and *mrf4* or herculin), in proteins involved in the development of the nervous system in *Drosophila*,[77,81] and immunoglobulin enhancer-binding proteins such as E12 and E47. A bHLH domain has also been identified in the *myc* oncoprotein. Like the bZIP proteins, the bHLH proteins form homo- or heterodimers. Dimerization is mediated through the hydrophobic interactions of the α helices, and the adjacent basic region interacts with the DNA. However, variants of the bHLH proteins have recently been discovered. These proteins have the bHLH portion but lack the basic amino acid region so that the protein can form dimers but cannot interact with the DNA. These variant proteins could act as negative regulators by titrating out the effector or positive regulator by forming heterodimers. A clear understanding of the expression of these proteins during growth or differentiation will be critical to the understanding of the functions of the positive and the negative regulators.

Homeodomain

Homeotic genes, as the name suggests, are the regulators of homeosis or the patterns of development.[8,20,57] A number of homeotic genes were first defined in *Drosophila* and subsequently isolated and characterized.[122] It was observed that most homeotic genes have conserved short stretches of DNA sequence (about 150 to 200 bp), which was initially called the homeobox and is now commonly referred to as the homeodomain. Structurally (Fig. 1E), most homeodomain proteins have a conserved amino-terminal region that in some proteins extends to 45 amino acids and is followed by a variable region. A small stretch of conserved amino acids, called the homeopeptide, lies between the homeodomain and the variable region. The carboxy-terminal end of the homeoproteins usually has acidic amino acids. The structure of the homeobox is not very different from the HTH proteins except that the homeobox has a third α-helical region and a fourth helical region very closely associated with the third helix in Antennapedia (Antp) protein. The sequences in the third helix are conserved like the first two helices and are considered to be the DNA recognition helix.

The homeodomain proteins bind to specific DNA sequences in vitro. However, unlike the prokaryotic HTH regulatory proteins, the HTH of homeodomain interacts with DNA as a monomer. Reasonably so, within given species, the third and fourth helical sequences are highly conserved.[30] The conserved amino acids and their interaction in the major groove have been analyzed by crystallographic studies.[56] The DNA-binding specificity has also been assessed by altering specific amino acids. For example, the *bicoid* (bcd) homeodomain protein has lysine in the recognition helix, while the Antp protein, a slightly modified version of this structure, has glutamine at a similar site. Mutating the amino acid from one to another changes the DNA-binding capacity of the proteins. This is in contrast to the prokaryotic HTH where different amino acids form the crucial recognition site. Sequences outside the DNA recognition helix also determine the specificity of interaction within families that have identical sequences in the recognition helix. This has been analyzed by homeobox swapping and deletion of the specific segments outside the homeobox region. Most of the homeobox proteins are thought to be transcription regulatory. A comprehensive view of the structure and DNA-binding specificity of homeodomain has recently been published.[18]

Pou/Homeodomain

These proteins were originally identified as octamer-binding proteins. The name "Pou" was defined after finding sequence homeology in three mammalian transcription factors and one nematode regulatory protein (Pit-1/GHF-1, Oct-1, oct-2, and Unc-56).[25,36,90,92,93] Subsequently, several other members of this family were identified and characterized. In most of these proteins, two distinct regions were commonly observed: 1) a N-terminal Pou domain followed by, 2) a Pou-specific homeodomain which is structurally not very different from the prototype homeodomain described above.

The 80-amino acid Pou-specific domain can be subdivided into two subdomains, A and B, as shown in Figure 1F. Both subdomains terminate with a sequence that presumably forms a helix. A cluster of basic amino acids is commonly seen upstream of the two helices, A and B, which possibly serve in high affinity DNA-binding by the Pou proteins. A cluster of acidic amino acids are located near both ends of the Pou domain. A poorly conserved 14 to 15 amino acid segment separates the Pou's domain from the 60-amino acid Pou homeodomain.

The Pou homeodomain consists of three helical regions with helix

2 and 3 forming the HTH motif. A stretch of basic amino acids upstream of helix 1 and the helix 3 are very well conserved. The third helix is the DNA recognition helix like most other HTH containing proteins. Functional analysis indicates that the Pou-specific domain is required for high affinity DNA-binding and also functions as low affinity-binding with relaxed specificity, and also protein-protein interactions. Disruption of the predicted first helix (helix A) in the Pou domain and helix in the Pou homeodomain abolishes the DNA-binding. Disruption of other helical regions does not seem to affect the DNA-binding function of the Pou homeodomain proteins.[97] Recently, a variant of the Pou homeodomain protein has been identified. This protein forms heterodimers with a specific cellular counterpart protein which prevents its biological function of transcription activation and is called inhibitor Pou (I-Pou).[112] Structurally, the protein is identical to other Pou homeodomain proteins except that it lacks two basic amino acids from the cluster of basic amino acids at the amino-terminus of the first helix in the Pou homeodomain region. The inhibition function of the proteins could very well be developmentally regulated, and remain to be further characterized.

Unclassified Structures

Liver-specific transcription factor HNF1 defines another form of homeodomain structure.[64] This protein is structurally related to the homeodomain proteins but has an unusual insertion of about 21 amino acids between the second and third helices. Although the function of this insert is not fully understood, since it is in the homeodomain, it is likely to be involved in specific interaction with either DNA or other cellular proteins. A second unusual feature of this protein is the presence of a dimerization motif in the amino-terminus which is similar to the myosin dimerization domain. Another unclassified domain is serine/threonine-proline-XX (S/TPXX), which is found commonly in proteins that bind DNA and regulate gene expression that includes homeotic gene products, segmentation gene products, steroid hormone receptors, and nuclear oncogene products (*myc, ski*).[107] The significance of these motifs is not clearly defined or understood. However, cell cycle dependent phosphorylation of these motifs in several proteins (Histone H1, H5) abolishes the DNA-binding activity of these proteins.[108,109] Further characterization of this motif and its role in gene expression is needed.

Action of Transcription Factors

Even though the transcription factors can be classified on the basis of their structure into three or four major groups, they can be classified into two groups on the basis of their function. The function may be activation or repression of transcription and will be discussed in the next section.

Direct Acting

This group of factors consists of proteins that do not need any intermediary modification for their action. The homeodomain proteins are a good example of this group.[57] It has been known that the homeodomain proteins can activate or repress transcription after directly interacting with the specific target sequences as monomers. Similarly, the Pou homeodomain proteins oct1 and oct2 can activate transcription after interacting with identical target octamer sequences. Oct1 is ubiquitously expressed, while Oct2 expression is restricted to the cells of lymphoid origin.[74,96] Oct2 interacts with the octamer-binding site and activates transcription of the immunoglobulin genes in B cells. Oct1, though expressed in every cell type, cannot activate gene expression from the immunoglobulin locus in non-B cells, suggesting that it must be activated or modified in order to be transcriptionally active.[118]

Some members of the zinc finger proteins can activate transcription without the help of other interactions. The Gal 4 gene product, which is a positive regulator of gene expression of galactose metabolism in yeast, activates transcription through its acidic carboxy-terminal domain. Another ubiquitously expressed transcription factor, SP1, has a glutamine-rich region as the activating domain in its carboxy-terminal. It was initially thought that the steroid hormone receptors (members of the zinc finger family of proteins) activate transcription on binding of the hormone.[4] Now there is growing evidence that these proteins are dimerized in order to be transcriptionally active.[98] An unclassified DNA-binding domain is found in CTF (CCAAT-binding transcription factor), and this protein has a proline-rich sequence at the carboxy-terminus that dictates the transcriptional activation domain. Most of the proteins described above can activate transcription without active association with other cellular factors and can be considered as direct acting.

Indirect Acting

This second group of transcription factors needs some kind of modification or interaction with other cellular factors in order to be active. The bZIP proteins are transcriptional activators that depend on dimerization. The best example is the interaction between the *fos* and *jun* oncogene products. The *jun* products can homodimerize and bind to their target sequences TGACTA (AP1 site) and activate transcription. The protein product of the *fos* gene cannot form homodimers but can form heterodimers with the *jun* proteins and can bind to the same AP1 site to activate transcription.[3,13,126] Similar examples are seen with the proteins that contain the bHLH domains. The *myc* oncogene protein has a bHLH domain followed by a bZIP-related region at the carboxy-terminus. Homodimers of the *myc* protein have been proposed, but heterodimers with other HLH proteins such as the E12, E47, and recently discovered *max/myn* are more readily formed. This dimerized complex then interacts with the common sequences identified for the bHLH proteins (CAXXTG or E box). Interaction of *myc* with *max-myn* seems to activate the transcription potential of the *myc* protein. This is because the heterodimer binds to the E box sequence with higher affinity than does either protein alone.[9,84]

These examples depend on the presence or absence of a cofactor in the cell and the effect of its association or dissociation to be transcriptionally active or inactive. Other possible mechanisms involved in activation are posttranslational modifications such as phosphorylation. cAMP response element-binding (CREB) protein is one of the best studied examples of a transcriptional factor that needs a posttranslational modification.[124] The protein belongs to the bZIP family and, by in vitro mutagenesis experiments, has been shown to bind to the target sequence only upon phosphorylation. Dephosphorylated forms exist as monomers and are inactive. CREB protein is activated by phosphorylation at a single site by protein kinase A without changing the DNA-binding affinity. The recently described inhibitory protein (IP) protein also must be dephosphorylated in order to be functionally active in repressing *fos-jun* function. The yeast gene SW15 product is essential for mating type switching.[103] The protein has zinc finger and undergoes a unique type of activation/inactivation process. It has been proposed that during cell cycle, the protein is phosphorylated and shuttled to the nucleus.[78] This is very much identical to the general transcription factors identified as nuclear factor kB (NFkB). The NFkB protein is held in the cytoplasm by inhibitor of kB (IkB) protein. Upon proper stimulus, the IkB gets phosphorylated, leading to the release of NFkB which is then transported to the nucleus.

Functions of Transcription Factors

It seems quite rhetorical to ask "what is the function of the transcription factors?" The presumed answer is that they activate transcription of specific genes. But then this is not always true, because there are many examples where these factors have been shown to be involved in repression of transcription. Here we will examine how different transcription factors activate or repress transcription through a few well-documented examples which have been reviewed recently.[85,86] But before we do that, let us remember that any transcription factor will have two major domains: a DNA-binding domain for the factor to bind to the specific target sequences, and a second domain to interact with the positive- or negative-acting cellular factors to activate or repress transcription.

Activation of Transcription

We have already, in brief, seen that the transcription activators interact directly or indirectly with DNA and active transcription. The Gal 4 protein involved in the regulation of yeast galactose metabolism system has been the most commonly used protein for studying the transcriptional activators. The amino-terminal region Gal 4 consists of a zinc cluster that recognizes the target sequences, whereas the acidic carboxy-terminus activates transcription.[105] In yeast, when the cells are growing in medium lacking galactose, the Gal 4 protein is inactive. This is through the interaction of the Gal 4 protein with the Gal 80 gene product, which suppresses the Gal 4 function. Upon growing cells in the galactose medium, the complex is dissociated and the Gal 4 protein activates the transcription of genes necessary for galactose utilization. The DNA-binding domain of the Gal 4 protein is well defined, and has been used to identify other proteins with transcriptional activation function. In these experiments, the sequences of the test protein are fused to the DNA-binding region of Gal 4. This chimeric protein is tested for transcription activation from the Gal 4-binding site. On the basis of such chimeric constructs, several different activating domains have been discovered. This approach has permitted the identification of the activation domains of transcriptional activators such as VP16, E1a, and Sp1 proteins.[17,65]

Herpesvirus protein VP16 has an acidic domain but lacks the DNA-binding domain. In mammalian cells, VP16 activates transcription only in cells that express another transcription factor, Oct1, which is an octomer-binding protein having a DNA-binding domain but no activation domain.[86] The VP16 protein and Oct1 together can have a DNA-binding domain and an acidic activation domain. This interacting complex thus becomes a positive regulator of gene expression. On further characterization of the chimeric Gal 4-VP16 protein, it was revealed that the complex can interact with the TFIIB and TFIID protein of the preinitiation complex. The experiments suggest that the acidic domain of a transcription factor can recognize the TFIID protein bound to the promoter. Therefore, when the Gal-VP16 fusion protein is overexpressed, a decrease in the cellular concentration of the TFIID protein may be observed. Such protein interaction can occur in the cytoplasm, and depletion of the essential transcription factor TFIID could result in the repression of other genes that require TFIID for transcription. Indeed, this was observed, and the process of removing the effector protein by these interactions has been termed squelching (Fig. 2).

The adenovirus E1a protein can activate as well as repress transcription, but has neither the specific DNA-binding domain nor the acidic activator domain described above.[24] How does this protein activate transcription? This is likely to be mediated through protein-protein interaction. If this is true, then one part of the E1a protein should interact with a protein(s) that can recognize a specific DNA sequence, and the other part of the E1a protein should interact with a protein that can activate transcription. It has been shown that the E1a protein interacts with sequence-specific DNA-binding transcription factors, ATF and Sp1.[119] Other proteins that can interact with the E1a protein are currently being characterized. Since the E1a protein has been known to activate or repress gene expression, it is possible that the second type of interaction could involve many different target proteins. Some experiments have been reported which indicate that the second protein does not have an acidic domain like that of the VP16 protein. Other experiments suggest that the contact point for both the E1a and VP16 proteins is the transcription factor TFIID, indicating that the TFIID protein is multifocal in nature.

Transcriptional activation by the steroid hormones introduces a

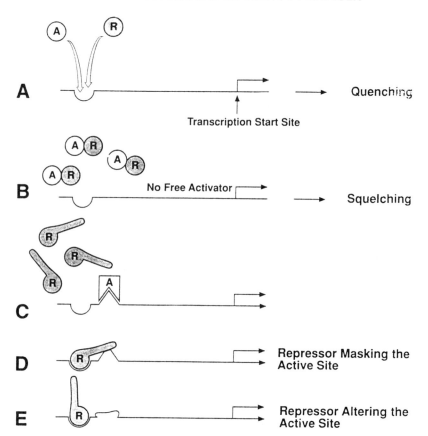

Figure 2. *Various interactions of activator (A) and repressor (R) proteins at the promoter/enhancer region of a gene. A: Competition for the same binding site. B: Physical association between the activator and repressor resulting in suppression of gene expression. C: Normal interaction of the activator protein that may be altered by binding of the repressor protein as shown below (D and E). D: Interaction of repressor resulting in masking of activator site or E: Modification of the activator site down-regulates gene expression.*

novel feature of synergism.[4,120] The strength of the steroid hormone response unit (HRU) is determined by both the receptor- and adjacent nonreceptor-binding sites. The best transcriptional activation is observed with two HRUs and other sequence-specific binding sites such as those of NFI, SpI, OctI, etc. How exactly the synergistic activation takes place is not fully understood.[34,75] Recent experimental evidence suggests that the progesterone and glucocorticoid receptors (GR) bound to HRU facilitate the binding of OTF-1 to the octamer motif in the MMTV promoter.[11]

Repression of Transcription

Transcription factors can mediate repression of expression.[39,43,58,61,89] We have already discussed the EIa protein as an activator or a repressor. There are multiple ways through which the repression can be brought about. Different models for the repression function have been proposed and some are shown in Figure 2. Two proteins, the activator and the repressor, can bind to the same target site or to adjacent nonoverlapping DNA sequences.[12,95] Analysis of the proliferin promoter suggests that the GR-binding might block the *fos-jun* from gaining access to its target sequence in the promoter. This is because the GR-binding site overlaps a cryptic AP1-binding site. Analogous to the above example is the response of osteoclastin gene promoter. The promoter is activated by a retinoic acid receptor and inactivated by AP1. The binding site for the two factors overlap, resulting in opposite effects on gene expression.[98] This is defined as quenching, which is different from the squelching described above. It is also possible that the repressor may directly bind to a sequence and interfere with the interaction of other transcription factors at the preinitiation complex by changing the conformation of the target DNA sequence. This has been observed for the members of steroid hormone receptors. For the steric hindrance mechanism of suppression of gene expression, the DNA-binding domain of the steroid receptor is necessary. However, another mechanism of repression has been described where the DNA-binding domain is not required. In this type of repression, addition of hormone leads to activation of the receptor and inactivation of some of the cellular transcription factors.[75,98] Two well-documented examples are glucocorticoid repression of the collagenase gene through inactivation of the transcription factor API and repression of the prolactin gene by the estrogen receptor through interaction with the pituitary transcription factor (pitI).

Another mode of repression that is currently receiving close attention is mediated through proteins with antitranscription function.[70] The first such gene product to be identified is the Id protein, which is a counterpart of MyoD, a muscle-specific protein.[7] MyoD belongs to the bHLH type of protein and interacts with the DNA through its basic amino acid region. Id protein is structurally similar to MyoD except that it lacks the basic amino acid region. A heterodimer between the MyoD and Id proteins inhibits the DNA-binding property of MyoD and suppresses its function. Other than the bHLH proteins, similar inhibitory proteins have been identified for the homeodomain protein, Cf1. Cf1 is a Pou homeodomain protein and is involved in a complex pattern of gene expression through the interaction of specific sequences. Recently, another protein was described, I-Pou, which forms a heterodimer with the Cf1 protein.[112] The I-Pou domain lacks the basic amino acids that are responsible for the interaction with the target sequences. Thus, a heterodimer of Cf1 and I-Pou inhibits the normal function of the Cf1 protein. A recently identified IP2 protein specifically blocks the *fos/jun*-induced transcription. The IP protein may be working as an antagonist through dimer formation with *fos* or *jun*. However, this remains to be proven.

Activation and Repression

While some proteins can only act as either activators or repressors of gene expression, there are proteins that have both functions.[38,47,48,125] The steroid hormone receptors and the E1a protein functioning as activators and repressors are well described. The inhibitory effect of GR on proliferin gene expression is through suppression of the cryptic Ap1 binding site. However, this effect depends on the presence or absence of cellular transcription factors. In the presence of c-*jun*, the GR asserts a positive effect. When both *fos* and *jun* are present, the GR shows a negative hormone dependent transcriptional regulation. Another set of proteins that can function in both directions are the homeodomain proteins. The most intriguing characteristic of the homeodomain proteins is their ability to recognize different target sequences.[100] This ability may be regulated by different protein interactions. Ultrabiothorax (Ubx) protein suppresses the basal activity of the Antp promoter that contains multiple Ubx-binding sites but at the same time activates its own promoter with similar sites. The *Drosophila* gap gene product, *Kruppel*, belongs to a member of the zinc family of proteins and can function both as a negative and positive regulation of transcription.[51,83,127] The protein seems to function as an activator at low concentratons and, on the same binding site, functions as a repressor at high concentrations.

These two functional activities have been mapped to different portions of the protein, indicating that other specific protein-protein interactions determine the functionality of the protein. Another zinc finger protein gene, *hunchback*, has been characterized by transient expression analyses. Like the *Kruppel* gene, the *hunchback* gene functions in a dose response fashion. Understanding these mechanisms and the role they play in the activation or repression of gene expression will be the focal point of transcription studies in years to come.

Specificity of Transcription Factors

It is clear that specific transcription factors can act and interact in different ways. Transcription factors regulate many target genes, and their own expression must be regulated by other factors. The homeodomain proteins can both autoregulate and also transregulate expression of other homeodomain proteins.[100] Some of these examples are described below. The product of *fos* gene can activate transcription on heterodimerization with the *jun* product through the AP1 recognition site. The same AP1 site is also found in the promoter of the *fos* gene. However, the *fos-jun* heterodimer does not activate transcription of the c-*fos* gene. This suggests that there is a specific interplay of various transcription factors.

Tissue-Specific Expression of Transcription Factors

Tissue-specific expression of the transcription factors in liver and brain has been well documented.[40,55,106,123] HNF1, C/EBP, and DBP are examples of the liver-specific transcription factors.[111] Apart from the most prominent tissue (liver), some of these proteins are also expressed in a few other tissues. HNF1 is also expressed in the kidney, stomach, and intestine, while C/EBP message is also found in the kidney, lung, and intestine. It has been commonly observed that the genes that are specifically expressed in the liver are also expressed in few other tissues.[64] It is possible that gene expression may be under an identical program in different tissues, but functionally the proteins may be active only in the target tissue. How different factors interact with the same target sequences is not fully understood. The functional activity in the target tissue could be specified by other interacting factors. Muscle-specific transcription factors such as MyoD, myogenin, etc., are expressed in muscle tissue, and their expression is stage-specific during development and differentiation.[81,94] The expression of the homeotic genes is the most tightly controlled during different stages of development. Any perturbations in their expression could be lethal. Nonspecific expression (i.e., expression of the gene in other than the normal tissue) could also lead to tumorigenesis.[16,116] Expression of growth hormone genes in the somatotrophic cells of the anterior pituitary is controlled by the growth hormone factor GHF1, also called Pit1. GHF1 or Pit1 expression is observed just two to three days prior to the expression of the growth hormone gene.[49] It would be interesting to determine how this tissue- or development-specific gene expression is regulated.[54]

Sequence Elements That Determine Specificity

Though not a perfect answer, a solution to this question is the presence of specific regulatory elements.[26,27,113] There are two types of regulatory elements that control transcription initiation by RNA pol II: promoters and enhancers.[21,22,73] There is not a major difference between these two types of elements, except that the promoter sequences are found near the TATA box and include the CAAT box. Both promoter and enhancer elements are stretches of 6 to 10 bp DNA sequences which are the targets for the binding of specific transcription factors. While the promoter sequences can act only in *cis* and only when in close proximity to the transcription preinitiation complex, the enhancer elements can be located far from the transcription start site and have also been shown to act in *trans* (although under artificial conditions). The enhancer elements have been located up to about 20 kb upstream of the transcription start site. Also, the promoter elements are restricted to the transcription start site, whereas the enhancer elements can be found either upstream, within introns or exons, or even downstream from the gene. Both promoter and enhancer sequences are regulated in a tissue- and development-specific manner. The liver-specific albumin promoter illustrates some of the characteristics described above. While it can be suggested that the transcription factors interacting at the promoter have an effect on the initiation of transcription, the effect of enhancers and enhancer-binding transcription factors located 5 to 15 kb upstream of the transcription start site cannot be easily explained. Two different models have been proposed. The first model suggests that the binding of the proteins to the enhancer facilitates looping out of the intervening DNA between the enhancer and the promoter. The other model suggests that after binding of the enhancer, the bound proteins facilitate the RNA polymerase to scan through the sequence before it reaches the promoter. However, neither model can satisfactorily explain the action of enhancers located in the introns or at the 3' end of the gene.

The tissue-specific or cell type-specific role of the enhancers in transcriptional control is observed for genes whose expression is likely to be deleterious outside of the specified tissue.[117] Thus, muscle-specific myosin genes are expressed in the skeletal muscle, while the cardiac muscle has its own tissue-specific promoter and enhancers for the regulation of expression of specific myosin heavy chains. One of the best studied examples of tissue- and development-specific expression of genes through the promoter and enhancer sequences is the *Fushi tarazu* (ftz) homeodomain-containing gene in *Drosophila*. This gene is expressed in the blastoderm and also during later stages of neurogenesis. Structurally, the ftz gene consists of a promoter element, an enhancer, and a neurogenic element between the promoter and enhancer. The promoter is recognized by two other homeodomain gene products for transcriptional activation. Once the ftz protein is synthesized in the early stage of development, the ftz gene product interacts with its own enhancer and activates its own transcription. This is a clear example of how sequential gene expression takes place during development.

Transcription Factors and Cell Cycle

We have already seen that expression of transcription factors is regulated during growth and differentiation and in a tissue-specific manner. Now there is growing interest in the field of cell and molecular biology to see if there are functional alterations or regulation of transcriptional factors during cell cycle.[66,72] There are at least two examples that relate to the functioning of transcriptional factors during the cell cycle. The Pou homeodomain protein Oct-1 is expressed ubiquitously. During cell cycle, the levels of Oct-1 protein remain unchanged. However, its activity is regulated by phosphorylation. A cAMP-dependent protein kinase A phosphorylates at a unique site in the Pou homeodomain just upstream of the helix 1. This site is conserved among the Pou homeodomain proteins and its phosphorylation during mitosis results in the inhibition of the binding of Oct-1 to cellular DNA targets.[99] This affects the transcriptional activation function of the Oct-1 protein and seems to correlate with general inhibition of transcription during mitosis. This hyperphosphorylation occurs during mitosis and is reversed as cells exit mitosis and enter the G1 growth phase of the cell cycle. Another example is transcription factor E2F. E2F is a cellular transcription factor that is present in low amounts when compared to other transcription factors like SP1, AP1, and AP2.[62] E2F-binding sites are found in a number of cellular genes that include oncogenes *myc* and *myb*, DHFR and EGF receptors. At least for c-*myc* and DHFR, the E2F sites have been shown to be important for transcriptional activity. During cell cycle, the E2F protein is kept in an inactive state by two of the cellular (nuclear) proteins; pRB (retinoblastoma) and P107.[14,19,102] These two nuclear proteins share structural similarities. During G1 phase of the cell cycle, the pRB protein associates with E2F, rendering it inactive. This complex dissociates during the G1-S boundary. At the S phase, the E2F protein is picked up by the other nuclear protein P107 in a complex that has cyclin and cdk2 kinase. In light of the interaction of E2F with cellular proteins, it becomes quite interesting that the transforming adenovirus (DNA virus) E1A protein interacts with both the nuclear proteins, pRB and p107. This interaction may lead to the release of free E2F protein leading to cellular transformation.

Oncogenic Transcription Factors

The study of oncogenes has played a pivotal role in our understanding of growth, development, and differentiation. Some of the nuclear oncogene products have been identified as transcription factors or subunits of transcription regulatory complex. A number of transcription factors belonging to various families have been implicated in different types of cancer (Table 1). The mechanisms by which they have been activated are also distinct.[31,60,63] In v-*jun*, the transforming counterpart of c-*jun* has a deletion in the region termed β. The presence of this Δ region in c-*jun* has a repressive effect and limits its transcriptional activity. As described, *jun* belongs to the bZIP family of transcription factors. Oncogenic proteins belonging to members of the zinc finger proteins have been characterized by studying the oncogene *erbA*. The c-*erb*A codes for thyroid hormone receptor. v-*erb*A is a

TABLE 1.
Oncogenic Transcription Factors

Oncogene	Family Type	Tumor/Species	Activation
fos	bZIP	osteosarcoma/mouse	overexpression truncation****
jun	bZIP	fibrosarcoma/avian	overexpression truncation
c-*myc*	bHLH	carcinoma, leukemia/avian	overexpression truncation
n-*myc**	bHLH	neuroblastoma/human	overexpression
l-*myc**	bHLH	small-cell lung carcinoma/ human	overexpression
*lyl***	bHLH	T-cell acute lymphoblastic leukemia/human	truncation
*scl/tal***	bHLH	T-cell acute lymphoblastic leukemia/human	truncation
*erb*A	zinc finger	erythroblastosis/avian	mutation
*myl/rar*α**	zinc finger	acute promyleocytic leukemia/human	truncation
*evi1**	zinc finger	myeloid leukemia/mouse	overexpression
*vav**	zinc finger	transfection/tissue culture	truncation
Gli1	zinc finger	glioblastoma/human	—
WT***	zinc finger	Wilms' tumor/human	deletion
Pbx*	homeobox	myeloid leukemia/mouse	truncation
Hox 2.4*	homeobox	PreB acute lymphoblastoid leukemia/human	ectopic
myb	unclassified	myleoblastosis/avian	truncation
rel	unclassified	lymphatic leukemia/ turkey	truncation
ets	unclassified	leukemia/avian	truncation
Spi-1 (*ets* related)	unclassified	mouse	—
*ski**	unclassified	transforming virus tissue culture/avian	overexpression
p53*/***	unclassified	carcinoma/ human	overexpression deletion, mutation
Rb*/***	classified	retinoblastoma/ human	deletion

*Transcriptional activation function: not confirmed

**Considered as transcriptional activators on the basis of similar functions of the other known family members.

***Possibly suppressors of transcription.

****Truncation refers to rearrangement of the gene leading to synthesis of a fusion product.

truncated version of c-*erb*A and has retained both the DNA-binding (zinc finger) and hormone-binding domain. However, the mutations in hormone-binding domains abolish the transcriptional activation function, and it is not surprising to observe v-*erb*A acting as a repressor. Translocation in the retinoic acid receptor, a member of the nuclear steroid hormone receptor family, leads to synthesis of a truncated transforming protein.[37,44] Members representing the bHLH have surfaced recently. Even though *myc* has been known for a long time to be activated by translocation and promoter insertion in B-cell lymphomas, the discovery of *scl* and *lyl* in adult T-cell leukemias signifies the importance of bHLH proteins in growth, normal or cancerous.[69] Both *scl* and *lyl* genes are overexpressed as a result of translocation in a cell type where they are not normally expressed.[6,15,45] Two homeobox containing proteins have also been recently implicated in oncogenesis. Retroviral insertions induces ectopic expression of Hox 2.4 in mouse myeloid leukemia and the *pbx* gene was found fused to the E2A gene[79] as a result of translocation in pre-B-cell acute lymphoblastoid leukemia. Pbx is a homeobox-containing protein, while E2A belongs with the bHLH family. These few examples clearly demonstrate the powerful role of transcription factors in oncogenesis.

Acknowledgment: I would like to thank Hilda Mausiodis for typing the manuscript. Research sponsored by the National Cancer Institute, DHHS, under contract No. NO1-CO-74101 with ABL.

References

1. Abel T, Maniatis T. Action of leucine zippers. Nature 1989; 341:24–25.
2. Auwerx J, Sassone Corsi P. IP-1: A dominant inhibitor of *fos/jun* whose activity is modulated by phosphorylation. Cell 1991; 64:983–993.
3. Bakkar O, Parker MG. CAAT/enhancer binding protein is able to bind to ATF/CRE elements. Nucl Acids Res 1991; 19:1213–1217.
4. Beato M. Gene regulation by steroid hormones. Cell 1989; 56:335–344.
5. Beckman H, Kadesch T. The leucine zipper of TFE-3 dictates helix loop helix dimerization specificity. Genes Dev 1991; 5:1057–1066.
6. Begley CG, Aplan PD, Denning SM, et al. The gene *scl* is expressed during early hematopoiesis and encodes a differentiation related DNA binding motif. Proc Natl Acad Sci USA 1989; 86:10128–10132.
7. Benezra R, Davies R, Lockshon D, et al. The protein Id: A negative regulator of helix loop helix DNA binding proteins. Cell 1990; 61:49–59.

8. Biggin MD, Tjian R. Transcription factors and the control of *Drosophila* development. Trends Genet 1989; 5:377–383.
9. Blackwood E, Eisenman RN. Max: A helix loop helix zipper protein that forms a sequence specific DNA binding complex with *myc*. Science 1991; 251:1211–1217.
10. Brenan RG, Mathews BW. Structural basis of DNA protein recognition. Trends Biochem Sci 1989; 14:286–290.
11. Bruggemeier U, Kalff M, Franke S, et al. Ubiquitous transcription factor Oct-1 mediates induction of the MMTV promoter through synergistic interaction with hormone receptors. Cell 1991; 64:565–572.
12. Budd PS, Jackson I. What do the regulators regulate? First glimpses downstream. Trends Genet 1991; 7:74–76.
13. Busch SJ, Sassone Corsi P. Dimers, leucine zippers and DNA binding domains. Trends Genet 1990; 6:36–40.
14. Cao L, Faba B, Dembski M, et al. Independent binding of the retinoblastoma protein and p107 to the transcription factor E2F. Nature 1992; 355:176–179.
15. Carroll A, Crist W, Ozanne B, et al. The *tal* gene undergoes chromosome translocation in T cell leukemia and potentially encodes a helix-loop-helix protein. EMBO J 1990; 9:411–424.
16. Cleary ML. Oncogenic conversion of transcription factors by chromosomal translocations. Cell 1991; 66:619–622.
17. Courey AJ, Tjian R. Analysis of SPI in vivo reveals multiple transcriptional domains, including a novel glutamine rich activation motif. Cell 1988; 55:887–898.
18. Deshchamps J, Meijlink F. Mammalian homeobox gene in normal development and neoplasia. Crt Rev Oncogenesis 1992; 3:117–174.
19. DeVoto SH, Mudrj M, Pines J, et al. A cyclin A-protein kinase complex possesses sequence specific DNA binding activity. p33^{cdk2} is a component of the E2F-cyclin A complex. Cell 1992; 68:167–176.
20. Dressler GR. An update on vertebrate homeobox. Trends Genet 1989; 5:129–131.
21. Dunn AR, Gough N. Tissue specific enhancers. Trends Biochem Sci 1984; 9:81–82.
22. Dynan WS. Modularity of promoters and enhancers. Cell 1989; 58:1–4.
23. El Baradi T, Picler T. Finger proteins: What we know and what we would like to know. Mech of Develop 1991; 35:155–170.
24. Ferguson B, Krippl O, Andrisane O, et al. Ela 13S and 12S mRNA products made in *E. coli* both function as nucleus localized transcription factors but do not directly bind DNA. Mol Cell Biol 1985; 2:2653–2661.
25. Finney M, Ruvkun G, Horvitz HR. The C. elegans cell lineage and differentiation gene unc-86 encodes a protein with a homeodomain and extended similarity to transcription factors. Cell 1988; 55:757–769.
26. Forsberg M, Westen G. Enhancer activation by a single type of transcription factor shows cell type dependence. EMBO J 1991; 10:2543–2551.
27. Frankel AD, Kim PS. Modular structure of transcription factors: Implications for gene regulation. Cell 1991; 65:717–719.
28. Fremont PS, Hansen IM, Trowsdale J. A novel cysteine rich sequence motif. Cell 1991; 64:483–484.

29. Freyd G, Kim SK, Horvitz HR. Novel cysteine rich motif and homeodomain in the product of the Caenorhabditis elegans cell lineage gene LIN II. Nature 1990; 344:876–879.
30. Gehring WJ, Muller M, Affolter M, et al. The structure of the homeodomain and its functional implications. Trends Genet 1990; 6:323–329.
31. Gilmore TD. Malignant transformation by mutant *rel* proteins. Trends Genet 1991; 7:318–322.
32. Greenblatt J. Roles of TFIID in transcriptional initiation by RNA polymerase II. Cell 1991; 66:1067–1070.
33. Ha I, Lane WS, Reinberg D. Cloning of a human gene encoding the general transcription factor IIB. Nature 1991; 352:689–694.
34. Harbomel P. Synergistic activation of eukaryotic transcription: The multireceptor target hypothesis. New Biol 1990; 2:1063–1070.
35. Harrison SC. A structural taxonomy of DNA binding domains. Nature 1991; 353:715–719.
36. Herr W, Sturm RA, Clerc RG, et al. The POU domain: A large conserved region in the mammalian pit-1, Oct-1, oct-2 and Caenorhabditis elegans unc-86 gene products. Genes Dev 1988; 2:1513–1516.
37. Hugues de The, Lavau C, Marchio A, et al. The PML-RARα fusion in RNA generated by the (C15;17) transformation in acute promyelocytes leukemia encodes a functionally altered RAR. Cell 1991; 66:677–684.
38. Jaynes JB, O'Farrell PH. Activation and repression of transcription by homeodomain containing proteins that bind a common site. Nature 1988; 336:744–749.
39. Jaynes JB, O'Farrell PH. Active repression of transcription by the engrailed homeodomain protein. EMBO J 1991; 10:1427–1433.
40. Johnson PF, McKnight SL. Eukaryotic transcriptional regulatory proteins. Ann Rev Biochem 1989; 58:799–839.
41. Johnson PF. Transcriptional activators in hepatocytes. Cell Growth Diff 1990; 1:47–51.
42. Jones N. Transcriptional regulation by dimerization: Two sides to an incestuous relationship. Cell 1990; 61:9–11.
43. Jones N. Complex inhibitions. Curr Biol 1991; 1:224–226.
44. Kakizuka A, Miller WH Jr, Umesono K, et al. Chromosomal translocation t(15;17) in human acute promyelocytic leukemic fuses RARα with a novel putative transcription factor, PML. Cell 1991; 66:663–674.
45. Kamps MP, Murre C, Sun XH, et al. A new homeobox gene contributes the DNA binding domain of the t(1;19) translocation protein in pre-BALL. Cell 1990; 60:547–555.
46. Kaptein R. Distinguishing features. Curr Biol 1991; 1:336–338.
47. Karin M. Complexities of gene regulation by cAMP. Trends Genet 1989; 5:65–67.
48. Karin M. Too many transcription factors; positive and negative interactions. New Biol 1990; 2:126–131.
49. Karin M, Castrillo JL, Theil LE. Growth hormone gene regulation: A paradigm for cell type specific gene activation. Trends Genet 1990; 6:92–96.
50. Karlson O, Thor S, Norberg T, et al. Insulin gene enhancer binding

protein ISL-1 is a member of a novel class of proteins containing both a homeodomain and a Cys-His domain. Nature 1990; 344:879–882.

51. Kerrigan L, Croston GE, Lira LM, et al. Sequence specific transcriptional antirepression of the *Drosophila* kruppel gene by the GAGA factor. J Biol Chem 1991; 266:574–582.

52. Koopman P, Ashworth A, Lovell Badge R. The ZFY gene family in humans and mice. Trends Genet 1991; 7:132–136.

53. Kouzaridis T, Ziff E. Behind the *fos* and *jun* leucine zippers. Cancer Cells 1989; 1:71–76.

54. Kuo CJ, Conley PB, Chen L, et al. A transcriptional hierarchy involved in mammalian cell type specification. Nature 1992; 355:457–461.

55. Lai E, Darnell JE Jr. Transcriptional control in hepatocytes: a window on development. Trends Biochem Sci 1991; 16:427–430.

56. Laughen A. DNA binding specificity of homeodomains. Biochemistry 1991; 30:11357–11367.

57. Levine M, Hoey T. Homeobox proteins as sequence specific transcription factors. Cell 1988; 55:537–540.

58. Levine M, Manley JL. Transcription repression of eukaryotic promoters. Cell 1989; 59:405–408.

59. Lewin B. Commitment and activation at pol II promoters: A tail of protein-protein interaction. Cell 1990; 61:1161–1164.

60. Lewin B. Oncogenic conversion by regulatory changes in transcription factors. Cell 1991; 64:303–312.

61. Licht JD, Grossel MJ, Figge J, et al. *Drosophila* kruppel protein is a transcriptional repressor. Nature 1990; 346:76–79.

62. Liu F, Freen MR. A specific member of the ATF transcription factor family can mediate transcription activation by the adenovirus E2a protein. Cell 1990; 61:1217–1224.

63. Lucibello FC, Muller R. Protooncogenes encoding transcriptional regulators: Unraveling the mechanisms of oncogenic conversion. Crt Rev Oncogenesis 1991; 2:259–276.

64. Mandel DB, Crabtree GR. HNF-1 a member of a novel class of dimerizing homeodomain proteins. J Biol Chem 1991; 266:677–680.

65. Martin KJ, Lillie JW, Green MR. Evidence for interaction of different eukaryotic transcriptional activators with distinct cellular targets. Nature 1990; 346:147–152.

66. McKinney JD, Heintz N. Transcriptional regulation in the eukaryotic cell cycle. Trends Biochem Sci 1991; 16:430–435.

67. McKnight S, Tijan R. Transcriptional selectivity of viral genes in mammalian cells. Cell 1986; 46:795–805.

68. McKnight SL. Molecular zippers in gene regulation. Scientific Amer 1991; 264:54–63.

69. Mellentin JD, Smith SD, Cleery ML. *lyl-1*, a novel gene altered by chromosomal translocation in T cell leukemia codes for a protein with a helix-loop-helix DNA binding motif. Cell 1989; 58:77–83.

70. Mendel DB, Khavari PA, Conley PB, et al. Characterization of a cofactor that regulates dimerization of a mammalian homeodomain protein. Science 1991; 254:1762–1767.

71. Mitchell PJ, Tijan R. Transcriptional regulation in mammalian cells by sequence specific DNA binding proteins. Science 1989; 245:371–378.
72. Moran E. Cycles within cycles. Curr Biol 1991; 1:281–283.
73. Muller HF, Schaffner W. Transcriptional enhancers can act in trans. Trends Genet 1990; 6:300–305.
74. Muller MM, Ruppert S, Schaffner W, et al. A cloned octomer transcription factor stimulates transcription from lymphoid specific promoters in non B cells. Nature 1988; 336:544–551.
75. Muller M, Renkawitz R. The glucocorticoid receptor. Biochem Biophys Acta 1991; 1088:171–182.
76. Murphy S, Moorfield B, Pielar T. Common mechanisms of promoter recognition by RNA polymerases II and III. Trends Genet 1989; 5:122–126.
77. Murre C, McCaw PS, Baltimore D. A new DNA binding and dimerization motif in the immunoglobulin enhancer binding, daughterless, MyoD and myc proteins. Cell 1989; 56:777–783.
78. Nasmyth K, Adolf G, Lydall D, et al. The identification of a second cell cycle control on the HO promoter in yeast: Cell cycle regulation of SW15 nuclear entry. Cell 1990; 62:631–647.
79. Nourse J, Mellentin JD, Galili N, et al. Chromosomal translocation t(1;19) results in synthesis of a homeobox fusion mRNA that codes for a potential chimeric transcription factor. Cell 1990; 60:535–545.
80. Nussinov R. Sequence signals in eukaryotic upstream region. CRC Rev Biochem Mol Biol 1990; 25:185–224.
81. Olson EN. MyoD family: A paradigm for development. Genes Dev 1990; 4:1454–1461.
82. O'Shea EK, Rutwoski R, Kim PS. Evidence that the leucine zipper is a coiled coil. Science 1989; 243:538–542.
83. Pankratz MJ, Seifert E, Gerwin W, et al. Gradients of Kruppel and Knirps gene products direct-pair-rule gene stripe patterning in the posterior region of the Drosophila embryo. Cell 1990; 61:309–317.
84. Prendergast GC, Lawe D, Ziff EB. Association of Myn, the murine homolog of Max, with cMyc stimulates methylation sensitive DNA binding and Ras cotransformation. Cell 1991; 65:395–407.
85. Ptashne M. How eukaryotic transcriptional activators work. Nature 1988; 335:683–689.
86. Ptashne M, Gann AAF. Activators and targets. Nature 1990; 346:329–331.
87. Ray A, LaForge KS, Sehgal PB. Repressor to activator switch by mutations in the first Zn finger of the glucocorticoid receptor: Is direct DNA binding necessary? Proc Natl Acad Sci USA 1991; 88:7086–7090.
88. Remerowski ML, Kellenbach E, Boclens R, et al. H NMR studies on DNA recognition by glucocorticoid receptor: Complex of the DNA binding domain with a half site response element. Biochemistry 1991; 30:11620–11624.
89. Renkawitz R. Transcriptional repression in eukaryotes. Trends Genet 1990; 6:192–196.
90. Robertson M. Homeoboxes, pou proteins and the limits to promiscuity. Nature 1988; 336:522–524.
91. Roeder RG. The complexities of eukaryotic transcription initiation: regu-

lation of preinitiation complex assembly. Trends Biochem Sci 1991; 16:402–408.

92. Rosenfeld MG. POU-domain transcription factors: pou-er-ful developmental regulators. Genes Dev 1991; 5:897–907.

93. Ruvkun G, Finney M. Regulation of transcription cell identity by pou domain proteins. Cell 1991; 64:475–478.

94. Sassoon D, Lyons G, Wright WE, et al. Expression of two myogenic regulatory factors, myogenin and MyoD1 during mouse embryogenesis. Nature 1989; 341:303–307.

95. Schaffner W. How do different transcription factors binding the same DNA sequence sort out their jobs? Trends Genet 1989; 5:37–39.

96. Scheiderit C, Cromlish JA, Gester T, et al. A human lymphoid specific transcription factor that activates immunoglobulin genes is a homeobox protein. Nature 1988; 336:551–557.

97. Scholer HR. Octamania: The POU factors in murine development. Trends Genet 1990; 1:323–329.

98. Schule R, Evans RM. Cross coupling of signal transduction pathways: zn fingers meet leucine zipper. Trends Genet 1991; 7:377–381.

99. Segil N, Roberts SB, Heintz N. Mitotic phosphorylation of the Oct-1 homeodomain protein and regulation of Oct-1 DNA binding activity. Science 1991; 254:1814–1816.

100. Serfling E. Autoregulation, a common property of eukaryotic transcription factors. Trends Genet 1989; 5:131–133.

101. Shaw PE. Multicompetant transcriptional factor complexes: The exception or the rule. New Biol 1990; 2:111–118.

102. Shirodkar S, Ewen M, DeCaprio JA, et al. The transcription factor E2F interacts with the retinoblastoma product and a p107-cyclin A complex in a cell cycle regulated manner. Cell 1992; 68:157–166.

103. Stillman DJ, Bankier AT, Sidden A, et al. Characterization of a transcription factor involved in mother cell specific transcription of the yeast HO gene. EMBO J 1988; 7:484–494.

104. Struhl K. Helix turn helix, Zn finger and leucine zipper motifs for eukaryotic transcriptional regulatory proteins. Trends Biochem Sci 1989; 4:137–140.

105. Struhl K. Acid connections. Curr Biol 1991; 1:188–191.

106. Sutcliffe JG, Milner RJ. Brain specific gene expression. Trends Biochem Sci 1984; 9:95–99.

107. Suzuki M. SPKK, a new nucleic acid binding unit of protein found in histones. EMBO J 1989; 8:797–804.

108. Suzuki M, Sohena H, Yazawa M, et al. Histone H1 kinase specific to the SPKK motif. J Biochem 1990; 108:356–364.

109. Suzuki M. The DNA binding motif, SPKK, and its variants. Nucl Acid Mol Biol 1991; 5:126–140.

110. Tabata T, Nakayama T, Mikami K, et al. HBP-1 and HBP-1b leucine zipper type transcription factors of wheat. EMBO J 1991; 10:1459–1467.

111. Tian JM, Schibler U. Tissue specific expression of the gene encoding hepatocyte nuclear factor 1 may involve hepatocyte nuclear factor 4. Genes Dev 1991; 5:2225–2234.

112. Treacy MN, He X, Rosenfeld MG. I-pou: A pou domain protein that inhibits neuron specific gene activation. Nature 1991; 350:577–584.
113. Umesono K, Evans RM. Determinants of target gene specifity for steroid thyroid hormone receptors. Cell 1989; 57:1139–1146.
114. Vallee BL, Coleman JE, Auld DS. Zinc fingers, zinc clusters and zinc twists in the DNA binding protein domains. Proc Natl Acad Sci USA 1991; 88:999–1003.
115. Vinson CR, Sigler PB, McKnight SL. Scissors grip model for DNA recognition by a family of leucine zipper protein. Science 1989; 246:911–916.
116. Visvader J, Begly CG. Helix loop helix genes translocated in lymphoid leukemia. Trends Biochem Sci 1991; 16:330–333.
117. Voss DS, Schlokat U, Gruss P. The role of enhancers in the regulation of cell type specific transcriptional control. Trends Biochem Sci 1986; 11:287–289.
118. Voss JW, Wilson L, Rosenfeld MG. Pou domain proteins pit-1 and Oct-1 interact to form a heteromeric complex and can cooperate to induce expression of the prolactin promoter. Genes Dev 1991; 5:1309–1320.
119. Weintraub SJ, Dean DC. Interaction of a common factor with ATF, Sp1 or TATAA promoter elements is required for these sequences to mediate transactivation by the adenoviral oncogene E1a. Mol Cell Biol 1992; 72:512–517.
120. Wieland S, Dobbeling U, Rusconi S. Interference and synergism of glucocorticoid receptors and octomer factors. EMBO J 1990; 10:2513–2521.
121. Wingender E. Transcription regulating proteins and their recognition sequences. Crt Rev Euk Gene Exp 1990; 1:11–48.
122. Wright CVE, Cho KWY, Oliver G, et al. Vertebrate homeodomain proteins: Families of region specific transcription factors. Trends Biochem Sci 1989; 14:52–56.
123. Xanthopoulos KG, Prezioso VR, Chan WS, et al. The different tissue transcription patterns of genes for HNF-1, C/EBP, HNF-3 and HNF-4 protein factors that govern liver specific expression. Proc Natl Acad Sci USA 1991; 88:3807–3811.
124. Yamamoto KK, Gonzalez GA, Biggs WH, et al. Phosphorylation induced binding and transcriptional efficacy of nuclear factor CREB. Nature 1988; 334:494–498.
125. Zappavigna V, Renucci A, Belmonte JCI, et al. Hox-4 genes encode transcription factors with potential acute and cross regulatory capacities. EMBO J 1991; 10:4177–4187.
126. Ziff EB. Transcription factors: A new family gathers at the cAMP response site. Trends Genet 1990; 6:69–72.
127. Zuo P, Stanogevic D, Colgan J, et al. Activation and repression of transcription by the gap proteins, hunchback and Kruppel, in cultured Drosophila cells. Genes Dev 1991; 5:254–264.

Chapter 9

Human Papillomaviruses

Kiranur N. Subramanian

Papillomaviruses are small DNA viruses belonging to a subdivision of the papovavirus family. Papillomaviruses induce papillomas or warts in a number of higher vertebrates including human beings. Infection by papillomaviruses is restricted to epithelial cells of the epidermis or squamous epithelial cells of the oral or genital mucosa. Infection is believed to occur by the entry of the virus into basal epithelial cells exposed by microlesions or local abrasions of the skin, or into proliferating cells which are exposed at the squamocolumnar border of the cervix uteri. Lesions induced by papillomaviruses are usually benign, but with certain types of these viruses and under certain conditions progression to malignancy occurs. Papillomaviruses are believed to infect basal epithelial cells and remain latent with no signs of infection detectable in those cells. When the infected keratinocytes start to differentiate and move upward to occupy suprabasal layers, a switch occurs from latency to productive infection, and newly synthesized viral mRNA, DNA, and proteins as well as virus particles are detectable, especially in the layer known as stratum granulosum. The identities of the signals causing this switch to virus production are unknown and are believed to be the same as or similar to those triggering the keratinocytes to differentiate.

There is as yet no known cell culture system for the vegetative propagation of any of the papillomaviruses. Despite this limitation, a great deal of research has been carried out, thanks to the advent of recombinant DNA technology. The approximately 7.9 kilobase pairs (kb) long viral DNA has been isolated from warts or other lesions,

From *The Molecular Basis of Human Cancer:* edited by B. Neel, M.D., Ph.D., R. Kumar, Ph.D. © 1993, Futura Publishing Co. Inc., Mount Kisco, NY.

cloned and sequenced. Viral DNA sequences have been analyzed to delineate open reading frames (ORFs) potentially capable of coding for viral proteins. Viral DNAs or segments thereof have been returned to cells to study the functions of the various ORFs and noncoding regions. Viral DNA sequences have been utilized to develop probes for the detection and typing of papillomaviruses in clinical specimens derived from lesions. A number of reviews have appeared on the pathology, biology, and molecular biology of papillomaviruses in the past.[17,67,103,138,164,165]

The most extensively studied member of the papillomavirus family is bovine papillomavirus type 1 (BPV-1). BPV-1 induces fibropapillomas in cattle and fibroblastic tumors in rodents, and transforms rodent cells in culture. BPV-1 DNA is usually present as a multicopy episome in the transformed cells.

Classification of Human Papillomaviruses

A total of 60 different types of human papillomaviruses (HPVs) have been isolated and characterized so far.[36] In order to be classified as a new type of HPV, the newly isolated DNA should be an approximately 7.9 kb closed circular, double stranded DNA exhibiting < 50% homology with any of the known HPV DNAs as detected by hybridization in liquid under high stringency conditions.[28] The known HPV DNAs typed in this fashion are listed in Table 1.

HPVs can be divided into roughly two major groups: those that cause cutaneous lesions and those that cause lesions of the oral or genital mucosa. Cutaneous lesions caused by HPVs include common warts or verruca vulgaris (e.g., HPV-2, HPV-4), plantar and palmar warts or verruca plantaris (e.g., HPV-1, HPV-4), flat and intermediate warts or verruca plana (e.g., HPV-3, HPV-10, HPV-28), and butcher's warts or common warts affecting meat and animal handlers (e.g., HPV-7). In addition to the above, a good number of cutaneous-type HPVs have been isolated from a rare skin disorder affecting young children known as epidermodysplasia verruciformis (EV). In some cases of EV the lesions remain benign, but in some other cases (e.g., those induced by HPV-5, HPV-8, HPV-14, HPV-17 and HPV-20) in about 30% of the patients the lesions progress into squamous cell carcinomas, especially in areas exposed to ultraviolet light.[100]

A majority of HPVs causing mucosal lesions have been found to be associated with lesions of the genital tract. These lesions include sharp anogenital warts known as condylomata acuminata (e.g., HPV-6, HPV-11), cervical intraepithelial neoplasia (CIN) (e.g., HPV-6, HPV-11, HPV-16, and HPV-18), penile intraepithelial neoplasia (PIN) or penile Bowenoid papulosis (e.g., HPV-39, HPV-40), and vulvar lesions (HPV-42 to -44, HPV-59). A number of HPVs which cause genital lesions primarily have also been found to be associated with lesions of the respiratory and digestive tract: e.g., HPV-6 and HPV-11 associated with laryngeal papilloma, HPV-30 associated with laryngeal carcinoma, and HPV-57 associated with inverted papilloma of the maxillary sinus. There are only two HPVs known which are exclusively associated with lesions of the oral mucosa. One of them, HPV-13, has only been detected in focal epithelial hyperplasia (FEH); the other, HPV-32, has been found in FEH as well as in oral papilloma. There are examples of HPVs associated with mucosal as well as cutaneous type lesions. For instance, HPV-57 which is primarily associated with lesions of the oral and genital mucosa, has also been detected in cutaneous lesions. HPV-2 which is associated with common hand warts has been detected in oral lesions. HPV-7 found in hand warts of meat handlers has often been detected in oral papillomas of patients infected with the human immunodeficiency virus (HIV). HPV-16, most commonly associated with CIN and cervical carcinomas has been isolated from a cutaneous lesion termed Bowen's disease.

Genome Organization

The papillomavirus particle (diameter = 55 nm) consists of an icosahedral outer shell or capsid made up of viral structural proteins enclosing a core that contains the viral DNA complexed with host histones forming a nucleosome structure similar to that of the host cellular DNA. Two viral proteins constitute the capsids of papillomaviruses: a major protein of molecular weight 55 kilo daltons (kd) which amounts to about 75% of the total viral protein, and a minor protein of 70 kd.

The genomes of several animal (BPV-1 and cottontail rabbit papillomavirus [CRPV]) and human (HPV-1, HPV-5, HPV-6, HPV-8, HPV-11, HPV-16, HPV-18, HPV-31, and HPV-33) papillomaviruses have been sequenced so far. Though the animal and HPV DNAs exhibit very little sequence homology, they exhibit a remarkable similarity in genome organization. There are approximately 10 pro-

TABLE 1.
HPVs Characterized and Lesions Associated with Them

Location	Lesions	HPV Types	Progression to Malignancy
Cutaneous	Plantar and palmar warts	1, 4	None
Cutaneous	Common warts	2, 4	None
Cutaneous	Butcher's warts	26, 27, 29, 57	Unknown
Cutaneous	Flat and intermediate warts	7	None
		28, 49	Unknown
Cutaneous	Isolated from macular lesions (EV); associated with EV (benign) or EV (squamous cell carcinoma)	3, 10	Rare
		5, 8, 17	High
		9, 12, 19	None
		22, 23, 24, 25	None
		46, 47, 50	None
Cutaneous	Iolated from flat warts (EV); associated with EV (benign) or EV (squamous cell carcinoma)	14, 20	High
		9, 15, 21, 50	None
Cutaneous	Isolated from actinic keratosis; associated with EV (benign)	36	None
Cutaneous	Isolated from keratoacanthoma	37	Unknown
Cutaneous	Isolated from malignant melanoma	38	Unknown
Cutaneous	Cutaneous squamous cell carcinoma	41, 48	High
Cutaneous	Isolated from epidermoid cysts	60	Unknown
Genital (and oral)	Condylomata acuminata	6, 11, 44, 54	None
Mucosa	Low grade cervical dysplasia; CIN;	6, 11	Rare
	laryngeal papilloma	6, 11	Rare

Location	Disease	HPV Types	Malignancy
Genital Mucosa	CIN; cervical carcinoma	16, 18, 31, 33, 35	High
		45, 51, 52, 56	High
Genital Mucosa	PIN; CIN; cervical carcinoma	39	High
Genital Mucosa	PIN; CIN	40, 55	Unknown
Genital Mucosa	Isolated from CIN	58	Unknown
Genital Mucosa	Isolated from normal cervical mucosa	53	Unknown
Genital Mucosa	Vulvar papilloma; CIN	42	None
Genital Mucosa	Vulvar hyperplasia; CIN	43	Rare
Genital Mucosa	Vulvar condyloma; CIN	44	Rare
Genital Mucosa	Vulvar intraepithelial neoplasia	59	Unknown
Genital Mucosa (also cutaneous)	Isolated from Bowen's disease (cutaneous); associated with CIN (genital)	34, 42	None
Genital and Oral Mucosa	Laryngeal carcinoma; CIN	16	High
		30	High
Oral and Genital Mucosa (also cutaneous)	Inverted papilloma of the maxillary sinus; CIN; common warts	57	Unknown
Oral Mucosa	FEH	13	None
Oral Mucosa	FEH and oral papilloma	32	None

EV: epidermodysplasia verruciformis; CIN: cervical intraepithelial neoplasia; PIN: penile intraepithelial neoplasia or penile Bowenoid papulosis; FEH: focal epithelial hyperplasia.

tein-coding regions or ORFs all of which are present on only one of the strands of the viral Dnas. The approximate number and respective positions of the different ORFs are similar for the different papillomaviruses, and have become a hallmark of their genome organization. The ORFs are further classified into early (E) or late (L) region ORFs. In the case of DNA viruses, the terms "early" or "late" regions refer to sectors of the viral DNA which are transcribed and translated prior to or after the onset of vegetative viral DNA replication, respectively. The early gene products usually have functions in replication, transcription, and transformation. The late gene products are viral structural proteins. Based on this definition, the E1 through E8 ORFs of BPV-1 are termed the early ORFs, and L1 and L2 are termed the late ORFs.

The genome maps of BPV-1 and four representative HPVs are illustrated in Figure 1. The maps show the positions of the various early region ORFs beginning with E6. They are followed by the late region ORFs L2 and L1. The L1 ORF coding for the major capsid protein is the most well-conserved among various papillomaviruses. The E1 ORF known to code for a replication protein (a la BPV-1) is also fairly well conserved. The E5 ORF, required for oncogenic transformation in BPV-1 but dispensable for this function in human papillomaviruses, is the least well-conserved. Upstream from the early region ORFs (or downstream from the L1 ORF) is located an approximately 0.4 to 1.0 kb region devoid of protein-coding capability. This region is termed by various investigators as the noncoding region (NCR), upstream regulatory region (URR), or long control region (LCR). This region contains upstream control elements for viral early and late mRNA transcription. In the case of BPV-1, this region has also been shown to contain the origin of DNA replication required for the maintenance of the viral DNA as an episome in mouse cells transformed by BPV-1. The term LCR will be used to refer to this region in this article.

Gene Expression and Regulation

Transcription of Viral mRNAs

An important feature of papillomavirus mRNA transcription is the presence of multiple promoters and splice and polyadenylation sites. In addition, the nature and relative amounts of the viral mRNAs

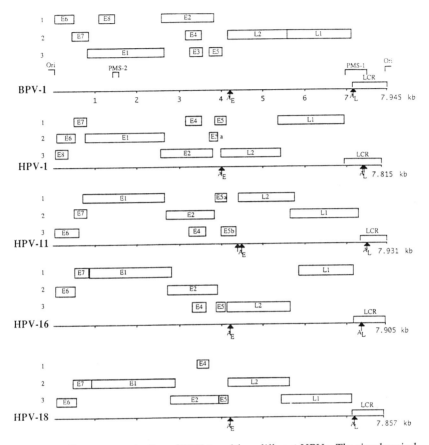

Figure 1. *Genome organization of BPV-1 and four different HPVs. The circular viral DNAs are shown in the linear form starting and ending at the unique HpaI restriction site in BPV-1 and homologous locations in the HPVs. The designations 1, 2, and 3 at the left indicate the three different reading frames on the coding strand of each viral DNA. The boundaries of the various ORFs are as predicted from the nucleotide sequences of the viral DNAs.[22,29,33,34,129] LCR (long control region) refers to the noncoding regulatory region containing cis-active sequences required for initiation of transcription of the viral mRNAs. PMS-1 and PMS-2 of BPV-1 refer to previously mapped plasmid maintenance sequences which were believed to be alternate origins of replication involved in episome maintenance.[76,79] Ori, which spans the HpaI restriction site, refers to the 60 bp BPV-1 minimal origin of replication identified recently by transient replication assays in vivo[151,152] and in vitro replication experiments.[160]*

vary depending upon the host cell type and the nature of the infection (viz productive or nonproductive). Subtle variations have also been noted between viruses that produce benign and malignant lesions. The structures of the mRNAs have been analyzed by a number of techniques: the S1 nuclease protection assay to quantitate mRNAs and to determine splice points; the primer extension technique to map mRNA 5' ends; the R-loop electron microscopic technique; preparation and sequence analysis of cDNAs by conventional techniques; and, more recently, cDNA production and sequence analysis by the polymerase chain reaction (PCR) technique.

In the case of BPV-1 a total of 18 different mRNAs have been mapped so far.[2,161] Twelve of these mRNAs have been detected in mouse C127 cells transformed by BPV-1; the remaining six have been detected in productively infected bovine fibropapillomas or warts. Sixteen of these mRNAs (including all ten from transformed rodent cells and four of the six detected in warts) encode early region products involved in regulation of viral mRNA transcription, viral DNA replication, and morphological transformation of cells. They all share a common 3' end at nucleotide (nt) 4203 which is specified by the polyadenylation signal A_E located at nt 4180 at the end of the early region ORFs (Fig. 1). The remaining two mRNAs, found exclusively in fibropapillomas, encode viral structural proteins. Their 3' ends are located at nt 7175 which is specified by the polyadenylation signal A_L located at nt 7156 at the end of the late region ORFs (Fig. 1).

The viral mRNAs are specified by seven different promoter elements. One of them, termed P_L or P_{7250}, operates exclusively in warts. (In papillomavirus terminology, promoters are designated by the letter P followed by the nucleotide postion of the 5' end of the most abundant mRNAs expressed from that promoter.) The six remaining promoters, termed P_{7185}, P_{7940}, P_{89}, P_{890}, P_{2443}, and P_{3080}, have been detected in mouse C127 cells transformed by BPV-1. Of these six promoters P_{89}, located immediately downstream from the LCR, is used most frequently. Another reason contributing to variety in viral mRNA structure is the use of alternative splice events; splice donor sites at nt 304, 864, 1234, 2505, 3764, and 7835 and acceptor sites at nt 528, 3225, 3605, and 5609 have been detected.

Regarding HPVs, information is available on the transcription of HPV-16 and HPV-18 mRNAs in cell-lines such as SiHa, CaSki, and HeLa derived from cervical carcinomas[125,134,135] and other cell-lines derived from low-grade cervical lesions,[39,132] HPV-6 and HPV-11 mRNAs in condylomata acuminata (genital warts),[25,113] and HPV-1 mRNAs in plantar warts.[101] In high-grade cervical lesions and in cervical carcinomas, the viral DNA is usually present integrated into the cell DNA with the integration occurring through the E2 or E1 ORFs (see below). The major viral mRNAs made in cervical carcinomas containing the oncogenic HPV-16 or HPV-18 are those that encode the E6 and E7 proteins which are both required for oncogenic transformation. In some cervical carcinomas mRNAs containing the E1 ORF are also made, but ORFs 3' to E1 (such as E2) are seldom transcribed. Viral mRNAs transcribed in cervical carcinomas usually contain adjoining cellular sequences located downstream at the site of integration.[125,134,135] In low-grade cervical lesions containing HPV-16, the viral DNA is usually present in episomal form. In such lesions and in a cell-line such as W12 derived from them, in addition to E6 and E7, the middle and 3' early region ORFs including E1, E2, E4, and E5, and even late region ORFs such as L1 appear in viral mRNAs (Table 2).[39,132]

The major promoters of HPV-16 and HPV-18 used in cervical carcinoma cells are termed P_{97} and P_{105}, respectively.[125,134,135] These promoters are equivalent to the major promoter P_{89} of BPV-1. The 5' ends of the most abundant mRNA species specified by the major HPV-16 and HPV-18 promoters are located immediately downstream from the viral LCR sequences similar to abundant mRNAs specified by P_{89} of BPV-1. In addition, minor mRNA initiation sites have been noted around nt 770 in the E7 ORF and nt 1260 in the E1 ORF of HPV-16 in the W12 cell-line derived from a low-grade cervical lesion indicating the presence of multiple promoters similar to that in BPV-1 (Table 2).[39]

The transcription of the nononcogenic HPV-6 and HPV-11 mRNAs has been studied in genital condylomata acuminata.[25] Transcription of HPV-11 has also been studied in xenografts of human foreskin epithelia which were productively infected with HPV-11 and implanted into the renal capsule of athymic (nude) mice.[113] Those implants develop into condyloma-like cysts indistinguishable from condylomata acuminata, and support the complete infectious cycle of HPV-11 giving rise to mature virions.[66] The pattern of transcription of the viral mRNAs in these cysts is similar to that in condylomata acuminata.[113] Transcripts produced by the cutaneous type virus HPV-1 have been investigated by preparation of a cDNA library from plantar warts and their sequence analysis.[101] Viral mRNAs encoding

TABLE 2.
Structures and Coding Potentials of HPV mRNAs

Virus	mRNA Species	5' End	Splice Donor/ Acceptor Sites	3' End	Coding Potential
HPV-11[113]	a	700	847/3325	4400	E1/E4
	b	700	1272/3325	4400	E1-M; E2-C
	c	700	—	4400	E1
	e	100	847/3325	4400	E6; E7; E1/E4
	f	100	847/2622	4400	E6; E7; E2
	g	700	847/2622	4400	E2
	h	1200	1272/3325	4400	E2-C
	j	700	847/3325; 3593/5771	7400	E1/E4; L1
	k	4400	—	7400	L2
HPV-16[39]	a	97	226/409; 880/3357	4213	E6*; E7; E1/E4; E5
	b	97	226/3357	4213	E6*; E5
	c	770	880/3357	4213	E1/E4; E5
	d	1260	1301/3357	4213	E2-C; E5
	e	1260	1301/5637	7260	L1
	f	1260	1301/3357; 3631/5637	7260	E2-M; L1
HPV-1[101]	a	750	827/3200	4000	E1/E4; E5a
	b	750	1231/3200	4000	E1-M; E2-C; E5a
	c	750	827/2545	4000	E2; E5a
	d	7800	827/3200	4000	E6; E7; E1/E4; E5a
	e	750	827/3200; 3592/5431	7431	E1/E4; L1
	f	7510	7710/3200; 3592/5431	7431	L1
	g	7510	7710/5431	7431	L1
	h	7510	7710/3200	7431	E5a; E5; L2
	i	750	827/3200	7431	E1/E4; E5a; E5; L2

The mRNAs for the analyses were isolated from the following sources: condyloma-like cysts produced from an HPV-11-infected human foreskin xenograft in an athymic mouse[66,113]; the W12 cell-line established from an HPV-16-induced low grade cervical lesion[39]; and, plantar warts induced by HPV-1.[101] The numbers shown are nucleotide positions based on the known nucleotide sequences of HPV-11,[34] HPV-16,[129] and HPV-1.[33] The 5' end of the HPV-11 mRNA termed 'k' at nt 4400 is probably created by truncation; the actual 5' end of this mRNA is not known.[113] The viral proteins that can be coded by the mRNAs are listed under "coding potential."

all the early region ORFs and the two late region ORFs have been detected in these systems (Table 2). The major promoter used in HPV-6 and HPV-11 is located around nt 700 within the E7 ORF bordering the E1 ORF. In addition, two other promoters are also used and are located around nt 100 downstream from the LCR and nt 1200 within the E1 ORF.[25] HPV-1 promoters around nt 750, 7800, and 7510 are active in plantar warts, with the most upstream one around nt 7510 being used preferentially for late mRNA transcription (Table 2).[101]

Similar to that in BPV-1, HPV mRNAs encoding the different viral proteins are produced by differential splicing (Table 2). An abundant mRNA in each case is produced by splicing a short 5′ portion of the E1 ORF with the E4 ORF, and encodes the E1/E4 protein, the most abundant viral protein in warts. Viral mRNAs coding for the other early and late viral proteins including two putative early proteins termed E2-C and E1-M are also produced. The putative E2-C protein would contain the carboxy-terminal half of the E2 ORF. A similar protein in BPV-1, termed E2-TR, has been found to exert negative regulation of BPV-1 transcription acting on the same E2-binding sites in the LCR recognized and bound to by the full-length E2 transactivator protein.[68] Another mRNA could code for a putative protein termed E1-M containing the amino-terminal sequences of the E1 ORF. A similar E1-M protein in BPV-1 was believed to exert negative regulation of viral DNA replication,[11] but that proposal has not been confirmed in a recent study.[151] All the early mRNAs have their 3′ ends located immediately downstream from the early region polyadenylation signal around nt 4000 to 4400 in the different HPVs. The late mRNAs have their 3′ ends determined by the polyadenylation signal located around nt 7260 to 7431 (Table 2).

An interesting feature unique to oncogenic genital HPVs such as HPV-16 and HPV-18 is that the major E6-encoding transcripts are spliced within the E6 ORF creating what is called the E6* gene.[125,135] The splicing occurs in two different ways: between nt 226 and 409 creating E6*I, and between nt 226 and 526 creating E6*II.[134] Since the E6 protein is initiated at the second AUG of the E6 ORF at nt 104, and 2 or 5 amino acids (aa) are added following the splice acceptor site in E6*I and E6*II, the putative E6*I or E6*II proteins would have sizes of 43 or 46 aa, respectively. (The complete E6 is a 158 aa protein.) The E6* proteins, however, have not been detected so far in cells infected or transformed by HPV-16 or HPV-18 (see below).

Regulation of Transcription

Two types of transcriptional enhancer elements have been identified in the LCR sequences of various papillomaviruses: conditional enhancer elements that respond to the viral E2 proteins, and constitutive enhancer elements that respond to cellular factors (Fig. 2). Regulation of transcription by E2 has been studied in detail in the case of BPV-1. The E2 ORF of BPV-1 gives rise to three proteins all of which have transcriptional regulatory properties. The full-length 48 kd E2 protein is a powerful transactivator of BPV-1 mRNA transcription.[57,58,140,141] Comparison of the amino acid sequences of the E2 proteins of various papillomaviruses indicates the presence of two conserved regions: a 220 aa amino-terminal region and a 100 aa carboxy-terminal region. The conserved amino-terminal region of the full-length E2 protein of BPV-1 is essential for its transactivation property,[85] and the conserved carboxy-terminal region is required for specific DNA-binding.[86] Between the amino- and carboxy-terminal regions is located a nonconserved hinge region. The amino-terminal region contains two amphipathic α helices (also termed "acid blobs") and a β strand. Mutations in the α helices, but not in the β strand, reduce transactivation by E2.[48,93] Negatively charged amphipathic α helices are present in many other eukaryotic and prokaryotic transactivator proteins and might mediate protein-protein interactions with the TATA box binding factor TFIID and RNA polymerase II to facilitate transcription.[47] The E2 ORF of BPV-1 is known to specify two other shorter proteins. One of them, initiated from an internal in-frame AUG and comprising the middle and the carboxy-terminal portions of the E2 ORF, is a 31 kd protein termed E2-TR. The other is a 28 kd protein produced by an RNA splice connecting the amino-terminal 11 aa of the E8 ORF with the carboxy-terminal portion of the E2 ORF. Both these smaller E2 proteins function as transcriptional repressors acting on the same E2-responsive conditional enhancer elements in the LCR as the full-length transactivator protein.[68] Binding to the same elements is to be expected since all three E2 proteins contain the carboxy-terminal conserved domain required for specific DNA-binding.

The E2 proteins of BPV-1 and other papillomaviruses bind as dimers to the sequence 5'-ACCN$_6$GGT-3', and the binding is most efficient to a subset of the above consensus sequence reading 5'-ACCGN$_4$CGGT-3'.[1,93] Sequences required for dimerization of E2 are

located in the carboxy-terminal conserved region.[85] Multiple copies of the E2-binding site appear in the LCRs of papillomaviruses (Fig. 2). In BPV-1 two E2-responsive enhancer regions termed $E2RE_1$ and $E2RE_2$ have been mapped.[140] $E2RE_1$, located immediately upstream from the P_{7940} and P_{89} promoters, is the stronger of these two enhancers and contains a pair of E2-binding sites at either end. E2-binding shows cooperativity, and a pair of E2 sites is needed for strong transcriptional activation.[57,58,60,139] E2-binding sites occur as a pair upstream from the major promoter of all papillomaviruses (Fig. 2). In BPV-1-transformed mouse C127 cells, the E2 repressor proteins (especially E2-TR) are present at much higher levels than the E2 transactivator protein, resulting in the maintenance of low levels of the BPV-1 mRNAs in those cells.[85]

The effect of the HPV E2 proteins on the HPV LCR sequences is much more complex. The full-length E2 proteins of HPVs as well as BPV-1 can activate transcription from the HPV LCR cloned upstream from heterologous promoters.[13,31,50,59,60,104,147] The two E2-binding sites located proximal to the major HPV LCR promoters (Fig. 2) are sufficient for this E2-mediated transactivation.[13,50,147] However, for the promoter contained in the HPV LCR, repression of transcription is observed in the presence of the full-length E2 protein.[13,147] It is likely that repression might be due to steric hindrance by the E2 protein with the binding of transcription factors to the CAAT and TATA motifs located between the E2-binding sites.

As seen from the foregoing, unlike the situation in BPV-1, HPV mRNA transcription is minimally dependent on transactivation by E2. Even under conditions in which transactivation is achieved, it is far lower quantitatively compared to transactivation of the BPV-1 LCR by the BPV-1 E2 protein. In this connection, it is worth noting that the BPV-1 E2 protein has a much higher affinity for the $5'$-$ACCGN_4CGGT$-$3'$-binding site than the HPV E2 proteins.[10] It appears that in HPVs the full-length E2 protein serves mainly as a repressor of viral mRNA transcription. This would explain why in malignant lesions the DNA of an oncogenic HPV such as HPV-16 or HPV-18 is almost always integrated into the cell DNA through the E2 or the E1 ORFs. Consequently the E2 ORF is either disrupted or separated from the HPV LCR promoter-enhancer region, and is not expressed. The absence of the E2 protein would result in high, derepressed levels of mRNAs containing the E6 and E7 ORFs which are required for oncogenic transformation. In benign, low-grade lesions the viral DNA is usually present as an episome. The E2 protein produced under these conditions will maintain a low level of E6 and E7 mRNAs through negative regulation.

HPV mRNAs, which encode the carboxy-terminal 45% of the E2 ORF, have been detected (Table 2). A shorter E2 protein, E2-C, could be the product of these mRNAs. The HPV-11 E2-C protein, expressed by placing the E2-C cDNA under the control of the Rous sarcoma virus (RSV) long terminal repeat (LTR) promoter-enhancer, has been found to be a competitive inhibitor of the full-length E2 protein-induced activation of transcription from a heterologous promoter fused with the HPV-11 LCR.[23] This finding would imply that the HPV-11 E2-C is a repressor similar to BPV-1 E2-TR. However, the protein product of the E2-C mRNA has never been found in cells harboring HPV-11 or any other HPVs.

In addition to the E2-responsive enhancer located proximal to the promoter elements, upstream regions of the HPV LCR sequences contain constitutive enhancers composed of motifs commonly present in other viral or cellular enhancers (Fig. 2). The constitutive enhancers of HPV-16, HPV-18, and HPV-11 contain several copies of the motif 5'-GCCAA-3' or its inverted form 5'-TTGGC-3', known to be the binding site of a well known, ubiquitous transcription factor called CAAT transcription factor/nuclear factor 1 (CTF/NF-1).[52,53] The HPV-18 and HPV-16 constitutive enhancers contain two copies of the motif 5'-TGACTC/AA-3' which is the binding site of a transcription factor termed activator protein 1 (AP-1).[21,46] The AP-1-binding sites in the HPV-18 LCR augment transcription from the P_{105} promoter, and are the targets for binding of a member of the AP-1 family present in keratinocytes but not in fibroblasts.[99] The AP-1-binding sites in HPV-16 are reported to mediate induction of transcription from the P_{97} promoter by phorbol esters.[21] In addition, all HPV LCRs examined so far contain a functional glucocorticoid responsive element (GRE) that confers strong inducibility by glucocorticoid hormones.[51] Another feature of the constitutive enhancers in the LCRs of HPV-18, HPV-16, and HPV-11 is the presence of the inverted form of the K motif 5'-AANCCAAA-3' which is known to occur in the promoters of many keratinocyte-specific genes.[14,34,146] It is interesting to speculate that the K motif is at least partly responsible for the increased activity of the enhancers of HPV-16, HPV-18, and HPV-11 in keratinocytes.[23,31,46] Support for this proposal comes from the finding that a keratinocyte-specific transcription factor binds specifically to the K motif in the HPV-18 constitutive enhancer.[53] However, there must also be other elements mediating keratinocyte cell specificity since the constitutive enhancer of HPV-11 lacking the K motif functions in keratinocytes in a cell-specific manner.[23] In addition to the enhancer elements present in the LCR, an enhancer termed the 3' distal enhancer has been identified downstream from the early region ORFs (and upstream from the late region ORFs) in BPV-1.[75] The function of this enhancer is not known.

Regulation of Transcription by Viral Proteins Other Than E2

In addition to E2, two other early gene products of HPVs have been found to exhibit transcriptional regulatory properties. One of them is the E7 protein of HPV-16,[105] which is important for the transforming functions of HPV-16 (see below). The HPV-16 E7 protein is a 21 kd phosphoprotein that exhibits sequence and functional similarities with the well-known adenovirus transactivator protein E1A. Similar to E1A, the HPV-16 E7 is capable of transactivation of the adenovirus early region 2 (E2) promoter. The elements of the adeno-virus E2 promoter mediating transactivation by the adenovirus E1A and HPV-16 E7 proteins are indistinguishable, indicating that the mechanism of transactivation by these two proteins might be the same.[105] The HPV-16 E7 protein has not been demonstrated to act on the HPV-16 (or other HPV) promoters. However, there is a report that the E6 protein of HPV-18 behaves as a transactivator protein capable of stimulation of transcription by acting on elements located within the HPV-18 LCR.[50]

Activation of Late mRNA Transcription

As mentioned above, mRNAs specifying the late proteins L1 and L2 are produced only in keratinocytes productively infected by papillomaviruses. The polyadenylation signal, termed A_L, which is located downstream from the L1 ORF (Fig. 1), is used to determine the 3' ends of the late mRNAs. In bovine keratinocytes productively infected by BPV-1, late mRNAs are initiated from a special promoter termed P_L or P_{7250}.[2] The binding of keratinocyte-specific transcription factors to sequence elements located in this promoter has been reported.[153] Viral late mRNAs are not produced in cells transformed by papillomaviruses. Possible reasons for that are attenuation of late mRNA synthesis before the transcription complex reaches A_L, and destabilization of late mRNAs by certain sequences located between the L1 ORF and A_L.[3] The early mRNAs produced in transformed cells utilize the early-specific polyadenylation signal A_E located between the end of the early region and the L2 ORF (Fig. 1). Since A_E intervenes between the late promoter and A_L (see Fig. 1), there must be mechanisms operating in productively infected keratinocytes to diminish the utilization of A_E and augment the use of A_L.

Episomal Replication of the Viral DNA

The mechanism of episomal replication of BPV-1 DNA in transformed rodent cells has been studied in detail. The full-length BPV-1 DNA as well as a 69% segment containing the LCR and the complete early region exist as stable, multicopy episomes in those cells, with the copy number ranging from 50 to 400 per cell.[41,69,70] After the introduction of the viral DNA into the cells, it is believed that there is an initial burst of replication resulting in multiple copies of viral DNA per cell which is followed by a slower, maintenance-type mode of replication.[11,76,111] The maintenance-type replication in transformed cells is believed to resemble the controlled replication of the viral DNA in basal, undifferentiated keratinocytes under conditions of latency.[19]

Cis and Trans Elements—Earlier Studies

The origin of Cairns-type replication was mapped in the LCR immediately downstream from the L1 ORF by electron microscopic analysis of DNA molecules produced as intermediates in replication.[155] The E1 and the E2 ORF functions were implicated in replication since mutants in these two ORFs failed to exist as episomes.[115] Further studies on BPV-1 DNA replication appeared in the literature between 1984 and 1986 from the laboratory of Michael Botchan.[11,12,76–79] In their initial study, defined fragments of BPV-1 DNA were cloned into a selectable plasmid vector containing the bacterial *neo* gene,[137] and the ability of the plasmids to persist as episomes in ID13 cells (BPV-transformed mouse C127 cells that produce all the *trans* functions necessary for replication) was investigated.[76] Two independent *cis*-active regions of BPV-1 DNA, termed plasmid maintenance sequences (or PMS elements), were mapped which could support extrachromosomal replication of the *neo* gene plasmids; one of them termed PMS-1 was mapped in the upstream portion of the LCR at or near the origin of Cairns-type replication mapped by other workers using electron microscopy,[155] and the other, termed PMS-2, was mapped between nt 1515 and 1655 within the E1 ORF.[76] Some sequence homology was noted between PMS-1 and PMS-2.[76] The PMS-1 element was reported to function as an origin in short-term (or transient) replication assays in ID13 cells.[79] The PMS-1 origin was reported to consist of two noncontiguous domains: domain 1 located between nt 6706 and 6793 in the L1 ORF (which was termed an enhancer of replication since it could be replaced by certain other viral transcriptional enhancers); and domain 2 located between nt 7116 and 7234 in the L1 ORF-proximal upstream portion of the LCR (which was believed to be the core region of replication).[79]

Regarding *trans* functions required for BPV-1 DNA replication, the E2 ORF was reported to be dispensable since a deletion mutant lacking the entire E2 ORF was found to be capable of replication, though at a reduced level.[77,79] The E1 ORF was subdivided into two complementation groups: the amino-terminal portion termed M having a replication inhibitor or modulator function, and the middle and carboxy-terminal portion termed R having an activator function absolutely required for replication.[11,77–79] Another complementation group called *cop* was identified in the E6 and E7 ORFs, since mutants in those two ORFs, though replication-competent, were reported to exhibit a copy number of about two orders of magnitude lower than the wild type.[11,77] When mouse C127 cells that already contained a *cop* mutant DNA were supertransfected with the wild type DNA, the wild type DNA was also found to be established with a low copy number of 1 to 5 per cell. However, when the *cop* mutant-harboring cells were supertransfected with a mutant in the E1-M gene, the E1-M mutant DNA was found to replicate efficiently and become established with a higher copy number of 50 to 400 per cell.[11,77] Based on the above results, the following model was proposed for replication and its regulation: 1) the E1-R protein is absolutely required for replication; 2) when the viral DNA is introduced into cells there is an initial burst of efficient replication giving rise to multiple copies of the viral DNA per cell; this amplification event requires E1-R and the products of the *cop* genes E6 and E7; and 3) following this initial amplification, the level of the E1-M protein increases and reaches a threshold inhibitory level; at that point, the E1-M protein would reduce the replication frequency to approximately once per cell cycle so that the amplified viral DNA copies are maintained at the same level thereafter.[11,77]

Cis and *Trans* Elements—Recent Revised Information

Except for the results of Sarver et al. that both the E1 and E2 ORF functions are required for BPV-1 DNA replication,[115] the majority of the results of the other studies described above have not been reproducible in more recent experiments, and crucial aspects of the model mentioned above have to be revised based on the new information. Using newly constructed mutants in the E6 and E7 ORFs as well as an E7 ORF mutant employed in one of the earlier studies referred to above,[77] Neary and DiMaio reported that the mutant DNAs replicate efficiently and establish a normal copy number of 50 to 400 per cell, indicating that the E6 and E7 proteins (the proposed *cop* gene products) are dispensable for replication and maintenance of normal copy number of the viral DNA.[97]

The existence of two separate complementation groups E1-M and E1-R within the E1 ORF proposed in the earlier model has now been found to be incorrect. Making use of previously used as well as newly constructed mutants, Ustav and Stenlund have demonstrated that mutations throughout the E1 ORF (including the amino-terminal portion) are defective for replication.[151] Thus, the entire E1 ORF corresponds to a single complementation group with a phenotype corresponding to what was proposed earlier for a putative two-thirds component termed E1-R. Also, though a 28 kd phosphoprotein believed to be the E1-M product has been identified in ID13 cells,[148] the new study has found no evidence for a separate E1-M-like maintenance function for replication.[151]

Another issue that remained controversial until recently is on the role of the transcription-modulating E2 proteins on BPV-1 DNA replication. Lusky and Botchan reported that the E2 ORF function is dispensable for replication based on their finding that a deletion mutant lacking the entire E2 ORF was replication-capable.[77,79] This conclusion was contrary to that reached by three other laboratories, based on analysis of other E2 ORF mutants, that the E2 ORF function is required for replication as well as regulation of transcription and oncogenic transformation.[38,55,108,115] This issue has now been resolved by Ustav and Stenlund who have demostrated that a plasmid containing the BPV-1 origin replicates in mouse C127 cells only if both the E1 and the E2 proteins are expressed in *trans*.[151] The requirement of both E1 and E2 for replication has also been reported under in vitro conditions by Yang et al.[160] Further evidence for this conclusion is provided by reports that the full-length E2 transactivator protein forms a complex with the full-length E1 protein.[15,91] The full-length E1 protein is a 68 to 72 kd ATP-binding phosphoprotein.[114,144] The E1 ORF exhibits significant homology with domains of the large tumor (T) antigens of SV40 and polyomavirus, which are required for the nuclear localization, DNA-binding, ATPase and DNA helicase activities of those proteins.[27] The E1 protein has been reported to bind specifically to a sequence in the BPV-1 minimal origin of replication.[152,160] How the E1 and the E2 proteins initiate replication remains to be elucidated.

Another controversial issue is the location of the BPV-1 origin of replication. Using the episome persistence assay, Lusky and Botchan reported the identification of two origins; one termed PMS-1 located in the upstream portion of the LCR, and another termed PMS-2 located within the E1 ORF.[76] An origin corresponding to PMS-2 has not been detectable by other methods for mapping origins of replication such as electron microscopy and two-dimensional gel electrophoresis performed with replicative intermediates,[126,155] or in transient replication assays.[151] The PMS-1 origin localization received initial support from electron microscopy,[155] but two-dimensional electrophoresis mapped the origin at a location 450 nucleotides downstream from PMS-1 at the $E2RE_1$ region containing the major E2-binding sites in the LCR.[159] Neither PMS-1 nor $E2RE_1$ has been found to function as an origin in transient replication assays in vivo; instead, the origin has been localized further downstream in the LCR spanning the *Hpa*I restriction site at nt 7945/1.[152] The sequence around the *Hpa*I site functions as an origin in in vitro replication assays also.[160] The minimal origin has been mapped to a 60 bp sequence located between nt 7915 and 29, and contains an $A + T$-rich sequence, an inverted repeat binding specifically to the replication protein E1, and an E2-binding site termed E2 BS 12.[152] Point mutations within E2 BS 12 do not affect replication, indicating that the binding of the second replication protein E2 to the origin is not required for replication.[152] It is believed that E2 would function in replication by binding to E1 with whom it is known to form a complex.[15,91] Further investigations are needed to determine whether this 60 bp sequence functions as an origin in the episome persistence assay also.

It is interesting to note that the newly mapped 60 bp minimal replication origin is immediately upstream from the major BPV-1 transcriptional promoter P_{89}, and might include some of the elements of that promoter. The overlapping of replication and transcription control elements in BPV-1 resembles a similar situation in the origin regions of papovaviruses.

Replication of HPV DNA

In contrast to the situation with BPV-1 outlined above, there is very little information on the cis-and trans-active elements required for HPV DNA replication. Keratinocyte cell-lines derived from human cervical lesions that harbor HPV DNAs as stable episomes have been described,[24,39,84] but the mechanism of episomal replication of the viral DNA in those cell-lines is not known. When newborn human foreskin keratinocytes in culture were infected with HPV-1, viral DNA was gradually lost with passage and was no longer detectable after the fifth passage of the cells, due to underreplication of HPV-1 DNA compared to the cell DNA.[109] HPV-6b DNA introduced into human foreskin keratinocytes by transfection was not found to replicate at all in a transient replication assay.[44] It has been suggested that the failed attempts to achieve HPV DNA replication in cultured cells are due to the inability to reconstitute a specific stage in keratinocyte differentiation which may be required for replication.

Sequences homologous with those present in the 60 bp BPV-1 minimal replication origin region are present in the corresponding portions of the LCRs of other papillomaviruses including HPVs.[152] The E1 ORFs of HPVs exhibit significant sequence homology with the E1 ORF of BPV-1. The full-length E2 proteins of HPVs and BPV-1 bind to the same consensus motif and exhibit trancription activation properties. Such a functional interchangeability may also apply to replication since it has been reported that the HPV-16 E2 protein can replace its BPV-1 counterpart in BPV-1 DNA replication.[152] These similarities between the cis and trans functions of BPV-1 and HPVs indicate that the mechanisms of replication of HPV and BPV-1 DNAs might be quite similar. Experimental evidence for this proposal is now awaited.

Oncogenic Transformation

Transforming Functions of BPV-1

Mouse C127 cells transformed by BPV-1 exhibit the characteristic features of morphological transformation including focus formation, loss of contact inhibition, anchorage independence, and tumorigenicity in nude mice.[41] As mentioned above, the viral DNA exists as a multicopy episome in those cells, though episomal existence is not a prerequisite for transformation. The transforming functions were found to be located in the early region of the genome since a 69% fragment of BPV-1 containing the LCR and the early region was transformation-competent.[74] By systematic mutagenesis of the various early region ORFs and analysis of their abilities to transform rodent cells in culture, two independent transforming functions of BPV-1 have been identified. One of these functions is specified by the E5 ORF,[55,120,162] and the other by the E6 and E7 ORFs.[119,161]

The E5 genes of papillomaviruses inducing fibropapillomas in their natural hosts (such as BPV-1) are highly conserved, while those of viruses whose targets are epithelial cells (such as HPVs) are not. The E5 gene is expressed very well in cells transformed by BPV-1. The E5 protein, with an apparent mass of 7 kd and comprised of 44 aa, is the smallest known native transforming protein. The E5 protein consists of two structural domains: a very hydrophobic domain comprising the amino-terminal two-thirds present in an α helical conformation, and a hydrophilic carboxy-terminal domain. The amino-terminal hydrophobic domain determines the membrane localization of the E5 protein.[122] The carboxy-terminal domain can function to induce cellular DNA synthesis when injected into quiescent cells.[54] The two cysteines in the carboxy-terminal domain mediate dimer formation, and are required for the transforming activity of E5.[18,62] Recent results indicate that the transforming activity of the E5 protein is related to its ability to activate receptors of growth factors such as epidermal growth factor, colony stimulating factor-1, and platelet-derived growth factor.[81,102]

Complete transformation of mouse C127 cell to anchorage independence and tumorigenicity in nude mice also requires the E6 and E7 ORF functions.[97,115] The E6 and E7 proteins are related in sequence to each other and to their counterparts specified by other papillomaviruses. They are believed to have evolved by duplication of a 33 aa core sequence containing the motif Cys-X-X-Cys (Cys refers to the amino acid cysteine and X refers to any amino acid) which is present in several zinc finger types of DNA-binding proteins. The 16 kd E6 protein of BPV-1 contains four copies of the Cys-X-X-Cys motif while the yet to be identified E7 protein contains two. The E6 protein is localized both in the nucleus and in the membrane fractions. The nuclear localization and the presence of the Cys-X-X-Cys repeats suggest that E6 may be a DNA-binding protein. Indeed the E6 and E7 proteins of several HPVs have been found to be zinc-containing, DNA-binding proteins.[6]

In addition to these three proteins, the E2 protein has also been found to be important for transformation by BPV-1.[38,55,108] However, the effect of E2 is indirect, acting by way of increasing the expression of E5, E6, and E7 genes through its transactivation function. If the transforming genes are expressed from strong heterologous promoter-enhancer sequences, there is no longer a requirement of E2 for transformation. There is also the suggestion that the E1 protein might exert a negative effect on transformation since mutants in the E1 ORF were found to exhibit an increased transforming activity, with the effect mediated by an increase in expression of the integrated viral genome in transformed cells.[66,118]

Transforming Functions of HPVs and Their Assays

The major interest in research on HPVs is the association of approximately 18 members of this group with anogenital cancers. Two prominent members of this group of viruses often associated with cervical cancer are HPV-16 and HPV-18. A few other members, most notably HPV-6 and HPV-11, also cause lesions of the genital tract; but those lesions very rarely undergo malignant conversion, unlike lesions associated with HPV-16 and HPV-18 where there is a much greater risk of progress to malignancy.

A number of techniques have been used to analyze and identify the transforming functions of oncogenic HPVs such as HPV-16 and HPV-18. One such assay is the morphological transformation of established or immortalized rodent cells such as NIH3T3 or Rat-1 cells in culture. This assay has been successfully used previously for the detection of certain viral and cellular oncogenes. Since HPV-16 and HPV-18 (and other oncogenic HPVs) are inefficient in transformation of established rodent cells, the technique has been modified by the introduction into the cells of the viral DNAs (or portions thereof) along with plasmids carrying dominant selectable marker genes such as the neomycin phosphotransferase (*neo*) gene.[137] Colonies selected for resistance to G418 are propagated and monitored for the transformed phenotype. Using this assay, the transforming functions of HPV-16 and HPV-18 were mapped initially to the E6-E7 region [9], and were pinpointed later to the E7 ORF.[63,105,145,154,163] HPVs transform rodent cells inefficiently as shown by the inability of HPV-16 and HPV-18 by themselves to transform primary rat embryo fibroblasts or baby rat kidney cells. However, these viruses can cooperate with the activated *ras* oncogene to transform primary rodent cells.[83] The viral immortalization function involved in this *ras* cooperation assay has been found to be the E7 protein.[8,105,143] In these assays, only those genital HPVs exhibiting a greater risk for malignant conversion (such as HPV-16, HPV-18, HPV-31, and HPV-33) are found to be active, while the low-risk genital HPVs (such as HPV-6 and HPV-11) are not.[143]

The transforming functions of HPVs have also been assayed using various human cells including fibroblasts, foreskin keratinocytes, and cervical squamous epithelial cells. Unlike rodent cells, human cells transformed by HPVs do not show certain characteristics of complete transformation including anchorage independence and tumorigenicity in nude mice. Instead, the assay measures the ability of the transformed human cells to proliferate and to offer resistance when challenged with signals for terminal differentiation.[40,64,106] Both the E6 and E7 ORFs of HPV-16 or HPV-18 are also required for transformation in this assay.[121,156] Since calcium ions facilitate differentiation, transfection procedures involving calcium phosphate coprecipitation of the DNA are not suitable for introducing the viral DNA into human keratinocytes. Instead the preferred ways of introducing the DNA into those cells appear to be via electroporation or lipofection. Using these techniques, it has been shown that only the oncogenic HPVs such as HPV-16 and HPV-18 produce truly immortal cell-lines which are refractory to differentiation-inducing signals.[121]

The HPV Transforming Protein E7

The E7 oncoprotein of HPV-16 and HPV-18 is necessary and sufficient for transformation of rodent cells by these viruses. The E7 protein is also the most abundant viral protein in cervical carcinomas and in cell-lines established from them such as SiHa, CaSki, and HeLa.[130,135,136] The HPV-16 E7 protein is 98 aa in length corresponding to a predicted size of 11 kd. However, in denaturing protein gels it behaves as a protein of 21 kd due to posttranslational modifications.[5] The E7 protein is phosphorylated at certain serine residues. It is localized mainly in the cytoplasm.

Though they are much smaller than the 289 aa E1A protein of human adenovirus, the E7 proteins of the oncogenic genital HPVs (viz. HPV-16, HPV-18, HPV-31, and HPV-33) show a striking similarity with the adenovirus E1A in being multifunctional proteins possessing transformation and transcription activation properties. Similar to E1A, the HPV-16 E7 protein transactivates the E1A-responsive adenovirus E2 promoter,[105] and cooperates with the activated *ras* oncogene protein to transform primary baby rat kidney cells.[8,105,143] The amino-terminal 37 aa portion of HPV-16 E7 possesses a striking sequence similarity with portions of conserved regions 1 and 2 of the adenovirus E1A protein.[105] Conserved regions 1 and 2 are essential for the transformation function of E1A, and are also required for its association with the 105 kd cellular tumor-suppressor protein p105-RB (mutations in which cause a predisposition to development of cancers such as retinoblastoma, osteosarcoma, breast carcinoma, and small cell lung carcinoma).[158] Homologous stretches of amino acids present in the SV40 large T-antigen are important for its transformation property and its association with the p105-RB protein.[35] Similar to E1A and large T-antigen, the E7 protein was also found to associate with p105-RB.[42] E7 proteins of genital HPVs with a higher risk for progression to malignancy (such as HPV-16 and HPV-18) bound more efficiently to p105-RB than E7 proteins of the lower risk genital HPVs (such as HPV-6 and HPV-11).[96] The E7 protein of BPV-1, whose amino-terminal sequence is unrelated to those of the HPV E7 proteins did not form a detectable complex with p105-RB.[96] Association between HPV-16 E7 and p105-RB was not only observed under in vitro conditions, but such a complex was also detected in an HPV-16-transformed human keratinocyte cell-line.[96]

The findings that the HPV E7, adenovirus E1A, and SV40 large T-antigen bind to the same cellular antioncogene protein (viz p105-RB) suggest that these viral oncoproteins might be using similar mechanisms for cellular transformation. The fact that the E7 proteins of genital HPVs belonging to both high-and low-risk types bind to p105-RB (albeit with different efficiencies) indicates that binding to p105-RB may not be sufficient for malignant transformation, but may be related to a property common to all genital HPVs such as induction of cell proliferation which occurs in both benign and malignant lesions.

The mechanism of transcriptional activation by the E7 proteins is not known. The Cys-X-X-Cys repeat which is present in the carboxy-terminal portion of E7 might be responsible for its transactivation function since this motif is also present in conserved region 3 of E1A which is required for its transactivation property.[92] The only promoter known to be transactivated by HPV E7 is the adenovirus E2 promoter. There is no evidence of modulation of transcription from the viral LCR by the E7 protein, nor is there any information regarding possible cellular targets of E7.

The HPV Transforming Protein E6

E6 is the second oncoprotein of HPVs. As mentioned above, both E7 and E6 are required for the immortalization of human squamous epithelial cells by HPVs. The HPV-16 E6 gene encodes an 18 to 19 kd protein. An important property of the E6 proteins of the high-risk oncogenic viruses HPV-16 and HPV-18 is their ability to associate in vitro with the cellular tumor-suppressor protein p53.[157] p53, which was recently established to be an antioncogene protein,[43,45] has previously been shown to form specific complexes with the adenovirus 55 kd E1B oncoprotein and the SV40 large T-antigen.[73] Thus, unlike SV40, adenoviruses and high-risk genital HPVs code for separate oncoproteins for interactions with p105-RB and p53. Since the E6 proteins of the high-risk but not the low-risk HPVs are capable of interaction with the cellular p53, it may be speculated that interaction with p53 might somehow be responsible for progression toward malignancy.

Though HeLa cervical carcinoma cells contain detectable quantities of translatable p53 mRNA, p53 protein could not be detected in those cells.[82] Also, while p53 is present in detectable quantities in primary human keratinocytes and keratinocytes transformed by SV40, it is lacking in human keratinocytes transformed by HPV-16.[117] These results prompted an investigation of the status of p53 upon association with the E7 proteins of HPV-16 and HPV-18. It has been found that the E7 proteins of HPV-16 and HPV-18 bind to p53 and engineer its degradation.[117] The E6-induced degradation of p53 is ATP-dependent, and is mediated by the ubiquitin-dependent protease system.[117] This is the first known example of the selective tagging and degradation of a cellular antioncogene protein by a dominant-acting viral oncoprotein, and amounts to a novel mechanism of carcinogenesis.

It should be noted that truncated E6 proteins corresponding to the E6* mRNAs (see the section above on transcription) have not been identified. Also, transformation experiments carried out with E6 or E6* cDNAs indicate that the truncated E6* could not satisfy the requirement of the full-length E6 ORF for the immortalization of human keratinocytes.[95]

The structural features, properties, and functions of the HPV proteins are summarized and listed in Table 3.

Involvement of Other Factors in Progression Toward Malignancy

In high-grade genital lesions and in cervical carcinomas, the oncogenic genital HPV DNAs are found integrated into the cell DNA, while in low-grade lesions that have not yet progressed to malignancy the viral DNA exists in episomal form.[40] In almost all cervical carcinomas, integration of the viral DNA occurs in such a way as to disrupt the E2 ORF or uncouple it from the E6 and E7 ORFs.[4,128] Since E2 functions as a repressor in the context of the intact LCR resulting in reduced transcription of the E6 and E7 mRNAs from the P_{97} or P_{105} promoters (in the case of HPV-16 or HPV-18, respectively),[147] the result is the continued high level expression of the E6 and E7 oncoproteins. However, the expression of E6 and E7 is by itself not sufficient for malignant transformation since the introduction and expression of E6 and E7 genes of HPV-16 or HPV-18 into primary human keratinocytes results only in immortalization of those cells.[40,64,96,106,121,156] In addition to the viral E6 and E7 proteins, other factors or assaults on the cells might be required for progression toward malignant transformation. One such factor could be the cellular c-*myc* protein. In HeLa cells, the site of integration of the HPV-18 DNA sequences is near the c-*myc* gene on chromosome 8.[71,107] Amplification and high level expression of c-*myc* has been observed in cervical carcinomas, especially in more advanced stages of the disease.[98,110]

A putative tumor-suppressor gene located on chromosome 11 might be involved in suppression of malignant transformation induced by HPV-16 and HPV-18. Tumorigenicity in nude mice of HeLa or SiHa cervical carcinoma cells (containing HPV-18 and HPV-16 sequences,

TABLE 3.
Properties and Functions of HPV Proteins

Protein	Size	Features and Properties	Functions
E6	18 to 19 kd	Contains four copies of the motif Cys-X-X-Cys; complexes with zinc and binds to DNA; E6 proteins of oncogenic genital HPVs (e.g., HPV-16 and HPV-18) form specific complexes with cellular antioncogene protein p53 and trigger its degradation *via* ubiquitination.	Required (along with E7) to transform primary human keratinocytes, and make them refractory to differentiation inducing signals. [Applies only to E6 and E7 of oncogenic genital HPVs].
E7	21 kd	Phosphorylated at certain serine residues; mainly cytoplasmic localization; contains two copies of the Cys-X-X-Cys motif, complexes with zinc, and binds to DNA; possesses homologies to the adenovirus E1A protein in sequence and functions such as transactivation of the adenovirus E2 promoter, cooperation with the activated *ras* oncogene protein to transform primary rodent cells, and formation of a specific complex with the cellular antioncogene protein p105-RB.	Required (along with E6) to transform primary human keratinocytes (see above); E7 of oncogenic genital HPVs is sufficient (E6 is not required) for transformation of established rodent cells, and for cooperation with activated *ras* to transform primary rodent cells.
E1	68 to 72 kd	Conserved fairly well among different papillomaviruses. *BPV-1:* ATP-binding phosphoprotein; exhibits homology with papovavirus large T antigen domains involved in nuclear localization, DNA-binding, ATPase and helicase activities; binds to minimal replication origin; forms a specific complex with the 48 kd E2 protein. *HPVs:* Homologous to BPV-1 E1; probably have similar properties.	Required in *trans* along with 48 kd E2 protein for replication of BPV-1; HPV E1 proteins are likely to have a similar function.
E2	*BPV-1:* 48 kd, 31 kd,	48 kd full-length protein possesses two conserved domains; a 220 aa amino-terminal transactivator domain containing two amphipathic alpha helices (or "acid blobs") followed	*BPV-1:* All three proteins bind to the same E2RE elements of the LCR, and cause activation (48 kd protein) or repression

and 28 kd *HPVs:* only 48 kd	by a beta strand; and a 100 aa carboxy-terminal domain required for dimerization and specific binding to the 5'-ACCN$_6$GGT-3' motif present as a repeat in the E2RE sequences of the LCRs; the two shorter repressor proteins of BPV-1 lack the amino-terminal transactivator domain, but contain the same carboxy-terminal domain as the full-length protein and bind to the same motif.	(31 and 28 kd proteins) of viral early mRNA transcription; required along with E1 for replication of viral DNA (48 kd protein). *HPVs:* The 48 kd full-length protein acts as transactivator or repressor of viral early mRNA transcription depending on the conditions.
E4 16 to 20 kd in various HPVs	Mainly cytoplasmic; associated with distinctive cytoplasmic inclusion granules; most abundant viral protein in warts; amounting to 30% of total protein in HPV-1 induced warts; acidic, multiply charged and able to form dimers; though classified as an early protein, produced mainly late in infection.	Not a virion structural protein (though produced in the late phase of infection); might aid virion maturation.
E5 7 kd	Conserved among papillomaviruses which infect (or transform) both fibroblasts and epithelial cells (such as BPVs, deer and elk papillomaviruses, etc.), but not those that affect only epithelial cells (such as HPVs). *BPV-1:* Amino terminal two-thirds are very hydrophobic (14 out of 30 amino acids are leucines) and are predicted to be in an alpha helical conformation; the carboxy terminal one-third is hydrophilic and contains a Cys-X-Cys motif; localized in the cell membrane; anchored into membrane through the hydrophobic domain and dimerizes through the cysteine residues of the carboxy-terminal domain located extracellularly; the cysteines are also required for oncogenic transformation by E5; increases the activity of receptors of growth factors such as EGF, CSF-1, and PDGF. *HPVs:* encode E5 with some structural similarities to that of the BPV-1 E5; properties not known.	*BPV-1:* Required (along with E6 and E7) for oncogenic transformation; transforms fibroblasts (e.g., mouse NIH 3T3 cells) more efficiently than epithelial cells (e.g., mouse C127 cells); responsible for the induction of fibroblastic tumors by BPV-1; carboxy-terminal hydrophilic domain can induce cell DNA synthesis upon injection into quiescent cells; transforming activity is perhaps related to activation of receptors involved in cell proliferation. *HPVs:* functions unknown; not known to have transforming activity which is not surprising since transformation by HPVs is restricted to epithelial cells.

(continued)

TABLE 3.
Properties and Functions of HPV Proteins (continued)

Protein	Size	Features and Properties	Functions
L1	55 kd	Transcribed and translated only in the most terminally differentiated keratinocytes; most highly conserved viral protein among papillomaviruses; carries the major antigenic determinants for group-specific cross-reactivity; highly glycosylated which contributes to stability of virus particle.	Major virion capsid protein.
L2	70 kd	Transcribed and translated only in the most terminally differentiated keratinocytes; not conserved well among papillomaviruses; antigenic determinants are very type-specific and do not crossreact even within the same group.	Minor virion capsid protein.

respectively) has been found to be suppressed by the introduction into those cells of the normal chromosome 11 via somatic cell hybridization with normal human fibroblasts.[65,116] This suppression has been attributed to a tumor-suppressor gene present on chromosome 11. Suppression of tumorigenicity has also been attributed to the inhibition of the HPV-18 E6 and E7 gene expression in HeLa X fibroblast hybrid cells by a putative cellular interference factor (CIF) specified by the normal chromosome 11 of the fibroblast.[16,112] Loss or mutation of either the tumor-suppressor gene or the CIF gene or both can be expected to lead to progression toward malignant transformation.

Certain physical and chemical agents could act as accomplices in the progression of HPV-associated lesions to malignancy. As mentioned earlier in this chapter, young children with a rare hereditary condition develop a skin lesion termed EV as a result of infection with certain types of HPV which do not affect the general population. In about 30% of the EV cases, especially those associated with HPV-5 or HPV-8, progression to squamous cell carcinoma occurs in areas exposed to ultraviolet light.[100] Tobacco smoking has been implicated as a risk factor in malignant conversion leading to cervical cancer.[26,150] Nicotine, which could give rise to the carcinogenic N-nitrosamines, can reach cervical cells as shown by its detection in vaginal fluids of smokers.[61] Exposure to other mutagens and carcinogens can also be expected to aid in malignant conversion of HPV-associated lesions.

The immune status of the host could also play a role in HPV infection and its malignant conversion. Transplant recipients are at a fivefold risk of developing cervical condyloma compared to the nonimmunosuppressed general population.[124] Immunosuppressed patients are also at a greater risk for malignant progression of genital lesions compared to the population in general.[133]

A number of physical, chemical, or biological agents or conditions determine progression towards malignancy. Infection by HPV, however, is an important step in this cascade as underscored by the presence of HPV sequences and their expression in those cancers, and by the fact that infections with only certain types of HPVs results in malignant conversion.

Detection of Human Papillomaviruses

Cervical carcinoma is a major type of cancer affecting women. Greater than 90% of cervical carcinomas and metastases are associated with high-risk HPVs such as HPV-16 (about 50% to 60%) and HPV-18 (about 20% to 30%). It is classified under sexually transmitted diseases, and its incidence is increasing especially in the younger population. Early detection and typing of the viral DNA would be of help in finding a cure and preventing further transmission. The most common method of detection has been by cytologic analysis of Pap smears. This technique requires confirmation by a more reliable and unequivocal method of detection. The condylomata acuminata induced by the low-risk genital HPVs HPV-6 and HPV-11 are sharp projections that are easier to recognize. In contrast, high-risk HPVs such as HPV-16 and HPV-18 induce flat warts which are more difficult to detect. There is no cell culture system available for propagation of virus samples for further analysis. Methods have been developed based on detection of HPV sequences using specific DNA probes by Southern or dot blot analysis of DNA isolated from cervical biopsies or cervical swabs,[87,123] but are time-consuming and are not very sensitive. An in situ hybridization procedure based on an RNA probe has been developed to detect HPV DNA and RNA sequences in condylomas and cervical carcinomas,[142] but requires prolonged autoradiography of up to four weeks.

These problems have been solved by methods developed recently using the PCR technique.[94] In the first study using PCR for the detection of HPV sequences, paraffin-embedded tissue specimens were used as the experimental material.[131] The specimens, which were randomly selected, were derived from patients with cervical squamous cell carcinoma, severe cervical dysplasia, or penile squamous cell carcinoma. The primers were designed based on a knowledge of the sequences of the E6 ORFs and of HPV-16 and HPV-18 DNAs, both of which are completely sequenced.[29,129] The 5' (or positive strand) primer used was common to both HPV-16 and HPV-18 (due to sequence homology in that location) while the 3' (or negative strand) primers were different in the two cases. The target size was 110 nucleotides. Amplified DNA was clearly detectable by dot blot hybridization using labeled oligonucleotide probes specific for the target regions after only 60 to 75 minutes of autoradiography. Hybridization to either the HPV-16 probe or the HPV-18 probe (but not to both) was observed. The majority of the DNA samples hybridized with the HPV-16 probe. Using template DNA produced from defined numbers of SiHa cervical carcinoma cells (which contain one to two copies of HPV-16 DNA per cell) for amplification, it was shown that the technique was sensitive enough to detect as few as 20 copies of the viral DNA, and that the whole assay could be carried out within 24 hours.[131]

Following this initial study, other studies of HPV detection using the PCR technique have been published.[32,89,90] In one of these studies, the presence of the high-(HPV-16, HPV-18 and HPV-33) and low-(HPV-6 and HPV-11) risk HPVs in clinical specimens including cervical scrapes and lavages, anal scrapes, and anogenital biopsies was examined by performing PCR using oligonucleotide primers derived from the E6 ORFs of these viruses.[32] The primers were designed such that different size amplification products were expected from the different viruses. The amplification products were fractionated by gel electrophoresis and detected by staining with ethidium bromide. The nature of the HPV infection was determined from the size of the amplification product and was confirmed by hybridization with virus-specific probes. As few as 10 copies of the viral DNA could be easily detected in this study.[32]

Another study was focused on male patients (as opposed to most studies which are carried out with female patients).[89] It was reasoned that HPV-16 and HPV-18 were associated with cervical as well as penile cancer,[88] and that condylomata acuminata associated mainly with HPV-6 or HPV-11 are found in both females[49] and males.[37] The screening of male patients was also deemed to be important due to the reported detection of genital HPVs in penile smears of 5.8% of apparently healthy males who were tested,[56] and the presence of HPV-2 and HPV-5 in semen from patients with severe chronic wart disease and EV, respectively,[7] indicating that semen could be a reservoir of HPV. Indeed, other reports indicate increased occurrence of cervical lesions in women whose sexual partners had condylomata acuminata of the penis.[7,20,72] For these reasons, urine samples from 17 male patients with condylomata acuminata in the meatus urethrae were tested for the presence of HPV-6 or HPV-11, with samples of 14 laboratory volunteers tested simultaneously as controls.[89] DNA was extracted from sediments produced by centrifugation of the urine and subjected to amplification by PCR using oligonucleotide primers located flanking the unique BamHI sites present in the L2 or L1 ORFs, respectively, in HPV-6 or HPV-11. (This approach was used to prevent amplification from recombinant plasmids containing HPV-6 and HPV-11 DNAs cloned through their BamHI sites into plasmid vectors, if those plasmids were accidentally contaminated with the experimental DNA samples.) The PCR products were fractionated by electrophoresis on agarose gels, blotted onto nitrocellulose filters, and hybridized with HPV-6-or HPV-11-specific radiolabeled probes. Fifteen of the 17 patients were found positive for HPV. Out of those 15, 8 were positive for HPV-6, 6 for HPV-11, and 1 for both; none from the control group of 14 tested positive for HPVs.[89] This study points to the possible transmission of HPV through urine and to the similar possibility of sexual transmission during ejaculation of HPV-infected cells present in the male genital tract, and underscores the importance of testing both females and their male cohorts.

Another dimension to the detection of HPVs by the PCR assay has been added by the development of consensus oligonucleotide primers that can amplify targets from up to 25 different genital HPVs belonging to both high-and low-risk groups.[80,149] The consensus primers were derived from the L1 ORF, since L1 (and to a less extent E1) ORFs are the most homologous among the different types of HPVs, and since the L1 ORF is never interrupted by the integration of HPV DNA into cell DNA in cervical carcinomas, while the E1 ORF could be interrupted in some cases under those conditions. Only one pair of 5' and 3' consensus primers were used, with the primers containing degeneracy at several positions (created by mixed base insertions at those positions during the synthesis of the primers), with the result that the primers were almost completely complementary to the five genital HPVs of known nucleotide sequence, viz HPV-16,[129] HPV-18,[29] HPV-33,[30] HPV-6,[127] and HPV-11.[34] Amplification by PCR resulted in a DNA band of approximately 450 bp in all these cases which could be detected by either a generic or a type-specific probe. The type specificity could also be ascertained by restriction analysis of the PCR products using differences in restriction sites present in the target sequence for amplification in each case. This approach is capable of identification and typing of up to 25 of the genital HPVs, and should prove to be valuable for the analysis of clinical specimens. The generic probe mix described in this study is now being improved to increase the spectrum of hybridization with the L1 ORF PCR products from different genital HPVs.[149] As the sequences of more HPV DNAs becomes available, additional probes could be designed for them. This method, like the other PCR-based methods described above, can detect as few as 10 copies of HPV DNA in a sample, and the type identification has been verified by other methods, such as in situ or Southern blot hybridization, to be accurate.[149]

Conclusions

Despite the limitation imposed by the inability to develop a cell culture system for the propagation of papillomaviruses, important advances have been made in this field during the last decade. Rapid and sensitive PCR-based methods have been developed for the detection and typing of genital HPVs in clinical specimens. Viral gene products having cell transformation properties have been identified. E6 and E7 are the oncoproteins of HPVs, and E5 also has transforming functions in BPV-1. Important differences have been noted between the transforming proteins of the high-and low-risk genital HPVs (regarding their interaction with cellular antioncogene proteins) which could provide at least a partial explanation of why the lesions lead to malignant conversion in one case but remain benign in the other. *Cis*-and *Trans*-acting functions required for viral mRNA transcription and its regulation have been identified. Transcription control mediated by the viral E2 gene products predominates in BPV-1, and less so in HPVs. Also, unlike in BPV-1 where the full-length E2 protein functions as a transcription activator and two shorter E2 proteins function as repressors, HPVs encode only the full-length E2 protein which functions to activate or repress transcription depending on the conditions. Possible collaborations between the viral E2 proteins and cellular factors have been proposed. *cis* and *trans* elements mediating the episomal replication of the viral DNA have been identified, but only in the case of BPV-1. A 60 bp minimal replication origin has been mapped, and both the E1 and E2 proteins have been found to be required in *trans* for replication. Further work is needed to understand the mechanism of vegetative DNA replication as well as other events occurring late in infection including late gene expression and virion assembly. Work in those areas would be greatly facilitated by the setting up of cell culture systems for virus propagation.

References

1. Androphy EJ, Lowy DR, Schiller JT. Bovine papillomavirus E2 *trans*-acting gene product binds to specific sites in papillomavirus DNA. Nature 1987; 325:70–73.
2. Baker CC, Howley PM. Differential promoter utilization by the papillomavirus in transformed cells and productively infected wart tissues. EMBO J 1987; 6:1027–1035.

3. Baker CC, Noe JS. Transcriptional termination between bovine papillomavirus type 1 (BPV-1) early and late polyadenylation sites blocks late transcription in BPV-1 transformed cells. J Virol 1989; 63:3529–3534.

4. Baker CC, Phelps WC, Lindgren V, et al. Structural and transcriptional analysis of human papillomavirus type 16 sequences in cervical carcinoma cell lines. J Virol 1987; 61:962-971.

5. Barbosa MS, Edmonds C, Fisher C, et al. The region of the HPV E7 oncoprotein homologous to adenovirus E1a and SV40 large T antigen contains separate domains for Rb binding and casein kinase II phosphorylation. EMBO J 1990; 9:153–160.

6. Barbosa MS, Lowy DR, Schiller JT. Papillomavirus polypeptides E6 and E7 are zinc binding proteins. J Virol 1989; 63:1404-1407.

7. Barrasso R, De Brux J, Croissant O, et al. High prevalence of papillomavirus-associated penile intraepithelial neoplasia in sexual partners of women with cervical intraepithelial neoplasia. N Engl J Med 1987; 317:916–923.

8. Bedell MA, Jones KH, Grossman SR, et al. Identification of human papillomavirus type 18 transforming genes in immortalized and primary cells. J Virol 1989; 63:1247–1255.

9. Bedell MA, Jones KH, Laimins LA. The E6-E7 region of human papillomavirus 18 is sufficient for transformation of NIH 3T3 and Rat-1 cells. J Virol 1987; 61:3635–3640.

10. Bedrosian CL, Bastia D. The DNA binding domain of HPV-16 E2 protein interaction with the viral enhancer: Protein-induced DNA binding and role of the nonconserved core sequence in binding site affinity. Virology 1990; 174:557–575.

11. Berg L, Lusky M, Stenlund A, et al. Repression of bovine papillomavirus replication is mediated by a virally encoded *trans*-acting factor. Cell 1986; 46:753–762.

12. Berg LJ, Singh K, Botchan MR. Complementation of a bovine papillomavirus low-copy-number mutant: Evidence for a temporal requirement of the complementing gene. Mol Cell Biol 1986; 6:859-869.

13. Bernard BA, Bailly C, Lenoir MC, et al. The human papillomavirus type 18 (HPV 18) E2 gene product is a repressor of the HPV 18 regulatory region in human keratinocytes. J Virol 1989; 63:4317–4324.

14. Blessing M, Zentgraf H, Jorcano JL. Differentially expressed bovine cytokeratin genes. Analysis of gene linkage and evolutionary conservation of 5' upstream sequences. EMBO J 1987; 6:567–575.

15. Blitz IL, Laimins L. The 68-kilodalton E1 protein of bovine papillomavirus is a DNA-binding phosphoprotein which associates with the E2 transcriptional activator in vitro. J Virol 1991; 65:649–656.

16. Bosch FZ, Schwarz E, Boukamp P, et al. Suppression in vivo of human papillomavirus type 18 E6-E7 gene expression in nontumorigenic HeLa x fibroblast hybrid cells. J Virol 1990; 64:4743–4754.

17. Broker TR, Botchan M. Papillomaviruses: Retrospectives and prospectives. Cancer Cells 1986; 4:17–36.

18. Burkhardt A, DiMaio D, Schlegel R. Genetic and biochemical definition of the bovine papillomavirus E5 transforming protein. EMBO J 1987; 6:2381–2385.

19. Burnett S, Kiessling U, Pettersson U. Loss of bovine papillomavirus DNA replication control in growth-arrested transformed cells. J Virol 1989; 63:2215–2225.
20. Campion MJ, Singer A, Clarkson PK, et al. Increased risk of cervical neoplasia in consorts of men with penile condylomata acuminata. Lancet 1985; i:943–946.
21. Chan WK, Chong T, Bernard HU, et al. Transcription of the transforming genes of the oncogenic human papillomavirus-16 is stimulated by tumor promoters through AP1 binding sites. Nucleic Acids Res 1990; 18:763–769.
22. Chen EY, Howley PM, Levinson AD, et al. The primary structure and genetic organization of the bovine papillomavirus type 1 genome. Nature 1982; 299:529–534.
23. Chin MT, Hirochika R, Hirochika H, et al. Regulation of human papillomavirus type 11 enhancer and E6 promoter by activating and repressing proteins from the E2 open reading frame: Functional and biochemical studies. J Virol 1988; 62:2994–3002.
24. Choo KB, Cheung WF, Liew LN, et al. Presence of catenated human papillomavirus type 16 episomes in a cervical carcinoma cell line. J Virol 1989; 63:782–789.
25. Chow LT, Nasseri M, Wolinsky SM, et al. Human papillomaviruses types 6 and 11 mRNAs from genital condylomata. J Virol 1987; 61:2581–2588.
26. Clarke EA, Morgan RW, Newman AM. Smoking as a risk factor in cancer of the cervix: Additional evidence from a case control study. Am J Epidemiol 1982; 115:59–66.
27. Clertant P, Seif I. A common function for polyomavirus large T and papillomavirus E1 proteins? Nature 1984; 311:276–279.
28. Coggin JR, Zur Hausen H. Workshop on papillomaviruses and cancer. Cancer Res 1979; 39:545–546.
29. Cole ST, Danos O. Nucleotide sequence and comparative analysis of the human papillomavirus type 18 genome. J Mol Biol 1987; 193:599–608.
30. Cole ST, Streeck RE. Genome organization and nucleotide sequence of human papillomavirus type 33, which is associated with cervical cancer. J Virol 1986; 58:991–995.
31. Cripe TP, Haugen TH, Turk JP, et al. Transcriptional regulation of the human papillomavirus-16 E6-E7 promoter by a keratinocyte-dependent enhancer, and by viral E2 transactivator and repressor gene products: Implications for cervical carcinogenesis. EMBO J 1987; 6:3745–3753.
32. Dallas PB, Flanagan JL, Nightingale BN, et al. Polymerase chain reaction for fast, nonradioactive detection of high-and low-risk papillomavirus types in routine cervical specimens and biopsies. J Med Virol 1989; 27:105–111.
33. Danos O, Katinka M, Yaniv M. Human papillomavirus 1a complete DNA sequence: A novel type of genome organization among papovaviridae. EMBO J 1982; 1:231–236.
34. Dartmann K, Schwarz E, Gissmann L, et al. The nucleotide sequence and genome organization of human papillomavirus type 11. Virology 1986; 151:124–130.
35. DeCaprio JA, Ludlow JW, Figge J, et al. SV40 large tumor antigen forms a specific complex with the product of the retinoblastoma susceptibility gene. Cell 1988; 54:275–283.

388   THE MOLECULAR BASIS OF HUMAN CANCER

36. De Villiers EM. Heterogeneity of the human papillomavirus group. J Virol 1989; 63:4898–4903.
37. Del Mistro A, Braunstein JD, Halwer M, et al. Identification of human papillomavirus types in male urethral condylomata acuminata by in situ hybridization. Hum Pathol 1987; 18:936-940.
38. DiMaio D, Settleman J. Bovine papillomavirus mutant temperature defective for transformation, replication and transactivation. EMBO J 1988; 7:1197–1204.
39. Doorbar J, Parton A, Hartley K, et al. Detection of novel splicing patterns in a HPV-16 containing keratinocyte cell line. Virology 1990; 178:254–262.
40. Durst M, Dzarlieva-Petruskova RT, Boukamp P, et al. Molecular and cytogenetic analysis of immortalized human primary keratinocytes obtained after transfection with human papillomavirus type 16 DNA. Oncogene 1987; 1:251–256.
41. Dvoretzky I, Shober R, Chattopadhyay SK, et al. A quantitative in vitro focus assay for bovine papillomavirus. Virology 1980; 103:369–375.
42. Dyson N, Howley PM, Munger K, et al. The human papillomavirus-16 E7 oncoprotein is able to bind the retinoblastoma gene product. Science 1989; 243:934–937.
43. Eliahu D, Michalovitz D, Eliahu S, et al. Wild-type p53 can inhibit oncogene-mediated focus formation. Proc Natl Acad Sci USA 1989; 86:8763–8767.
44. Farr A, McAteer JA, Roman A. Transfection of human keratinocytes with pRSVcat and human papillomavirus type-6 DNA. Cancer Cells 1987; 5:171–177.
45. Finlay CA, Hinds PW, Levine AJ. The p53 proto-oncogene can act as a suppressor of transformation. Cell 1989; 57:1083-1093.
46. Garcia-Carranca A, Thierry F, Yaniv M. Interplay of viral and cellular proteins along the long control region of human papillomavirus type 18. J Virol 1988; 62:4321–4330.
47. Gill G, Ptashne M. Mutants of gal 4 protein altered in an activation function. Cell 1987; 51:121–126.
48. Giri I, Yaniv M. Study of the E2 gene product of the cottontail rabbit papillomavirus reveals a common mechanism of transactivation among the papillomaviruses. J Virol 1988; 62:1573–1581.
49. Gissmann L, Wolnik L, Ikenberg H, et al. Human papillomavirus types 6 and 11 DNA sequences in genital and laryngeal papillomas and in some cervical cancers. Proc Natl Acad Sci USA 1983; 80:560–563.
50. Gius D, Grossman S, Bedell MA, et al. Inducible and constitutive enhancer domains in the noncoding region of human papillomavirus type 18. J Virol 1988; 62:665–672.
51. Gloss B, Bernard HU, Seedorf K, et al. The upstream regulatory region of the human papillomavirus-16 contains an E2 protein-independent enhancer which is specific for cervical carcinoma cells and regulated by glucocorticoid hormones. EMBO J 1987; 6:3735–3743.
52. Gloss B, Chong T, Bernard HU. Numerous nuclear proteins bind the long control region of human papillomavirus type 16: A subset of 6 of 23 DNase I protected segments coincides with the location of the cell-type specific enhancer. J Virol 1989; 63:1142-1152.

53. Gloss B, Yeo-Gloss M, Meisterernst M, et al. Clusters of nuclear factor I binding sites identify enhancers of several papillomaviruses but alone are not sufficient for enhancer function. Nucleic Acids Res 1989; 17:3519–3533.
54. Green M, Loewenstein PM. Demonstration that a chemically synthesized BPV-1 oncoprotein and its C-terminal domain function to induce cellular DNA synthesis. Cell 1987; 51:795–802.
55. Groff DE, Lancaster WD. Genetic analysis of the 3' early region transformation and replication functions of bovine papillomavirus type 1. Virology 1986; 150:221–230.
56. Grussendorf-Conen EI, De Villiers EM, Gissmann L. Human papillomavirus genomes in penile smears of healthy men. Lancet 1986; i:1092.
57. Haugen TH, Cripe TP, Ginder GD, et al. Transactivation of an upstream early gene promoter of bovine papillomavirus-1 by a product of the viral E2 gene. EMBO J 1987; 6:145–152.
58. Hawley-Nelson P, Androphy EJ, Lowy DR, et al. The specific DNA recognition sequence of bovine papillomavirus E2 protein is an E2-dependent enhancer. EMBO J 1988; 7:525–531.
59. Hirochika H, Broker TR, Chow LT. Enhancers and *trans*-acting E2 transcriptional factors of papillomaviruses. J Virol 1987; 61:2599–2606.
60. Hirochika H, Hirochika R, Broker TR, et al. Functional mapping of the human papillomavirus type 11 transcriptional enhancer and its interaction with the *trans*-acting E2 protein. Genes Dev 1988; 2:54–67.
61. Hoffmann D, Hecht S, Haley S, et al. Tumorigenic agents in tobacco products and their uptake by chewers, smokers and nonsmokers. J Cell Biochem 1985; 9c(suppl):33.
62. Horwitz BH, Burkhardt AL, Schlegel R, et al. The 44 amino acid E5 transforming protein of bovine papillomavirus requires a hydrophobic core and specific carboxy terminal amino acids. Mol Cell Biol 1988; 8:4071–4078.
63. Kanda T, Furuno A, Yoshiike K. Human papillomavirus type 16 open reading frame E7 encodes a transforming gene for rat 3Y1 cells. J Virol 1988; 62:610–613.
64. Kaur P, McDougall JK. Characterization of primary human keratinocytes transformed by human papillomavirus type 18. J Virol 1988; 62:1917–1924.
65. Koi M, Morita H, Yamada H, et al. Normal human chromosome 11 suppresses tumorigenicity of human cervical tumor cell line SiHa. Mol Carcinogen 1989; 2:12–21.
66. Kreider JW, Howett MK, Leure-Dupree AE, et al. Laboratory production in vivo of human papillomavirus type 11. J Virol 1987; 61:590–593.
67. Lambert PF, Baker CC, Howley PM. The genetics of bovine papillomavirus type 1. Annu Rev Genet 1988; 22:235–258.
68. Lambert PF, Spalholz BA, Howley PM. A transcriptional repressor encoded by BPV-1 shares a common carboxy terminal domain with the E2 transactivator. Cell 1987; 50:68–78.
69. Lancaster WD. Apparent lack of integration of bovine papillomavirus DNA in virus-induced equine and bovine tumor cells and virus-transformed mouse cells. Virology 1981; 108:251–255.
70. Law MF, Lowy DR, Dvoretzky I, et al. Mouse cells transformed by bovine

papillomavirus contain only extrachromosomal viral DNA sequences. Proc Natl Acad Sci USA 1981; 78:2727–2731.

71. Lazo PA. Rearrangement of both alleles of human chromosome 8, one of them as a result of papillomavirus DNA integration. J Biol Chem 1988; 263:360–367.

72. Levine RV, Crum CP, Herman E, et al. Cervical papillomavirus infections and intraepithelial neoplasia: A study of male sexual partners. Obstet Gynecol 1984; 64:16–20.

73. Linzer DIH, Levine AJ. Characterization of a 54 K dalton cellular SV40 tumor antigen present in SV40-transformed cells and uninfected embryonal carcinoma cells. Cell 1979; 17:43–52.

74. Lowy DR, Dvoretzky I, Shober R, et al. In vitro tumorigenic transformation by a defined sub-genomic fragment of bovine papillomavirus DNA. Nature 1980; 287:72–74.

75. Lusky M, Berg L, Weiher H, et al. Bovine papillomavirus contains an activator of gene expression at the distal end of the early transcription unit. Mol Cell Biol 1983; 3:1108–1122.

76. Lusky M, Botchan MR. Characterization of the bovine papillomavirus plasmid maintenance sequences. Cell 1984; 36:391-401.

77. Lusky M, Botchan MR. Genetic analysis of bovine papillomavirus type 1 trans-acting replication factors. J Virol 1985; 53:955–965.

78. Lusky M, Botchan MR. A bovine papillomavirus type 1-encoded modulator function is dispensable for transient viral replication but is required for establishment of the stable plasmid state. J Virol 1986; 60:729–742.

79. Lusky M, Botchan MR. Transient replication of bovine papillomavirus type 1 plasmids: cis and trans requirements. Proc Natl Acad Sci USA 1986; 83:3609–3613.

80. Manos MM, Ting Y, Wright DK, et al. The use of polymerase chain reaction amplification for the detection of genital human papillomaviruses. Cancer Cells 1989; 7:209–214.

81. Martin P, Vass WC, Schiller JT, et al. The bovine papillomavirus E5 transforming protein can stimulate the transforming activity of EGF and CSF-1 receptors. Cell 1989; 59:21–32.

82. Matlashewski G, Banks L, Pim D, et al. Analysis of human p53 proteins and mRNA levels in normal and transformed cells. Eur J Biochem 1986; 154:665–672.

83. Matlashewski G, Schneider J, Banks L, et al. Human papillomavirus type 16 DNA cooperates with activated ras in transforming primary cells. EMBO J 1987; 6:1741–1746.

84. Matsukura T, Koi S, Sugase M. Both episomal and integrated forms of human papillomavirus type 16 are involved in invasive cervical cancers. Virology 1989; 172:63–72.

85. McBride AA, Byrne JC, Howley PM. E2 polypeptides encoded by bovine papillomavirus 1 form dimers through the carboxy-terminal DNA binding domain: Transactivation is mediated through the conserved amino terminal domain. Proc Natl Acad Sci USA 1989; 86:510–514.

86. McBride AA, Schlegel R, Howley PM. The carboxy-terminal domain shared by the bovine papillomavirus E2 transactivator and repressor proteins contains a specific DNA binding activity. EMBO J 1988; 7:533–539.

87. McCance DJ, Campion MJ, Singer A. Non-invasive detection of cervical papillomavirus DNA. Lancet 1986; i:558.
88. McCance DJ, Kalache A, Ashdown K, et al. Human papillomavirus types 16 and 18 in carcinomas of the penis from Brazil. Int J Cancer 1986; 37:55–59.
89. Melchers WJG, Schift R, Stolz E, et al. Human papillomavirus detection in urine samples from male patients by the polymerase chain reaction. J Clin Microbiol 1989; 27:1711–1714.
90. Melchers W, Van den Brule A, Walboomers J, et al. Increased detection rate of human papillomavirus in cervical scrapes by the polymerase chain reaction as compared to modified FISH and Southern blot analyses. J Med Virol 1989; 27:329–335.
91. Mohr IJ, Clark R, Sun S, et al. Targeting the E1 replication protein to the papillomavirus origin of replication by complex formation with the E2 transactivator. Science 1990; 250:1694-1699.
92. Moran E, Matthews MB. Multiple functional domains in the adenovirus E1a gene. Cell 1987; 48:177–178.
93. Moskaluk C, Bastia D. The E2 "gene" of bovine papillomavirus encodes an enhancer-binding protein. Proc Natl Acad Sci USA 1987; 84:1215–1218.
94. Mullis KB, Faloona FA. Specific synthesis of DNA in vitro via a polymerase-catalyzed chain reaction. Methods Enzymol 1987; 155:335–350.
95. Munger K, Phelps WC, Bubb V, et al. The E6 and E7 genes of the human papillomavirus type 16 together are necessary and sufficient for transformation of primary human keratinocytes. J Virol 1989; 63:4417–4421.
96. Munger K, Werness BA, Dyson N, et al. Complex formation of human papillomavirus E7 proteins with the retinoblastoma tumor suppressor gene product. EMBO J 1989; 8:4099–4105.
97. Neary K, DiMaio D. Open reading frames E6 and E7 of bovine papillomavirus type 1 are both required for full transformation of mouse C127 cells. J Virol 1989; 63:259–266.
98. Ocadiz R, Sauceda R, Cruz M, et al. High correlation between molecular alterations of the c-*myc* oncogene and carcinoma of the uterine cervix. Cancer Res 1987; 47:4173–4177.
99. Offord EA, Beard P. A member of the activator protein 1 family found in keratinocytes but not in fibroblasts required for transcription from a human papillomavirus type 18 promoter. J Virol 1990; 64:4792–4798.
100. Orth G. Epidermodysplasia verruciformis: A model for understanding the oncogenicity of human papillomaviruses. In: Papillomaviruses— Symposium No. 120, CIBA Foundation Symposium. New York, John Wiley & Sons 1986; pp. 156–174.
101. Palermo-Dilts DA, Broker TR, Chow LT. Human papillomavirus type 1 produces redundant as well as polycistronic mRNAs in plantar warts. J Virol 1990; 64:3144–3149.
102. Petti L, Nilson LA, DiMaio D. Activation of the platelet-derived growth factor receptor by the bovine papillomavirus E5 transforming protein. EMBO J 1991; 10:845–855.
103. Pfister H. Human papillomaviruses and genical cancer. Adv Cancer Res 1987; 48:113–147.

392 THE MOLECULAR BASIS OF HUMAN CANCER

104. Phelps WC, Howley PM. Transcriptional transactivation by the human papillomavirus type 16 E2 gene product. J Virol 1987; 61:1630–1638.
105. Phelps WC, Yee CL, Munger K, et al. The human papillomavirus type 16 E7 gene encodes transactivation and transformation functions similar to adenovirus E1a. Cell 1988; 53:539–547.
106. Pirisi L, Yasumoto S, Feller M, et al. Transformation of human fibroblasts and keratinocytes with human papillomavirus type 16 DNA. J Virol 1987; 61:1061–1066.
107. Popescu NC, DiPaolo JA, Amsbaugh SC. Integration sites of human papillomavirus 18 DNA sequences on HeLa cell chromosomes. Cytogenet Cell Genet 1987; 44:58–62.
108. Rabson MS, Yee C, Yang YC, et al. Bovine papillomavirus type 1 3' early region transformation and plasmid maintenance functions. J Virol 1986; 60:626–634.
109. Reilly SS, Taichman LB. Underreplication of human papillomavirus type-1 DNA in cultures of foreskin keratinocytes. Cancer Cells 1987; 5:159–163.
110. Riou G, Barrois M, Le MG, et al. C-myc proto-oncogene expression and prognosis in early carcinoma of the uterine cervix. Lancet 1987; i:761–763.
111. Roberts JM, Weintraub H. Negative control of DNA replication in composite SV40—bovine papillomavirus plasmids. Cell 1986; 46:741–752.
112. Rosl F, Durst M, Zur Hausen H. Selective suppression of human papillomavirus transcription in non-tumorigenic cells by 5-azacytidine. EMBO J 1988; 7:1321–1328.
113. Rotenberg MO, Chow LT, Broker TR. Characterization of rare human papillomavirus type 11 mRNAs coding for regulatory and structural proteins using the polymerase chain reaction. Virology 1989; 172:489–497.
114. Santucci S, Androphy EJ, Bonne-Andrea C, et al. Proteins encoded by the bovine papillomavirus E1 open reading frame: Expression in heterologous systems and in virally transformed cells. J Virol 1990; 64:6027–6039.
115. Sarver N, Rabson MS, Yang YC, et al. Localization and analysis of bovine papillomavirus type 1 transforming functions. J Virol 1984; 52:377–388.
116. Saxon PJ, Srivatsan ES, Stanbridge EJ. Introduction of human chromosome 11 via microcell transfer controls tumorigenic expression of HeLa cells. EMBO J 1986; 5:3461–3466.
117. Scheffner M, Werness BA, Huibregtse JM, et al. The E6 oncoprotein encoded by human papillomavirus types 16 and 18 promotes the degradation of p53. Cell 1990; 63:1129–1136.
118. Schiller JT, Kleiner E, Androphy EJ, et al. Identification of bovine papillomavirus E1 mutants with increased transforming and transcriptional activity. J Virol 1989; 63:1775–1782.
119. Schiller JT, Vass WC, Lowy DR. Identification of a second transforming region in bovine papillomavirus DNA. Proc Natl Acad Sci USA 1984; 81:7880–7884.

120. Schiller JT, Vass WC, Vousden KH, et al. The E5 open reading frame of bovine papillomavirus type 1 encodes a transforming gene. J Virol 1986; 57:1–6.
121. Schlegel R, Phelps WC, Zhang YL, et al. Quantitative keratinocyte assay detects two biological activities of human papillomavirus DNA and identifies viral types associated with cervical carcinoma. EMBO J 1988; 7:3181–3187.
122. Schlegel R, Wade-Glass M, Rabson M, et al. The E5 transforming gene of bovine papillomavirus encodes a small, hydrophobic polypeptide. Science 1986; 233:464–467.
123. Schneider A, Oltersdorf T, Schneider V, et al. Distribution of human papillomavirus 16 genome in cervical neoplasia by molecular in situ hybridization of tissue sections. Int J Cancer 1987; 39:717–721.
124. Schneider V, Kay S, Lee HM. Immunosuppression as a high risk factor in the development of condyloma acuminata and squamous neoplasia of the cervix. Octa Cytol 1983; 27:220–224.
125. Schneider-Gadicke A, Schwarz E. Different human cervical carcinoma cell lines show similar transcription patterns of human papillomavirus type 18 early genes. EMBO J 1986; 5:2285–2292.
126. Schvartzman JB, Adolph S, Martin-Parras L, et al. Evidence that replication initiates at only some of the potential origins in each oligomeric form of bovine papillomavirus type 1 DNA. Mol Cell Biol 1990; 10:3078–3086.
127. Schwarz E, Durst M, Demankowski C, et al. DNA sequence and genome organization of genital human papillomavirus type 6b. EMBO J 1983; 2:2341–2348.
128. Schwarz E, Freese UK, Gissmann L, et al. Structure and transcription of human papillomavirus sequences in cervical carcinoma cells. Nature 1985; 314:111–114.
129. Seedorf K, Krammer G, Durst M, et al. Human papillomavirus type 16 DNA sequence. Virology 1985; 145:181–185.
130. Seedorf K, Oltersdorf T, Krammer G, et al. Identification of early proteins of human papillomaviruses type 16 (HPV 16) and type 18 (HPV 18) in cervical carcinoma cells. EMBO J 1987; 6:139-144.
131. Shibata DK, Arnheim N, Martin WJ. Detection of human papillomavirus in paraffin-embedded tissue using the polymerase chain reaction. J Exp Med 1988; 167:225–230.
132. Shirasawa H, Tomita Y, Sekiya S, et al. Integration and transcription of human papillomavirus type 16 and 18 sequences in cell lines derived from cervical carcinoma. J Gen Virol 1987; 68:583–591.
133. Sillman F, Stanek A, Sedlis A, et al. The relationship between human papillomavirus and lower genital intraepithelial neoplasia in immuno-suppressed women. J Obstet Gynecol 1984; 150:300–308.
134. Smotkin D, Prokoph H, Wettstein FO. Oncogenic and nononcogenic genital papillomaviruses generate the E7 mRNA by different mechanisms. J Virol 1989; 63:1441–1447.
135. Smotkin D, Wettstein FO. Transcription of human papillomavirus type 16 early genes in a cervical cancer and a cancer-derived cell line and identification of the protein. Proc Natl Acad Sci USA 1986; 83:4680–4684.

394   THE MOLECULAR BASIS OF HUMAN CANCER

136. Smotkin D, Wettstein FO. The major human papillomavirus protein in cervical cancers is a cytoplasmic phosphoprotein. J Virol 1987; 61:1686–1689.
137. Southern P, Berg P. Transformation of mammalian cells to antibiotic resistance with a bacterial gene under the control of the SV40 early region promoter. J Mol Appl Genet 1982; 1:327-341.
138. Souza R, Dostatni N, Yaniv M. Control of papillomavirus gene expression. Biochim Biophys Acta 1990; 1032:19–37.
139. Spalholz BA, Byrne JC, Howley PM. Evidence for cooperativity between E2 binding sites in E2 transregulation of bovine papillomavirus type 1. J Virol 1988; 62:3143–3150.
140. Spalholz BA, Lambert PF, Yee CL, Howley PM. Bovine papillomavirus transcriptional regulation: Localization of the E2-responsive elements of the long control region. J Virol 1987; 61:2128–2137.
141. Spalholz BA, Yang YC, Howley PM. Transactivation of a bovine papillomavirus transcriptional regulatory element by the E2 gene product. Cell 1985; 42:183–191.
142. Stoler MH, Broker TR. In situ hybridization detection of human papillomavirus DNAs and messenger RNAs in genital condyloma and a cervical carcinoma. Hum Pathol 1986; 17:1250–1258.
143. Storey A, Pim D, Murray A, et al. Comparison of the in vitro transforming activities of human papillomavirus types. EMBO J 1988; 7:1815–1820.
144. Sun S, Thorner M, Lentz M, et al. Identification of a 68-kilodalton nuclear ATP-binding phosphoprotein encoded by bovine papillomavirus type 1. J Virol 1990; 64:5093–5105.
145. Tanaka A, Noda T, Yajima H, et al. Identification of a transforming gene of human papillomavirus type 16. J Virol 1989; 63:1465–1469.
146. Thierry F, Heard JM, Dartmann K, Yaniv M. Characterization of a transcriptional promoter of human papillomavirus 18 and modulation of its expression by simian virus 40 and adenovirus early antigens. J Virol 1987; 61:134–142.
147. Thierry F, Yaniv M. The BPV1-E1 *trans*-acting protein can be either an activator or a repressor of the HPV 18 regulatory region. EMBO J 1987; 6:3391–3397.
148. Thorner L, Bucay N, Choe J, Botchan M. The product of the bovine papillomavirus type 1 modulator gene (M) is a phosphoprotein. J Virol 1988; 62:2474–2482.
149. Ting Y, Manos MM. Detection and typing of genital human papillomaviruses. In: PCR Protocols: A Guide to Methods and Applications, Innis MA, Gelfand DH, Sninsky JJ, et al, eds. San Diego, Academic Press 1990; pp. 356–376.
150. Trevathan E, Layde P, Webster LA, et al. Cigarette smoking and dysplasia and carcinoma in situ of the uterine cervix. J Am Med Assoc 1984; 250:499–502.
151. Ustav M, Stenlund A. Transient replication of BPV-1 requires two viral polypeptides encoded by the E1 and E2 open reading frames. EMBO J 1991; 10:449–457.
152. Ustav M, Ustav E, Szymanski P, et al. Identification of the origin of

replication of bovine papillomavirus and characterization of the viral origin recognition factor E1. EMBO J 1991; 10:4321–4329.

153. Vande Pol SB, Howley PM. A bovine papillomavirus constitutive enhancer is negatively regulated by the E2 repressor through competitive binding for a cellular factor. J Virol 1990; 64:5420–5429.

154. Vousden KH, Doninger J, DiPaolo JA, et al. The E7 open reading frame of human papillomavirus type 16 encodes a transforming gene. Oncogene Res 1988; 3:167–175.

155. Waldeck S, Rosl F, Zentgraf H. Origin of replication in episomal bovine papillomavirus type 1 DNA isolated from transformed cells. EMBO J 1984; 3:2173–2178.

156. Watanabe S, Kanda T, Yoshiike K. Human papillomavirus type 16 transformation of primary human embryonic fibroblasts requires expression of open reading frames E6 and E7. J Virol 1989; 63:965–969.

157. Werness BA, Levine AJ, Howley PM. Association of human papillomavirus types 16 and 18 E6 proteins with p53. Science 1990; 248:76–79.

158. Whyte P, Buchkovich KJ, Horwitz JM, et al. Association between an oncogene and an antioncogene: The adenovirus E1a proteins bind to the retinoblastoma gene product. Nature 1988; 334:124–129.

159. Yang L, Botchan M. Replication of bovine papillomavirus type 1 DNA initiates within an E2-responsive enhancer element. J Virol 1990; 64:5903–5911.

160. Yang L, Li R, Mohr IJ, et al. Activation of BPV-1 replication in vitro by the transcription factor E2. Nature 1991; 353:628–632.

161. Yang YC, Okayama H, Howley PM. Bovine papillomavirus contains multiple transforming genes. Proc Natl Acad Sci USA 1985; 82:1030–1034.

162. Yang YC, Spalholz BA, Rabson MS, Howley PM. Dissociation of transforming and transactivating functions for bovine papillomavirus type 1. Nature 1985; 318:575–577.

163. Yutsudo M, Okamoto Y, Hakura A. Functional dissociation of transforming genes of human papillomavirus type 16. Virology 1988; 166:594–597.

164. Zur Hausen H. Papillomaviruses as carcinomaviruses. Adv Viral Oncol 1989; 8:1–26.

165. Zur Hausen H, Schneider A. The role of papillomaviruses in human anogenital cancer. In: The Papovaviridae, Volume 2, Papillomaviruses, Howley PM, Salzman NP, eds. New York, Plenum 1987; pp. 245–263.

Chapter 10

Transgenic Mouse Models of Cancer

Michael P. Rosenberg

Genetics and Cancer: Model Systems

The use of mice to study cancer has its roots in the development of inbred strains of mice to study genetics.[49] These studies also launched two new areas of research, immunogenetics and retrovirology. The field of immunogenetics arose because of attempts by Little and his colleagues to transplant tumors between animals, and was more fully investigated by George Snell at the Jackson Laboratory. The discovery that retroviruses in mammals can cause cancer was pioneered by Bittner during his efforts to discover the milk agent involved in mammary tumors in strain C3H/He, eventually shown to be the mouse mammary tumor virus (MMTV).

It was soon demonstrated that each inbred strain has its own characteristic frequency, type, and time of onset of tumors.[48] It was also realized that various gene defects can affect the type of tumors or their frequency. For example, mice carrying the dominant spotting locus W, recently shown to be the c-kit tyrosine kinase receptor for the $Steel$ (Sl) growth factor, develop specific neoplasias depending on the mutant alleles present.[101,132] Other genetic loci influence or enhance formation of tumors, such as the lethal yellow (A^y) or viable yellow (A^{vy}) alleles at the $agouti$ (A) locus.[115,133] Development of two inbred strains that have high frequency of ovarian teratomas or testicular teratocarcinomas[100] enabled Roy Stevens at the Jackson Laboratory to

From *The Molecular Basis of Human Cancer:* edited by B. Neel, M.D., Ph.D., R. Kumar, Ph.D. © 1993, Futura Publishing Co. Inc., Mount Kisco, NY.

trace not only the developmental origin of these tumors to partheno-
genetic oocytes or fetal germ cells, respectively, but also to the
development of embryonic-like cells in culture. With the genetic basis
of cancer etiology and the diversity of genes in specific inbred strains
firmly established, it was perhaps not totally surprising to find that
human cancers likewise may have a genetic origin (see Chapter 2).

Over the past five years the use of mice in cancer research has
focused on mice genetically engineered to carry specific segments of
cloned genes encoding one of several classes of proto-oncogenes or
oncogenes, linked to promoters capable of directing expression to
specific tissues and cells. These genetically engineered mice are called
transgenic mice, and the artificial genes they carry are called transgenes. These transgenic mice can develop cancer with a predictable
time course and frequency, and they can transmit this trait to
subsequent generations in a Mendelian manner. The other value of
these transgenic mice is that they develop tumors that are, in many
cases, rare in both mice and humans or for which no animal model
exists. The most prevalent technique used to generate these mice
involves microinjecting cloned recombinant DNA sequences into the
pronuclei of newly fertilized mouse zygotes (Fig. 1). The entire
procedure is illustrated in Figure 2 and is more fully described by
Brinster et al.[18,90]

Transgenic mice have allowed investigators to address basic
questions of mechanisms in cancer which cannot be addressed by the

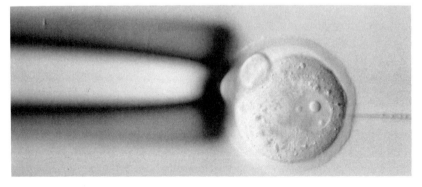

Figure 1. *Injection of DNA into a mouse zygote. On the left is a blunt glass pipet
attached to a hydraulic syringe device that provides suction. The mouse zygote with
two pronuclei visible is held in place by the translucent ring-like structure called the
zona pullicida or fertilization membrane. Entering the zygote on the right is a finely
drawn micropipet attached to another syringe hydraulic device that is used to inject a
DNA fragment into the pronuclei.*

Construction of Transgenic Mice

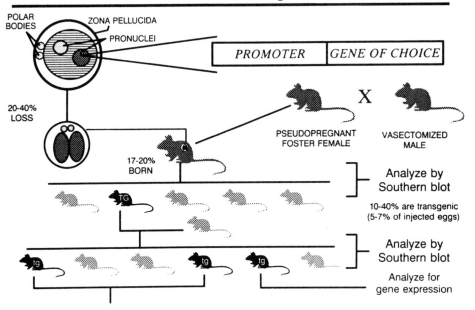

Figure 2. *Summary of the procedure used to develop a transgenic mouse. A DNA construct containing a promoter linked to a gene of interest is injected into a newly fertilized egg. The injected eggs are cultured overnight to the two-cell stage and then transferred to a psuedopregnant foster female. This mouse is derived by mating a female to a vasectomized male mouse. After an 18 to 19 day gestation the mice are born, and when the mice are old enough (2 to 3 weeks) a biopsy of the tail is taken to determine which mice have successfully taken up the DNA. Various methods are used to detect the inserted transgene such as Southern blots or the polymerase chain reaction (PCR). The transgenic mice (N_O generation) are then mated to nontransgenic mice to propagate the lines and to generate mice for the analysis of transgene expression. The overall efficiency of the procedure is 5%, but between 10% and 45% of the liveborn may be transgenic depending on the DNA construct and other technical factors.*

use of tissue culture model systems. In many cases use of tissue-specific promoters has allowed researchers to assay oncogenicity, while use of promoters promiscuous in their tissue specificity has created the potential for discovering whether a proto-oncogene or oncogene is capable of transforming a variety of cell types. The expression of a gene construct in a tissue-specific manner resulting in tumors has allowed investigators to establish in culture these cells that were otherwise difficult to cultivate in vitro.

Hyperplasia and Neoplasias

While hyperplasia usually precedes neoplasias, expression of oncogenes in mice often leads to hyperplastic growth that does not progress to neoplastic states. In fact, expression of an oncogene in a specific tissue may not lead to hyperplasia or cancer. In other cases a long latency occurs before hyperplasia and neoplasia, and still other cases are found where more than one oncogene is required to cause any growth abnormality. The development from a prehyperplastic to hyperplastic, dysplastic, and then neoplastic state can be followed in transgenic mice because these mice develop neoplasia along a predictable time course. A fuller discussion of transgenic mice as a model system to decipher the sequential progression from hyperplasia to neoplasia can be found in a review by Hanahan.[42]

Hyperplasia

The MMTV-long terminal repeat (LTR) contains regulatory sequences directing gene expression primarily to the mammary gland, but also to the harderian and salivary glands[52,71,74,118,124] and epididymal tissue,[52,71,74,85] among others. When linked to the MMTV-LTR expression of either a human c-*myc*, N-*ras*, mouse c-*ret*, *int*-1, *int*-2, or c-*neu* genes in transgenic mice leads to hyperplasia of the harderian gland, salivary glands, or epididymis. Expression of either the mouse c-*mos* proto-oncogene or v-*mos* oncogene from a truncated Maloney sarcoma virus (MSV) LTR also results in hyperplastic lesions of the harderian gland which appears multifocal in origin.[95] To date progression from hyperplasia to neoplasia has not been observed in any of these tissues with any of the different oncogenes expressed. Failure of these hyperplastic growths to progress to neoplasia may be an intrinsic property of these tissues.

Several studies suggest that cell surface glycoproteins and interleukins can act as local autocrine regulators of cellular proliferation and differentiation. Aberrant expression of the developmentally regulated cell surface glycoprotein Thy-1.2 under the transcriptional regulation of the immunoglobulin heavy chain (IgH) enhancer (Eμ) results in lymphoid hyperplasia.[22] The Thy-1.2 protein is expressed in both the bone marrow B-cell progenitor and mature B lymphocytes. Thus, the Thy-1 cell surface antigen may mediate signals to normal marrow cells to leave the cell cycle and differentiate. Constitutive overexpression of the cytokine IL-5 using the promoter of the human CD-2 gene results in an abnormal proliferation of eosinophils.[27] Thus it is possible that eosinophils require IL-5 for growth and maturation. Overexpression of another growth factor, granulocyte-macrophage colony stimulating factor (GM-CSF), from the Maloney murine leukemia viral (MoMuLV) LTR also leads to uncontrolled proliferation of macrophages.[67,82] These lines of transgenic mice eventually succumb to the macrophages' infiltration of tissues and the subsequent autolysis of the tissues.

Inappropriate expression of either the viral oncogene *fps* tyrosine-kinase receptor[137] or SV40 large T-antigen[12] leads to a controlled overproliferation of cardiac cells resulting in cardiomegaly. Cardiomegaly was also found in one transgenic line expressing a metallothionein/polyoma large T-antigen transgene.[21] Markedly enlarged cells mixed with normal cells were found in the latter case, and mice succumbed to thrombus formation and cardiac failure at approximately 160 days. An atrial natriuretic factor (ANF)/SV40 T-antigen transgene resulted in asymmetrical growth of the right atrium leading to cardiac arrythymias and eventual death.[33] In another example the overexpression of a human growth hormone-releasing factor gene in the pituitary led to pituitary hyperplasia.[77] Hyperplasia presumably resulted from a paracrine feedback mechanism and not because the releasing factor is oncogenic.

The expression of a proto-oncogene or growth factor/receptor can result in aberrant development in addition to proliferation. This is more fully discussed below (see Oncogenesis and Development). When a truncated c-*ski* cDNA was expressed from a MSV-LTR, several of the transgenic mice demonstrated a hypertrophy of skeletal muscle.[120] This is not the same as hyperplasia since the growth was not aberrant. The c-*ski* proto-oncogene is normally expressed in developing muscle cells, and although its function is not known, it is involved in the growth and differentiation of muscle cells. The hypertrophy is limited to the type II fast fibers which are the fibers found in adult animals, suggesting that expression is restricted to either developing cells or to differentiating fibers causing a limited round of proliferation before terminal differentiation.

Two other examples of aberrant gene expression also appear to lead to benign hyperplastic lesions.[14,104] In both cases, ectopic expression of either a H2-K^d histocompatability promoter/c-*fos*[104] or a hypothalamic peptide growth hormone-releasing factor/SV40 large T-antigen transgenes[14] resulted in an alteration of thymic epithelial cells. This alteration likely resulted in the inappropriate expression of T-cell growth regulating factors, affecting the self-renewal and differentiation of T cells.

These studies indicate that hyperplasia does not automatically lead to neoplasia, and other events must occur or certain constraints removed for the progression of hyperplastic tissues to become tumors. Other constraints may include release from various controls on the rate of cellular division or the "dedifferentiation" of these tissues. Some of these issues have been addressed by Hanahan[42] and will not be considered further. In the examples presented below, the progression from a hyperplastic to a neoplastic state seems to involve a second genetic defect, i.e., activation of another gene. Except for one example of overexpression of the *neu* gene in a line of transgenic mice,[114] expression of a single oncogene does not appear to be sufficient for transformation. In many cases, overexpression of certain oncogenes in a tissue may not even be sufficient to obtain hyperplasia.[76,108,135] (see also Oncogenesis and Development).

Neoplasia

Hematopoeitic tumors

The most dramatic demonstrations of tumorigenesis in transgenic mice are those of the hematopoietic system, as recently reviewed by Adams and his colleagues.[1,44] Most of these studies involve the overexpression of those cellular or activated oncogenes that are predominantly expressed in human hematologic malignancies, such as c-*myc*, N-*ras*, *abl*, or the *bcr/abl* fusion genes.[45] Frequently, genetic alterations found in human malignancies involve the rearrangements of oncogenes with the IgHEμ. Consequently, this regulatory sequence is used in many studies targeting expression to T and B cells.[2,62] Expression of IgHEμ enhancer/*myc* constructs in transgenic mice results in T-cell lymphomas or myeloid tumors.[5] Transgenic mice carrying both an Eμ-enhancer-SV40-promoter/N-*ras* and an Eμ/*myc* transgene developed early B lymphoid tumors and the neoplastic B cells failed to undergo IgH arrangements.[109] Therefore these cells represent tumors of an intermediate or immature B-cell type.[109] This experiment also demonstrates that alteration of promoter/enhancer activity can result in changes in lineage range and timing of expression. Deregulated expression of c-*myc* from the MMTV-LTR results in mast cell, pre-B-cell, B-cell, and T-cell neoplasias, suggesting that autocrine regulation of these cells is affected by changes in the proliferative capacity of precursor cells.[71] Interestingly, cloned Eμ-c-*myc* B cells can be induced to differentiate into macrophages upon infection with a virus carrying the v-*raf* oncogene.[61] This developmental switch suggests that expression of various oncogenes may be involved in shifting cells to alternate developmental pathways.

Overexpression of the v-*abl* oncogene from an Eμ-enhancer-SV40-promoter did not result in a B-cell lymphoma as expected from the above studies, but instead resulted in plasmacytomas after a long latency.[44] Presumably transformation with v-*abl* requires secondary events (see Oncogene Cooperativity) or a promoter active in pre-B cells. Two groups have successfully produced transgenic mice carrying a chimeric *bcr*/c-*abl*[45] or v-*abl*[44,57] gene that developed leukemia, reminiscent of the Philadelphia chromosome translocation found in some human patients with acute lymphoblastic leukemia. In both cases investigators have found that mice succumb to acute myeloid or lymphoid leukemia between 10 and 77 days after birth. This work points to a direct causal relationship between overexpression of an activated oncogene resulting from a translocation in humans with the development of a cancer. Both studies also point to common pathways or lineages between B and T cells and myeloid cells.

Attempts to induce tumors of the myeloid lineage using the *fps* nonreceptor protein tyrosine kinase, which is normally expressed in this lineage, have met with variable success.[37,135] Transgenic mice carrying a 13 kilobase genomic fragment containing the human c-*fps* gene expressed *fps* mRNA appropriately in macrophages, but failed to demonstrate any abnormalities in hematopoiesis. However, ectopic expression of a v-*fps* oncogene encoding a *gag-fps* fusion protein, from either 5′ human globin or 5′ and 3′ human globin regulatory sequences resulted in a variety of tumors, but most consistently caused T-cell lymphomas.[135] *fps* mRNA expression was also found in heart, brain, lung, and testes, but no malignancies developed in these tissues. Histocytic lymphomas were also induced by ectopic expression of a human IgH-SV40 promoter/*myc* construct.[119]

Another hematopoietic cancer that occurs in humans for which there was no mouse model is acute thrombocythemic myeloproliferative disease. A model for this disease has been created not in transgenic mice but by using a recombinant MoMuLV carrying a polyoma DNA tumor virus middle T gene.[35] Infection of mice with this virus induced disease 7 to 15 days after inoculation. Unlike transgenic mice which contain the transgene in every cell whose expression is limited to the tissue specificity of the promoter, expression in retrovirally transducted mice is limited to those tissues that have been successfully infected and where the provirus has been integrated into the genome.

Mammary tumors

One of the most interesting models for human tumor systems is that of mammary adenomas which are one of the most prevalent types of cancer among women. Creation of transgenic mice that develop mammary tumors has relied on directing expression of various proto- and oncogenes to the mammary gland using either the MMTV-LTR, whose expression is restricted to a few tissues including the mammary gland, or the murine whey acidic protein (WAP) promoter which is highly tissue-specific for the mammary gland. Both promoters are subject to hormonal regulation during pregnancy, and the MMTV-LTR promoter can also be regulated by glucocorticoid hormones.

Transgenic mice carrying MMTV-LTR enhancer/promoter linked to c-myc,[71,118] v-Ha-ras,[114,124] an activated human N-ras oncogene,[74] an activated neu oncogene,[15,85] the mouse Wnt-1 (int-1) proto-oncogene,[78,125] the mouse int-2 proto-oncogene,[84] or a human ret-transforming gene[52] have been created. In addition, the WAP promoter linked to c-myc or Ha-ras has been used to obtain transgenic mice with oncogenes expressed in the mammary gland.[7,110] It is now established that the MMTV can initiate tumors in the murine mammary gland by insertional mutagenesis of oncogenes. The integration of the provirus can occur in close proximity to a proto-oncogene, which can cause expression of the affected oncogene in the mammary gland using the viral LTR regulatory sequences. Several genes, initially named int for integration, have been molecularly cloned using the viral genome as a molecular tag. The int-1 gene (renamed Wnt-1 because of its homology to the Drosophila wingless locus) encodes a growth factor. The integration of the virus twins on the expression of the int-1 gene in the mammary gland resulting in the development of mammary tumors. Proof for the causal role of these genes in mammary tumorigenesis was provided by expressing either the int-1 gene[78,125] or the int-2 gene[84] from the MMTV-LTR in transgenic mice.

The human neu oncogene encodes a receptor tyrosine kinase and is expressed in many human mammary adenocarcinomas. Transgenic mice expressing *ras* or *neu* in the mammary gland could be considered for a model of human mammary adenocarcinomas. Mammary adenocarcinomas arose in MMTV/c-*myc* female mice (see above) only after undergoing several pregnancies, but arose much earlier in MMTV/v-H-*ras* and MMTV/*neu* transgenics. This indicates that expression of any of these genes alone is insufficient to lead to transformation, and that a second activation step must take place for tumor progression. This was demonstrated when Sinn et al.[114] mated two different oncogene bearing transgenic mice carrying either a MMTV/c-*myc* or a MMTV/v-H-*ras* transgene. The resulting mice expressed both oncogenes in the mammary gland and had a much shorter latency for tumor formation. This study demonstrates that two oncogenes can cooperate to give rise to a tumor.

The overexpression of an activated *neu* oncogene from the MMTV promoter results in mammary adenocarcinomas with prolonged latency,[15,85] but in one exceptional case there was no latency of tumor formation.[85] In this line, immature and mature nonbreeding female and male mice developed hyperplasia of the epithelium in each gland that was synchronous and polyclonal in origin. Since the mammary anlagen atrophies in male mice in the first week postnatally, it is unusual that MMTV/*neu* male mice developed mammary adenomas. While mammary expression of a *neu* oncogene was sufficient for multiple tumor formation in these transgenics, expression of the oncogene in the epididymis only caused hyperplasia. The epididymis may be refractory to progression to neoplasia because of the differentiated state, whereas the cycle of proliferation that mammary epithelium undergoes with each pregnancy may predispose that tissue to transformation. The fact that *neu* expression led to transformation and progression with no latency only in one transgenic line of mice is an exception rather than the rule.[15] Further work is needed to determine the molecular mechanisms of one step carcinogenesis in these mice.

Transforming growth factor-α (TGF-α) is a potent mitogen that is expressed in a variety of tissues in the embryo and adult. Because TGF-α is produced in the mammary epithelia it was a candidate to test for its ability to cause tumors when linked to the MMTV-LTR.[77] Overexpression of the MMTV/TGF-α transgene only resulted in hyperplasia and progression to tumors in mammary glands and not in many other tissues where the MMTV-LTR is active. Although this suggests a selective or restricted action of TGF-α in mammary epithelia, it is possible that the other tissues and organs are unable to process the precursor protein to its active form. Alternatively, TGF-α

has been shown to act through the epidermal growth factor receptor (EGFR), which is upregulated in the mammary glands expressing the transgene. One cannot exclude the fact that the cells of some organs may lack the EGFR, or that there is a failure to induce the receptor.

Neural tumors

Transgenic mice carrying neural tumors in a variety of neuronal cell types, i.e., sympathetic, parasympathetic, or sensory neurons have been created. Tumors have also been derived from the adrenal medulla which originates from the neural crest, or the choroid plexus which is derived from neuroepithelium. Production of mice carrying a mouse metallothionein promoter-SV40 enhancer linked to the SV40 Tantigen results in the development of choroid plexus tumors.[17,81,91] Tissue specificity in this construct was dependent on the 72 bp SV40 enhancer,[91] which also directed expression to the thymus and kidney. Additionally, tumors of the choroid plexus showed alteration or amplification of the transgene compared to nontumor tissue.[17] Deletion of the mouse metallothionein promoter with the retention of the SV40 72 bp enhancer resulted in peripheral neuropathy of unknown cause, and thus is of interest for study in human diabetic patients who develop peripheral autonomic and sensory neuropathy.[91] The cells of the choroid plexus expressed the SV40 T-antigen gene several weeks prior to development of the tumor and some subsets of cells express the gene but fail to progress to tumors, further evidence for a two-step process in carcinogenesis.[81] In these studies it was not clear whether hyperplasia preceded neoplasia.

Multiple neuroblastomas of the central and peripheral nervous system result from the position-dependent expression of a thymidine kinase/polyoma middle T-antigen construct.[4] Preneoplastic lesions formed in sympathetic ganglia and the adrenal medulla. Similar to the human tumors, they express characteristic markers of neuroblastomas and have high expression of the N-*myc* proto-oncogene. These tumors could not be grown in culture but could be transplanted into nude mice. Both the human JC and BK DNA tumor viruses, which are similar to the SV40 virus, have been implicated in human neuropathologies; for example, the JC virus is associated with a fatal demyelinating disease progressing to multifocal leukoencephalopathy. The production of transgenic mice harboring copies of either virus resulted in a variety of neoplasias.[116] Five transgenic mice bearing the JC transgene died soon after birth, and an additional four mice, subsequently shown to be mosaic for the transgene, developed adrenal medullary neuroblastomas.[116]

Mouse models for neuroblastoma, pineal cell tumors, and medulla blastomas of humans were obtained in two studies. Ectopic site-dependent expression of a MMTV/human adenovirus type 12 E1A and E1B transgene in a line of transgenic mice resulted in an olfactory neuroblastoma by 6 to 9 months of age.[64] In the second study, primitive neuroectodermal tumors were derived from transgenic mice carrying the SV40 T-antigen gene under the control of the MSV-LTR enhancer or the SV40 regulatory sequences.[66] In these tumors both the S-antigen and Rod-Opsin proteins were detected. These antigens are expressed in human pineal cell tumors and medullablastomas.

Two sets of transgenic mice may be models for myelinated nerve tumors and develop tumors that share similarities to Schwannomas or neurofibromas. The first involved the inappropriate expression of the v-*fps* nonreceptor tyrosine kinase oncogene linked to the human μ globin promoter, which resulted in the enlargement of the trigeminal nerve. These mice subsequently displayed tremors[137] most likely due to altered nerve conductance. Expression of the *tax*-1 gene from the human T-cell lymphotrophic virus-1 (HTLV-1) LTR results in a characteristic set of tumors that were defined as neurofibromatomas.[51] However, since neurofibromatomas closely resemble Schwannomas in mice, and none of the characteristic cytologic markers (e.g., S-100) were used to define the tumors, this diagnosis is tenuous. In another study a similar construct, when expressed in the transgenic mice, resulted in tumors of the same tissue, but these tumors were defined as Schwannomas.[94] In this case, tumors were positive for the S-100 antigen characteristic of Schwann cells. Tumors in both cases were observed within 2 weeks after birth. Since the *tax*-1 gene is thought to encode a transcriptional protein, it is possible that more than one cellular oncogene is activated in these animals, resulting in an immediate progression of the tumor with little or no latency.

Transgenic mice expressing the SV40 large T-antigen under the control of the promoter of the human phenylethanolamine N-methyltransferase gene develop pheochromacytomas and retinal tumors.[41] Retinal neurons were established in culture from these mice. These cells expressed phenotypic characteristics of retinal cells, all three neurofilament subunits, and the axon growth protein GAP43.[41] Establishment of a true neuronal cell type will be useful for studying growth and differentiation of neuronal cells.

Production of transgenic mice carrying the c-*mos* proto-oncogene linked to 800 bp of 5' flanking sequence and the MSV LTR resulted in several neuronal defects[96] (see below). In addition, on rare occasions mice carrying this proto-oncogene also develop astrocytomas by 10 to 14 months of age.[96] Since the spontaneous occurrence of this type of tumor is extremely rare, the transgene may have indirectly caused the neoplasia in these animals.

Liver and kidney tumors

Hepatocellular carcinomas are common in humans, especially in China. One possible causative agent is the hepatitis B virus, which could lead to cirrhosis and hepatocellular carcinomas. Transgenic mice that overproduce the hepatitis B virus large envelope polypeptide and surface antigen within hepatocytes develop a syndrome leading to neoplasia. These mice represent a model for hepatitis B-induced carcinoma.[23] In these mice, hepatocytes show severe pathological changes including inflammation, hyperplasia, and aneuploidy. The incidence of hepatocellular carcinoma is influenced by the genetic background and sex. Thus, the cellular and molecular pathogenesis leading to these carcinomas can be studied in these mice.

Transgenic mice bearing a variety of transforming genes, including SV40 T-antigen,[8,29,91,93,113] JC virus large T-antigen,[116] Ha-*ras* and c-*myc*,[108] or the TGF-α[54] genes also developed hepatocellular carcinomas or adenomas. In the best characterized report of liver tumor development, three different oncogenes were linked to the mouse albumin (Alb) promoter sequences[108] and used to create transgenic mice. Expression of each oncogene resulted in a specific pattern of hepatocellular pathology. Transgenic mice expressing high levels of the Ha-*ras* oncogene have atypical architecture of pleomorphic cells and die several days after birth. Low expressing Ha-*ras* transgenics have hepatic dysplasia, but no hyperplasia; these mice die of lung tumors. Alb/SV40 T-antigen expressing transgenics have hepatic dysplasia and a latency ranging from 3 to 7 months. Transgenics expressing the Alb/c-*myc* gene also develop hepatic dysplasia to varying degrees and focal hepatic adenomas with multinucleated cells. In all of these cases no metastases were observed. Intercrosses between the various oncogene bearing transgenic mice generally result in a shorter period of latency in the formation of tumors (see below). Most notable is that coexpression of *ras* and SV40 large T-antigen resulted in a twofold enlargement of the liver by 6 days postnatally, focal lobar necrosis, hepatomegaly, hyperplasia, and dysplasia.

Interestingly, two different research groups have used almost identical gene constructs (mouse metallothionein promoter/TGF-α) to create transgenic mice, but have obtained widely different results.[54,106] In one study, the expression of human TGF-α resulted in multifocal, well-differentiated hepatocellular carcinomas.[54] However, expression of a rat TGF-α gene or even a human TGF-α minigene containing several introns (presumably to increase the level of expression) resulted only in liver hyperplasia.[106] Clearly secondary events, such as genetic background, may influence the progression from hyperplasia to dysplasia to neoplasia.

The mouse major urinary protein (MUP) gene is expressed in a variety of tissues, including the sebaceous gland of the skin, preputial gland, and the liver. This gene is regulated by androgens and its product is secreted in the urine. When the promoter of this gene was linked to the SV40 large T-antigen, the transgenic mice consistently developed liver hyperplasia which lead to neoplasia.[46] Curiously, the expression of the transgene in the liver suppressed the endogenous liver MUP mRNA levels but not other liver-specific mRNAs. These results indicate a novel control, presumably involving MUP-specific transcriptional proteins.

Expression of several different oncogenes have resulted in models of kidney neoplasias. Ectopic expression of a chimeric human-mouse Thy-1 promoter fortuitously linked to SV40 T-antigen gene resulted in abnormal proliferation of proximal tubule cells. These abnormal cells could be established in culture, and when injected into nude mice resulted in the development of tumors.[65] Transgenic mice carrying renin/SV40 large T-antigen also resulted in proximal kidney tumors.[113,117] Renal adenocarcinomas found in transgenic mice expressing the BK virus early region developed only after amplification of the BK sequences.[26,116] This indicates that increased levels of transcription may have been required for transformation. These transgenic mice could be useful in studying Wilm's tumor, a human hereditary cancer.

Tumors of the endocrine and paracrine system

The very first tumor bearing transgenic mice studied carried the SV40 T-antigen linked to the rat insulin promoter. These studies underscore the usefulness of the transgenic mouse system in studying human neoplasia and demonstrate that cellular transformation in vivo mimicked spontaneous tumors. The formation of pancreatic B-cell tumors in transgenic mice with the rat insulin promoter/SV40 large T-antigen gene has recently been reviewed.[42] These tumors were highly differentiated and produced insulin.[30] Similar to the transgenic mice described above that coexpressed two oncogenes from the alb promoter,[108] hyperplastic but not neoplastic islets were found in these mice. All of the hyperplastic islets expressed high levels of the p53 recessive oncogene product[31]; and while it suggests that expression of p53 did not prevent hyperplasia,[122] it was possible that a point mutation in the p53 gene occurred rendering the protein ineffective. Developmental studies revealed that T-antigen was expressed transiently in neural crest cells, in pancreatic bud cells, and in non-β islet cells when they first appeared, leading Hanahan to propose that pancreatic cells share a common precursor with neuronal cells.[6] However, the role of insulin as a growth factor for the fetus cannot be ruled out.

A line of transgenic mice ectopically expressing the SV40 small and large T-antigen gene developed several different tumors including pancreatic β islet cells.[80] Mice carrying this construct developed islet adenomas accompanied by weakness and paralysis shortly before death. A detailed study of these mice revealed that the neuropathy is due to acute axonal degeneration coincident with hyperinsulinemia and hypoglycemia.[28] These data indicate a causal link between the incidence of peripheral neuropathy in humans treated for diabetes mellitus that experience transient hyperinsulinemic periods with similar peripheral nerve disorders in patients with insulinomas.[28]

In contrast to these studies, expression of a rat insulin II promoter/H-*ras* mutant oncogene in transgenic mouse islets results in destruction of islet cells within 3 to 5 months of age.[32] Only male mice developed this syndrome. Clinical manifestations included hyperglycemia, glycosuria, and reduced plasma insulin levels. The molecular mechanism for islet cell destruction is not clear. It is also unusual that female mice expressing the mutant *ras* oncogene did not develop tumors. Similar constructs using the same promoter linked to either the polyoma small T-antigen or the SV40 large T-antigen genes did not cause this phenotype.[99] In addition, the latter transgenic mice developed endoderm-derived tumors of the gut and pancreas.[99] This study poses many unanswered questions regarding specificity of an oncogene for a cellular target.

The class I H-2 K^b enhancer and part of the SV40 regulatory sequences to SV40 T-antigen gene were used to create transgenic mice.[98] Class I histocompatability genes are expressed in a variety of cells and tissues to varying extents, but not in neuronal tissue, and at very low levels in the liver. Many mice had multiple tumors including benign thymomas, and the majority of the mice had tumors of the lung, heart, liver, intestine, kidney, muscle, salivary gland, and ovary. The microscopic benign tumors were myocardial myomas, neuroblastomas, and rhabdomyosarcomas. Significantly, six founder transgenic mice showed neoplasias of several endocrine tissues including pancreas, thyroid, adrenal cortex and medulla, and testicular interstitial Leydig cells. The analysis of the types of cells involved was not reported, so it is not known what types of neoplasias were present in these tumors. This unique approach indicates that the SV40 T-antigen is capable of transforming a variety of tissues and cells.

Pancreatic acinar cell tumors have been induced in transgenic mice using either the rat elastase I (EL1)[89,97] or amylase 2.2 promoter[22] linked either to an activated human c-H-*ras*[97] SV40 T-antigen[20,89] or to the c-*myc*[107] gene. An ELl/proto-*ras* gene construct also failed to induce tumors, but instead led to aberrant differentiation of acinar cells.[97] Because this promoter is active by day 14 of gestation, transgenic mice bearing the mutant EL1/*ras* or EL1/SV40 T-antigen transgenes had hyperplastic changes by 16 to 17 days in utero. All but four mice bearing the mutant *ras* construct died soon after birth with acinar cell tumors; the remaining four animals were shown to be mosaic and had tumors of some acinar cells, but did not die as a result of the tumor. Since the mosaic mice had some normal acinar tissue and the other mice did not, these data indicate that the tumors per se did not kill the mice, but rather disrupted normal acinar cell functions. Therefore, one might be led to believe that it is not tumorigenesis that is lethal, but loss of essential functions necessary for survival that results from transformation. This area is largely unexplored and has great implications for treatment of patients with chemotherapeutic agents.

Mice bearing the EL1/SV40 T-antigen gene had a longer latency for tumorigenesis compared to the EL1/*ras* transgenics. This suggests that the expression of an activated *ras* gene is sufficient for neoplasia, whereas the SV40 T-antigen needed other genes to be activated for progression from hyperplasia to neoplasia in acinar cells. In contrast, ELl/c-myc transgenic mice showed a greater variability in latency, ranging between 2 to 7 months. The pathology was variable and included pancreatic masses with the remainder of the pancreas atrophied. Why the remainder of the pancreas had atrophied is curious, but may, in part, be due to an autoimmune reaction or a blockage of ducts and failure to secrete pancreatic enzymes. This, again, will bear further investigation as a disease mechanism. Microscopically, the masses were acinar cell carcinomas, acinar-like and duct-like cells embedded in stroma, squamous metaplasia, or adenosquamous carcinoma. Many of these findings may relate to the role of c-myc in maintaining cells in a state of continued proliferation, and the timing of expression during differentiation of the gland.

Tumors of the cardiovascular system

Certain oncogenes will show a predilection to transforming specific tissues in various organs. In an earlier example, the SV40 large T-antigen was expressed in a variety of cells and organs using a Class I histocompatability enhancer, but only specific tissues showed hyperplastic or a transformed phenotype.[98] The reason for this selection is not understood, but is probably dependent on several factors. DNA tumor viruses are selective in the tissues they are capable of infecting and transforming. The polyoma virus (PyV) is related to SV40; however, it differs in host range, gene sequence, gene function, and the ability to transform. Polyoma is indigenous to mice and causes multiple tumors. Transgenic mice carrying one of the two transforming genes of PyV develop tumors in different tissues depending on the promoter used.

Transgenic mice derived from embryonic stem (ES) cells transformed with a defective murine leukemia virus (MLV) carrying polyoma middle T gene develop endothelial tumors or hemangiomas.[131] These tumors developed in utero and the fetuses subsequently died. Transgenic mice were generated carrying the PyV middle T gene or large T gene driven by polyoma early gene regulatory sequences.[42] Unlike a viral infection of mice in which only cells expressing the virus receptor are capable of being infected, tumors should develop in a wider range of tissues because every cell carries the gene. Mice carrying the large T-antigen failed to develop tumors until they were crossed with a line of transgenic mice carrying an insulin/SV40 large T-antigen gene (see previous section). Mice that carried the middle T gene, however, also developed hemangiomas of endothelial origin.[10] In both studies it was possible to establish cell-lines from the tissues. One cell-line could make von Willebrand's factor,[131] a marker of endothelial cells. Such cell-lines will be invaluable for the study of angiogenesis, as well as for the production of therapeutic products active on endothelial cells.

Ectopic expression of the v-*fps* oncogene linked to the human μ globin promoter also led to hemangiomas as well as angiosarcomas.[135] The v-*fps* gene in this case was also expressed in a variety of other tissues without consequence. However, some selection was shown in that all of the tumors that developed in these mice were mesenchymal in origin.

Ectopic expression of a mouse protamine promoter/SV40 large T-antigen transgene also led to rhabdomyosarcomas of the right atrium of the heart,[12] as did an ANF/SV40 large T-antigen transgene.[33] The mouse protamine 1 gene is normaily expressed only during the haploid phases of spermatogenesis. Thus it is highly unusual to be expressed in the heart, whereas ANF is specific for endothelial cells.

Skin tumors

The papilloma viruses are the causative agents of warts and papillomas, and have been implicated in the formation of genital tumors. The E5 and E6 genes of papilloma viruses have been shown to be important to tumor formation. Introduction of a Bovine Papilloma Virus (BPV) T-antigen clone in transgenic mice resulted in multiple independent papillomas and the production of virus particles.[42] This points to a causal relationship between papilloma viruses and cancer. Tumors did not form until wounding occurred, and thus expression of the viral genome was the initiation step while expression of genes involved in wounding repair caused progression to neoplasia.

In addition to the BPV gene construct,[42] a mouse fetal Δ-globin/Ha-*ras*,[70] K10 Ha-*ras*,[9] and v-*jun*[111] transgenes have all produced papillomas or tumors after wounding. Only in the case of the keratin promoter linked to Ha-*ras* gene construct did spontaneous papillomas result, and then only in specific locations, e.g., behind the ears. Thus, the expression of these genes was insufficient for the production of tumors, but could initiate tumors. Progression in these cases could require expression of genes involved in wound healing which could act as tumor promoter-like agents.

Expression of the mutant human Ha-*ras* oncogene using the human keratin K10 promoter, which directs gene expression suprabasally in the epidermis and some other stratified epithelia, resulted in stunted growth and hyperkeratinosis in the absence of hyperplasia.[9] Epithelial hyperplasia and hyperkeratinosis were also observed in transgenic mice bearing the *tat* gene from the human immunodeficiency virus (HIV),[68,94] or the *tax*-1 gene of the HTLV-1 driven by a metallothionein promoter.[94] The expression of HIV-*tat* appeared to lead to a syndrome similar to Kaposi's sarcoma in male but not female transgenics.[128] Curiously, these Kaposi-like sarcomas arose only after the mice were 16 months of age, and were likely to resolve spontaneously. In contrast, ectopic expression of a human fetal globin promoter/Ha-*ras* oncogene[70] or a v-*jun* oncogene[111] in the skin of transgenics did not show any abnormalities prior to progression to occult tumors.

Recently, Mintz and her colleagues have developed models for melanomas[16,59] by the introduction of a tyrosinase promoter/SV40 large T-antigen construct into the germ line of mice. In these transgenics the gene is developmentally expressed in pigmented epithelia of the retina at day 10 to 11 in utero, and these mice developed aggressive eye tumors very soon after birth. The occurrence of melanomas in the human eye is common, and these transgenics may model this type of melanoma. In these transgenics the development of melanoblasts was altered, since the mice appeared lighter in color than their littermates. Interestingly, changes in the appearance and color of precancerous moles precede the development of melanoma in humans.

Mesenchymal tumors: osteosarcomas and fibrosarcomas

The Fos transcription factor appears to have a role in the development of many mesenchymal tissues, including the bone.[79] Expression of a c-*fos* transgene in developing bone led to osteoclast hyperplasia visible as a mass on x-ray examination of the mice.[102] Approximately 15% of these lesions progressed to osteosarcomas with a latency of 9.5 months,[103] and the osteoclasts were capable of being established in cell culture.[36] Analysis of the bones and tumors showed that several markers of osteoclast differentiation were absent, leading to the suggestion that c-*fos* acts by disrupting terminal differentiations of osteoblasts.[36]

The α *Amylase*-1 (*Amy*-1ᵃ) gene of mice contains a bipartite promoter with early and late expression regions regulating expression at different times in development. One transgenic line bearing the *Amy*-1ᵃ late promoter linked to the SV40 T-antigen gene developed osteosarcomas at multiple sites with a latency of over one year.[63] In contrast, the early promoter, when linked to SV40 T-antigen, resulted in hibernomas, or brown fat tumors, with a short latency.[34] The long latency for tumors to form is suggestive of secondary activation of another proto-oncogene during progression. The differences in tissue specificity between the early and late *Amy* promoters are also interesting because these are abnormal sites for expression of the endogenous gene; hence these promoter elements when separated show an unusual pattern of expression and suggest a novel *cis*-dependency of sequences. Bilateral osteosarcomas were observed in transgenic mice carrying a protamine/SV40 T-antigen gene.[12] This is another example of ectopic expression of an oncogene resulting in a rare type of tumor in mice.

Expression of a BPV genome in a tandem array caused fibromatoses, and fibrosarcomas were induced in mice after a latency of 8 to 9 months.[42] Progression from fibromatomas to fibrosarcomas appeared to involve abnormalities of chromosomes 8 and 14.[72] Ectopic expression of the v-*fps* protein-tyrosine kinase under the control of the human μ globin promoter and 3' regulatory sequences led to the development of fibrosarcomas in ears, body wall, tail, and paws.[135] Expression of the oncogene in some tissues did not lead to hyperplastic or neoplastic changes. The wide range of neoplastic, neurological, and cardiac abnormalities that developed in these mice[135] makes it probable that other secondary events as well as epigenetic events must occur for transformation to progress. It would be informative to examine these mice for the presence of chromosomal abnormalities and to determine if they are the same as in the BPV transgenic mice. This information would help to identify a genetic loci involved in the progression from preneoplastic lesions to tumors.

Eye tumors

The expression of oncogenes in lenticular and nonlenticular sites of the eye has resulted in interesting effects on eye development.[129]

Spontaneous neoplasia of the ocular lens of mice has never been described. However, tumors developed when the SV40 T-antigen gene fused to the α-A-crystallin promoter is expressed in transgenic mice.[73,86] Expression of the polyoma T-antigen c-mos and SV40 T-antigen genes, in contrast, led to perturbation of normal lens fiber cell differentiation.[39,96,123] Interestingly, the cells derived from these transgenic mice proliferate in vitro in the absence of basic fibroblast growth factor,[38] which is thought to be necessary for the growth of fetal lens cells.

Transgenic mice overexpressing a GM-CSF transgene develop blindness.[67] The loss of vision was the result of aberrant proliferation of macrophages in the eye leading to tissue destruction. Some component or peculiarity of eye structure must make it more susceptible for the autolysis of tissue occurring in these mice. It is possible that the immune system might somehow be activated against spontaneously occurring tumors of the eye.

Hereditary retinoblastomas arise early in humans as multifocal bilateral tumors with high penetrance of the inherited mutant retinoblastoma (Rb) gene. Sporadic nonhereditary retinoblastomas result from spontaneous inactivation mutations in Rb with subsequent loss of heterozygosity, and the tumors are unilateral and unifocal. Cases of hereditary bilateral retinoblastoma with midline intracranial malignancies involving the pineal gland or supracellular or paracellular regions have been found and termed trilateral retinoblastoma.[88,134] Ectopic expression in a single line of transgenic mice bearing a human Leutinizing hormone/SV40 T-antigen transgene resulted in tumors that are morphologically very similar to those found in trilateral retinoblastoma patients. Penetrance of the retinoblastomas in these mice is 100%, thus acting as a dominant mutation, while only 15% develop midline tumors. Demonstration that the integration of the transgene in this line is not in the mouse Rb locus precludes the tumors arising from an insertional mutation. However, association of the T-antigen with Rb protein suggests a functional loss of the Rb gene product. These mice will prove to be important for tracing the developmental history of this hereditary cancer.

Tumors of the reproductive system

Tumors of the reproductive system in transgenic mice have been confined to the nongerminal component. Most reproductive organ tumors result from the expression of an oncogene using the MMTV-LTR. In some cases hyperplasia and dysplasia have been erroneously characterized as tumors,[52] but these "tumors" fail to grow in nude mice. Epididymis, vas deferens, and seminal vesicles were found to be enlarged in these animals, and sterility was a secondary observation.[52,85,114] In one case, a Sertoli cell tumor was found.[71] In addition to these tumors, transgenic mice expressing TGF-α developed hyperplasia and dysplasia of the coagulation gland, with focal characteristics of a carcinoma.[106] The embryologically related prostate gland was not affected, indicating that response to TGF-α is restricted to certain epithelial cells. As yet, similar reproductive tract tumors in female mice have not been found.

Oncogene Cooperativity

Gain of Function

Progression from hyperplastic to dysplastic to frank tumors, in all but one transgenic mouse line (bearing an MMTV/*neu* transgene[85]), requires a variable latency period. This progression suggests a stochastic mechanism, implying the activation of additional oncogenes. The two activated genes work in a cooperative manner to achieve progression. Alternatively, the activation of an oncogene followed by inactivation or mutation of a recessive oncogene or antioncogene can likewise result in transformation, as has been shown for *ras* p53 in vitro.[50,92]

The first transgenic study to demonstrate cooperativity was the intercross of mice bearing either a MMTV/v-H-*ras* oncogene or MMTV/*myc* oncogene.[114] Multiple tumors arose in the appropriate tissues. However, the latency of tumor formation was significantly shorter than that for either transgene alone. Because there were multiple tumors, one could not rule out physiological abnormalities that would result in a shorter latency. However, Groner and his colleagues[40] have found similar results using the mammary gland-specific WAP promoter.

myc-ras oncogene cooperativity was also shown for liver tumor-specific Alb promoter.[108] Coexpression of an Alb/SV40 T-antigen and Alb/*ras* oncogenes resulted in a liver phenotype different from either gene alone or in other combinations. Neonates displayed enlarged livers with a prominent ductile pattern similar to bile duct. The authors suggest that the bile duct epithelial cells were more susceptible to transformation by this combination of oncogenes. The lack of a latency was interpreted as indicating that SV40 T-antigen potentiated the action of *ras* through some rate limiting pathway or, more likely, by the direct action on complementary pathways in transformation. While all hepatocytes in Alb/*ras* + Alb/*myc*, or Alb/SV40 + Alb/*myc* double transgenics expressed the two oncogenes, not all the cells were transformed. Second, *myc*-SV40 transgenics had a very short latency and died before three weeks of age with focal tumors containing hyperplastic and dysplastic hepatocytes, but not neoplastic lesions. Both Alb/*myc* + Alb/*ras* and MMTV/*myc* + MMTV/*ras* transgenics showed accelerated multifocal tumor development. But Alb/*myc* transgenic animals did not develop tumors. Thus the *myc* gene may act by causing some cells to retain their proliferative capacity. One interpretation of this data would be that additional events must occur, beyond the activation of two oncogenes, to allow for the progression from hyperplasia to tumor. These additional events may include the loss of expression of tumor-suppressor genes, activation of other proto-oncogenes, and loss of a differentiated function.

Infection of mice with MLV frequently results in T-cell lymphomas. When these tumors were analyzed for common sites of proviral integration, it was found that a serine/threonine protein kinase named *pim*-1 was frequently activated. Transgenic mice carrying an IgHEμ enhancer/promoter/*pim*-1 construct developed T-cell lymphomas at a 10% to 15% frequency.[127] Because only very few mice developed tumors, it can be concluded that activation of *pim*-1 alone was insufficient for transformation.

The idea that expression of *myc* predisposes cells to transformation has been tested. The *pim*-1 transgenic mice were injected with MLV at birth.[126] T-cell lymphomas developed in the infected mice with a latency of 7 to 8 weeks compared to 22 weeks for infected nontransgenic mice. Twenty-one of 26 tumors examined had proviral inserts into the c-*myc* locus, and the remaining five tumors had inserts into the N-*myc* locus. In contrast, three out of nine tumors in nontransgenic mice had an insert into c-*myc*, one in the N-*myc*, and one in both the c-*myc* and N-*myc* loci. Spontaneous lymphomas in *pim*-1 transgenics had no rearrangements in c-*myc* or N-*myc*, but all had overexpression of c-*myc* and not N-*myc*. These data point to a cooperative action between *pim*-1 and c-*myc* in T-cell lymphogenesis. These data were confirmed and extended in transgenic mice bearing both $E\mu/myc$ and $E\mu/pim$-1; transgenics showed an acceleration in development of pre-B-cell leukemias, often developing the cancer in utero.[127]

In a similar experiment, Adams and coworkers[60] infected $E\mu/myc$ transgenic mice (see above) with retroviruses expressing the v-*raf* oncogene. It had been previously shown that infection of bone marrow cells with v-*myc* and v-*raf* retroviruses resulted in B- and T-cell lymphomas. However, when cells were propagated in culture some clones converted into macrophages. These results indicate that the v-*myc* + v-*raf* combination may disrupt the developmental program of committed B cells, resulting in their switch to myeloid lineage. It was therefore not surprising that infection of transgenic mice changed cloned pre-B and B cell-lines into mature and immature macrophages. Furthermore, cells ceased expressing the *myc* transgene in the more differentiated cells that remained tumorigenic, indicating that the transgene expression is not required for maintenance of the capacity to divide.

As a model for viral oncogene transformation resulting from infection of cells and tissues by SV40, transgenic mice were created expressing either the SV40 large T-antigen or large and small t-antigens under the control of the MMTV-LTR promoter/enhancer.[25] While transgenic mice bearing either transgene develop lymphomas, only mice bearing *both* large and small t-antigen had ductile epithelial adenocarcinomas in the lung and/or kidney by 4 months of age. Similar analyses have been carried out using PyV T-antigens.[11] These results indicate that although SV40 and polyoma large T-antigen are capable of causing hyperplasia, small t-antigens supply an accessory function for transformation.

Loss of Function

Aberrant function or loss of activity by several proteins can lead to tumorigenesis (see Chapter 2). One such protein is the p53 gene product which has been shown to bind to other oncoproteins.[50] When a mutant p53 allele that bound to *ras* and exhibited cooperativity[50] was introduced into the germ line of mice, several types of tumors formed, including tumors of the lung, bone, and lymphoid system.[69] Efrat and Hanahan were able to show that the p53 protein was associated with SV40 large T-antigen in pancreatic β-cell tumors of transgenic mice, and that p53 was expressed at higher than normal levels.[31] Similarly,

T-antigen expressed in the retina also bound to the Rb gene product resulted in a loss of function of this protein.[88,134] Intercrossing the p53 transgenic mice carrying activated oncogenes expressed in various tissues can reveal how recessive oncogenes may cause tumors upon their mutation or loss.

Genetics and Cancer

Immunity

Tumor cells often express several antigens which are normally expressed during embryogenesis. As the tumor progresses and becomes centrally necrotic, novel tumor antigens are then exposed to the immune system. Such novel antigens are sometimes expressed on tumor cells including the p97 protein on melanoma cells.[19] The SV40 large T-antigen expressed in mice from a transgene can act as a non-H-2 histocompatability antigen.[55,130] Syngeneic mice immunized with transgenic splenocytes mount a cytotoxic T-cell response. Because the mice differ only in the expression of SV40 large T-antigen the results indicate that this nuclear protein is expressed on the surface of splenocytes. It is possible that tumor cells may escape immune surveillance by expressing targets for an immune reaction on the cell surface, conditioning the immune system to recognize the antigen as self.

In contrast, Hanahan and colleagues[43] have found that expression of the SV40 large T-antigen resulted in autoimmunity in some, but not all, of the transgenic mice thet have studied. Transgenic mice bearing a rat insulin promoter linked to SV40 large T-antigen gene developed insulinitis, which was characterized by increased vascularization and 55% to 80% lymphocytic infiltration. This was also found to be the case when mice were immunized with exogenous large T-antigen. One line of mice showed tolerance to the antigen and failed to develop insulinitis. Autoimmune response preceded tumor formation, and was independent of the development of tumors. The development of self-tolerance in some of these lines of mice may be due to either the timing of expression of the gene or the development of the tumor. Regulation of T-helper cell function and killing in these mice remains to be analyzed. Similar effects may also be noted in other tumors; for example, the unusual appearance of acinar cell tumors in EL1/*ras* and EL1/*myc* transgenics[97,107] (see previous section). The inability to mount a proper immune response against tumor antigens may be due to certain combinations of the Major Histocompatability complex (MHC) locus, and may be an essential key for future treatment paradigms.

Effect of Genotype on Tumorigenesis

Identification of the genes that affect multistep carcinogenesis in humans is extremely difficult. Experiments directed to answering this question can be undertaken in transgenic mice by backcrossing transgenes into different genetic background. In one experiment, continued backcross of Eµ/c-*myc* mice to C57BL/6J X SJL/J F1 (B6SJLF1) hybrid mice insured heterogeneity for either C57BL/6J or SJL/J genetic backgrounds, and the resulting mice were observed to have different life spans depending on the genetic background.[112] Ten backcrosses to the C57BL/6 strain resulted in a lifespan of 134 days, while three backcrosses to SJL/J resulted in a lifespan reduction to 82 days. Backcrossing the C57BL/6 Eµ/c-*myc* transgenics to the BALB strain also reduced the lifespan from 134 days to 99 days. This is suggestive of a limited number of dominant-acting genes that affect lymphoma formation. This approach holds great promise that these genes might be identified using recombinant inbred mice, and subsequently their mode of action can be deduced.

Additional evidence for dominant and recessive modifiers of multistep carcinogenesis comes from other studies. Transgenic mice bearing SV40 regulatory sequences linked to large T-antigen gene developed choroid plexus papillomas. These tumors contained elevated amounts of the p53 gene product, which was complexed to the T-antigen.[75] Transgenic mice of the C57BL/6J genetic background developed tumors by 80 to 90 days of age, and 100% of the mice were dead by 125 days.[24] These mice were mated to different strains of mice such as C57BL/10SnJ, C3H/HeJ, AKR/J, and NZW/lacJ mice to create F1 hybrids. The C57BL/10SnJ mice were similar to the C57BL/6J mice in terms of survival, while F1 mice with C3H/HeJ and AKR/J mice died by 140 to 160 days. In contrast, F1 hybrids with NZW/lacJ mice had a lifespan almost twice as long as the parental C57BL/6J mice. At 120 to 125 days when 100% of the C57BL/6J mice were dead, 90% of the F1 hybrids were still alive. Northern blot analysis of RNA from these hybrids demonstrated that the onset of large T-antigen expression in F1 hybrid mice was delayed. Thus, the NZW/lacJ mice may carry an allele of a gene that acts in a dominant-negative fashion to regulate large T-antigen expression and to suppress tumor formation. These studies indicate that secondary effects resulting in variable latencies may be caused by mutations in such dominant alleles.

Tumorigenesis and Metastases

Tumorigenesis

A recurring theme of oncogenesis in transgenic mice is that the expression of the transgene does not necessarily lead to tumor formation. This may be due, in part, to the inability of the particular oncogene to have an effect on the replication machinery in that particular cell. In some cases the expression of a transgene may lead to the failure of the cells to properly differentiate. For example, the expression of a variety of oncogenes linked to the EL1 promoter causes aberrant duct formation.[8,31,108] Transgenic mice carrying oncogenes can be induced to tumorigenesis by several different means. Therefore, these mice can be used as a test system for evaluating agents that accelerate carcinogenesis.

The introduction of human Ha-*ras* oncogenes into mouse embryos results in the formation of tumors that cause lethality during embryogenesis.[56] In other experiments transgenic mice were created that carried a human Ha-*ras* gene with a mutation in the last intron. This mutation resulted in a high level of transcription of the gene.[105] This transgenic experiment was designed to test whether overexpression of the unmutated gene could also result in tumor formation.[105] Fifty percent of the mice developed tumors in some, but not all, of the tissues overexpressing the human gene by the time they were 85 months old. Thus overexpression of *ras* was insufficient for tumorigenesis in all tissues. The tumors, but not the normal tissues, contained *ras* genes that had acquired a mutation either in the 12th or 61st codon of the transgene, the same mutation which is found in human bladder cancers.[105] Therefore, this study demonstrates that overexpression is not sufficient to cause tumors, but the acquisition of mutations coupled with overexpression will cause tumorigenesis.

Ectopic expression of a mouse fetal globin promoter/v-H-*ras* transgene in the skin has created an invaluable model for evaluating tumor promoters.[70] Because these mice contain an activated *ras* gene, they have in effect undergone the initiation step. When these mice are treated with tumor promoters such as phorbol esters, the formation of multiple papillomas resulted, some of which progressed to squamous cell carcinomas and underlying sarcomas. The effect of phorbol esters could be antagonized by retinoic acid treatment.[70] These mice will prove useful for assaying tumor promoting agents and pharmacological agents that can inhibit or slow tumor proliferation.

Metastasis

Metastasis is the process of the spreading of cancerous cells from their origin to other sites. Metastasis occurs with a high frequency in certain melanomas, osteosarcomas, and small cell lung carcinomas. The process occurs in discrete steps including one in which the tumor cells invade a capillary wall and migrate through the blood system. Metastases in spontaneous and transgenic mouse tumors is a rare event. One reason for this rarity is the long period of latency of the tumor. Another possibility is that whereas in humans metastases often follow treatment of the primary tumor, the tumor bearing mice are often sacrificed before metastasis can develop. To date, six reports have appeared in which metastases had been found in transgenic mice developing tumors. These include mammary tumors,[52] hybridomas,[34] acinar cell tumors,[22] pancreatic tumors,[98] fibrosarcomas,[135] and adrenal neuroblastomas.[116] These tumors involve six different oncogenes, the *ret* oncogene,[52] SV40 large T-antigen,[20,34,98] the JC tumor antigen,[116] and the viral v-*fps*.[135] In all but one involving fibrosarcomas,[135] all of the tumor cells were well differentiated. Thus metastases in these cases is not restricted to a specific differentiated state of the cell or the type of oncogene. The ability of a tumor cell to metastasize could depend on the cell type of the transformed cell. In two noted exceptions this was not the case. Pancreatic acinar cell tumors created using the tissue-specific EL1 promoter did not metastasize. When different MMTV-LTR linked oncogenes were compared, only the *ret* oncogene-derived tumors were found to be metastatic.

Oncogenesis and Development

The relationship between cancer and development has long been recognized. Misexpression of oncogenes during development of the mouse might be expected to result in developmental aberrations in transgenic mice.[87,121] The expression of proto-oncogenes or DNA tumor virus oncogenes in the eye lens cells during postnatal development resulted in aberrant lens formation.[129] The c-*mos* proto-oncogene[58] and the SV40 large T-antigen gene[123] under the control of MSV LTR lead to perturbation of the ability of the lens fiber cells to enucleate and clear, resulting in a cataract-like lens abnormality. In one study, lenticular tumors were observed,[129] and it is possible that this is due to expression of the oncogene while the cells still have a proliferative capacity. In the other cases, aberrations of the lens resulted from the expression of the transgene after the lens cells had become committed to cease dividing and differentiate.

Transgenic mice bearing a MSV/c-*mos* transgene also displayed severe behavioral and neurological defects.[96] The behavioral abnormalities ranged from hyperactivity with head bobbing to rapid circling and ataxia. Neurological defects included axonal degeneration, gliosis, and Purkinje cell degeneration. In addition, defects were observed in the hair cells and spiral ganglions of the inner ear that resulted in deafness. Older mice also showed a severe neuro-inflammatory reaction presumably caused by an unusually high number of mast cells associated with neurons. These mice could be invaluable for studying neuro-pharmacological agents that can inhibit the inflammatory response.

Transgenic mice carrying c-*myc* linked to an elastase promoter showed expression in pancreatic acinar cells.[107] Pancreatic masses in these mice were characterized by the presence of both ductile epithelia and acinar cell tumors. The close association of these cells suggested to the authors that one type of cell can differentiate into another. Similar relationships were observed when transgenic mice carrying Alb promoter linked transgenes were created to direct expression of the oncogene to the liver.[108] This is particularly true for the Alb/*ras* transgene which induced morphological changes throughout the fetal liver. Interestingly, expression of an activated *ras* gene under the control of a heat shock inducible promoter in *Drosophila* results in profound morphological alterations of the eye.[13]

The expression of c-*fos* gene using the H2-K[b] promoter affects T-cell development.[104] In these animals, there is an increased number of mature monocytes and an altered distribution of T-cell subsets. One possible explanation for this phenotype is that fetal T cells originate in the fetal thymus, and that in these mice the transition to the marrow is impaired. Interestingly, both B- and T-cell functions in these mice were affected.

Transgenic mice bearing an MSV/*ski* transgene show abnormal proliferation of myocytes resulting in greater muscle mass.[120] This is not strictly due to a hyperplasia of tissue since muscle development is not perturbed. Instead, this may result from additional rounds of proliferation of myoblasts before their fusion. The c-*myc* proto-oncogene is thought to be involved in cardiac myocyte proliferation. The *myc* protein may be involved in regulating the proliferative capacity of a number of different cells. Constitutive overexpression of a c-*myc* transgene in the heart during embryogenesis resulted in the enlargement of the heart.[53] Therefore it may be possible to modify the size of certain tissues and organs in transgenic animals of commercial value by selectively expressing proto-oncogenes during development.

Prospects for Drug Design

Transgenic mice can be used as models for the human cancer. Many potential therapeutic agents can be tested in mice to determine their toxicity, efficacy, and stability. For example, monoclonal antibodies directed against specific tumor antigens can be coupled to various toxic agents or radionuclides and tested in vivo in the mice for their ability to attack the tumor. Expression of human tumor antigens with tissue-specific promoters in transgenics would be invaluable in testing immunotherapy regimens.[47]

A second aspect of anticancer therapy is drug resistance. Resistance to drugs in many cases is due to the P-glycoprotein product encoded by the multidrug resistance (MDR) locus. P-glycoprotein functions as a transporter protein that cycles different types of hydrophobic chemotherapeutic agents from the cancer cell before they can have an effect. Resistant cells often overexpress MDR transcripts. Mickisch and his colleagues created a transgenic mouse model to investigate MDR. In this model the MDR1 gene was expressed using the chicken β actin promoter.[83] The product of the transgene in the MDR protein was shown to be active. These results can be extrapolated to human gene therapy trials in the future.

References

1. Adams JM, Harris AW, Langdon WY, et al. c-*myc*-induced lymphogenesis in transgenic mice and the role of the Pvt-1 locus in lymphoid neoplasia. Rev Curr Top Microbiol Immunol 1986; 132:1–8.

2. Adams JM, Harris AW, Pinkert CA, et al. The c-*myc* oncogene driven by immunoglobulin enhancers induces lymphoid malignancy in transgenic mice. Nature 1985; 318:533–538.

3. Adams TE, Alpert S, Hanahan D. Non-tolerance and autoantibodies to a transgenic self antigen expressed in pancreatic μ cells. Nature 1987; 325:223–228.

4. Aguzzi A, Wagner EF, Williams RL, et al. Sympathetic hyperplasia and neuroblastomas in transgenic mice expressing polyoma middle T antigen. The New Biol 1990; 2:533–543.

5. Alexander WS, Schrader JW, Adams JM. Expression of the c-*myc* oncogene under control of an immunoglobulin enhancer in Eμ-*myc* transgenic mice. Mol Cell Biol 1987; 7:1436–1444.

6. Alpert S, Hanahan D, Teiteman G. Hybrid insulin genes reveal a developmental lineage for pancreatic endocrine cells and imply a relationship with neurons. Cell 1988; 53:295–308.

7. Andres A-C, Schonenberger C-A, Groner B, et al. Ha-*ras* oncogene expression directed by a milk protein gene promoter: Tissue specificity, hormonal regulation, and tumor induction in transgenic mice. Proc Natl Acad Sci USA 1987; 84:1299–1303.

8. Araki K, Miyazaki J-I, Hino O, et al. Expression and replication of hepatitis B virus genome in transgenic mice. Proc Natl Acad Sci USA 1989; 86:207–211.

9. Bailleul B, Surani MA, White S, et al. Skin hyperkeratosis and papilloma formation in transgenic mice expressing a *ras* oncogene from a suprabasal keratin promoter. Cell 1990; 62:697–708.

10. Bautch VL, Toda S, Hassell JA, et al. Endothelial cell tumors develop in transgenic mice carrying polyoma virus middle T oncogene. Cell 1987; 51:529–538.

11. Bautch VL. Effects of polyoma virus oncogenes in transgenic mice. Mol Biol Med 1989; 6:309–317.

12. Behringer RR, Peschon JJ, Messing A, et al. Heart and bone tumors in transgenic mice. Proc Natl Acad Sci USA 1988; 85:2648–2652.

13. Bishop JG III, Corces VG. Expression of an activated *ras* gene causes developmental abnormalities in transgenic *Drosophila* melanogaster. Genes & Dev 1988; 2:567–577.

14. Botter FM, van der Putten H, Wong DF, et al. Unexpected thymic hyperplasia in transgenic mice harboring a neuronal promoter fused with simian virus 40 large T antigen. Mol Cell Biol 1987; 7:3178–3184.

15. Bouchard L, Lamarre L, Tremblay PJ. Stochastic appearance of mammary tumors in transgene mice carrying the MMTV/c-*neu* oncogene. Cell 1989; 57:931–936.

16. Bradl M, Klein-Szanto A, Porter S, et al. Malignant melanoma in transgenic mice. Proc Natl Acad Sci USA 1991; 88:164–168.

17. Brinster RL, Chen HY, Messing A, et al. Transgenic mice harboring SV40 T-antigen genes develop characteristic brain tumors. Cell 1984; 37:367–379.

18. Brinster RL, Chen HY, Trumbauer ME, et al. Factors affecting the efficiency of introducing foreign DNA into mice by microinjecting eggs. Proc Natl Acad Sci USA 1985; 82:4438–4442.

19. Brown JP, Nishiyama K, Hellstrom I, et al. Structural characterization of human melanoma-associated antigen p97 with monoclonal antibodies. J Immun 1981; 127:539–546.
20. Ceci JD, Kovatch RM, Swing DA, et al. Transgenic mice carrying a murine 2.2/SV40 T antigen fusion gene develop pancreatic acinar cell and stomach carcinomas. Oncogene 1990; 6:323–332.
21. Chalifour LE, Gomes ML, Wang N-S, et al. Polyomavirus large T-antigen expression in heart of transgenic mice causes cardiomyopathy. Oncogene 1990; 5:1719–1726.
22. Chen S, Botteri F, van der Putten H, et al. A lymphoproliferative abnormality associated with inappropriate expression of the Thy-1 antigen in transgenic mice. Cell 1987; 51:7–19.
23. Chisari FV, Klopchin K, Morlyama T, et al. Molecular pathogenesis of hepatocellular carcinoma in hepatitis B virus transgenic mice. Cell 1989; 59:1145–1156.
24. Cho HJ, Seiberg M, Georgoff I, et al. Impact of the genetic background of transgenic mice upon the formation and timing of choroid plexus papillomas. J Neurosci Res 1989; 24:115–122.
25. Choi Y, Lee I, Ross SR. Requirement for the simian virus 40 small tumor antigen in tumorigenesis in transgenic mice. Mol Cell Biol 1988; 8:3382–3390.
26. Dalrymple SA, Beemon KL. BK virus T antigens induce kidney carcinomas and thymoproliferative disorders in transgenic mice. J Virol 1990; 64:1182–1191.
27. Dent LA, Strath M, Mellor AL, et al. Eosinophilia in transgenic mice expressing interleukin 5. J Exp Med 1990; 172:1425–1431.
28. Dyer KD, Messing A. Peripheral neuropathy associated with functional islet cell adenomas in SV40 transgenic mice. J Neuropathol & Exp Neurol 1989; 48:1399–412.
29. Dyer KR, Messing A. Metal-inducible pathology in the liver, pancreas, and kidney of transgenic mice expressing SV40 early region genes. Am J Pathol 1989; 135:401–410.
30. Efrat S, Hanahan D. Evidence for threshold effects in transformation of pancreatic μ cells by SV40 T antigen in transgenic mice. Curr Topics Microbiol & Immun 1989; 144:89–95.
31. Efrat S, Baekkeskov S, Lane D, et al. Coordinate expression of the endogenous p53 gene in X cells of transgenic mice expressing hybrid insulin-SV40 T antigen genes. EMBO J 1987; 6:2699–2704.
32. Efrat S, Fleischer N, Hanahan D. Diabetes induced in male transgenic mice by expression of human H-ras oncoprotein in pancreatic X cells. Mol Cell Biol 1990; 10:1779–1783.
33. Field LJ. Atrial natriuretic factor—SV40 T antigen trangenes produce tumors and cardiac arrhythmias in mice. Science 1988; 239:1029–1033.
34. Fox N, Crooke R, Hwang L-H, et al. Metastatic hibernomas in transgenic mice expressing an α-amylase-SV40 T antigen hybrid gene. Science 1989; 244:460–463.
35. Fusco A, Portella G, Grieco M, et al. A retrovirus carrying the polyomavirus middle T gene induces acute thrombocythemic myeloproliferative disease in mice. J Virol 1988; 62:361–365.

36. Goralczyk R, Closs EI, Ruther U, et al. Characterization of *fos*-induced osteogenic tumors and tumour-derived murine cell lines. Differentiation 1990; 44:122–131.
37. Greer P, Maltby V, Rossant J, et al. Myeloid expression of the human c-*fps/fes* proto-oncogene in transgenic mice. Mol Cell Biol 1990; 10:2521–2527.
38. Griep AE, Westphal H. Differentiation versus proliferation of transgenic mouse lens cells expressing polyoma large T antigen: Evidence for regulation by an endogenous growth factor. New Biol 1990; 8:727–738.
39. Griep AE, Kuwabara T, Lee EJ, et al. Perturbed development of the mouse lens by polyomavirus large T antigen does not lead to tumor formation. Genes & Dev 1989; 3:1075–1085.
40. Groner B, Schonenberger C-A, Andres AC. Targeted expression of the *ras* and *myc* oncogenes in transgenic mice. TIG 1987; 3:306–308.
41. Hammang JP, Baetge EE, Behringer RR, et al. Immortalized retinal neurons derived from SV40 T-antigen-induced tumors in transgenic mice. Neuron 1990; 4:775–782.
42. Hanahan D. Dissecting multistep tumorigenesis in transgenic mice. Annu Rev Genet 1988; 22:479–519.
43. Hanahan D. Transgenic mouse models of self-tolerance and autoreactivity by the immune system. Ann Review Cell Biol 1990; 6:493–537.
44. Harris AW, Langdon WY, Alexander WS, et al. Transgenic mouse models for hematopoietic tumorigenesis. Rev Curr Top Microbiol Immunol 1988; 141:82–93.
45. Heisterkamp N, Jenster G, ten Hoeve J, et al. Acute leukaemia in *bcr/abl* transgenic mice. Nature 1990; 344:251–253.
46. Held WA, Mullins JJ, Kuhn NJ, et al. T antigen expression and tumorigenesis in transgenic mice containing a mouse major urinary protein/SV40 T antigen hybrid gene. EMBO J 1989; 8:183–191.
47. Hellstrom I, Hellstrom KE. Cancer vaccines for therapy. In: Accomplishments in Cancer Research, Fortner JF, Rhoads JE, eds. Philadelphia, J.P. Lipincott 1988; pp. 319–333.
48. Heston WE. Cancer: A comprehensive treatise. In: Genetics: Animal Tumors, Becker FF, ed. New York, Plenum Press 1975; Vol. 1, p. 33.
49. Heston WE. Development and utilization of inbred strains of mice for cancer research. In: Mammalian Genetics and Cancer, Russell ES, ed. New York, Alan R. Liss 1981; pp. 279–290.
50. Hinds P, Finlay C, Levine AJ. Mutation is required to activate the p53 gene for cooperation with the *ras* oncogene and transformation. J Virol 1989; 63:739–746.
51. Hinrichs SH, Nerenberg M, Reynolds RK, et al. A transgenic mouse model for human fibromatosis. Science 1987; 237:1340–1343.
52. Iwamoto T, Takahashi M, Ito M, et al. Oncogenicity of the *ret* transforming gene in MMTV/*ret* transgenic mice. Oncogene 1990; 5:535–542.
53. Jackson T, Allard MF, Sreenan CM, et al. The c-*myc* proto-oncogene regulates cardiac development in transgenic mice. Mol Cell Biol 1990; 10:3709–3716.
54. Jhappan C, Stahle C, Harkins RN, et al. TGF overexpression in transgenic

mice induces liver neoplasia and abnormal development of the mammary gland and pancreas. Cell 1990; 61:1137-I146.

55. Juretic A, Knowles BB. SV40 T antigen acts as a minor histocompatability antigen of SV40 T antigen tolerant transgenic mice. Immunogenetics 1989; 29:366–370.

56. Katsuki M, Kimura M, Hata J, et al. Embryonal tumors from transgenic mouse zygotes carrying human activated c-Ha-*ras* genes. Mol Biol Med 1989; 6:567–572.

57. Kelliher MA, McLaughlin J, Witte ON, et al. Induction of a chronic myelogenous leukemia-like syndrome in mice with v-*abl* and BCR/ABL. Proc Natl Acad Sci USA 1990; 87:6649–6653.

58. Khillan JS, Oskarsson MK, Propst F, et al. Defects in lens fiber differentiation are linked to c-*mos* overexpression in transgenic mice. Genes & Dev 1987; 1:1327–1335.

59. Klein-Szanto A, Bradl M, Porter S, et al. Melanosis and associated tumors in transgenic mice. Proc Natl Acad Sci USA 1991; 88:169–173.

60. Klinken SP, Alexander WS, Adams JM. Hemopoietic lineage switch: v-*raf* oncogene converts Eμ-*myc* transgenic B cells into macrophages. Cell 1988; 53:857–867.

61. Klinken SP, Alexander WS, Adams JM. Hemopoietic lineage switch: v-*raf* oncogene converts Eμ-*myc* transgenic B cells into macrophages. Cell 1988; 53:857–867.

62. Knight KL, Spieker-Polet H, Kazdin DS, et al. Transgenic rabbits with lymphocytic leukemia induced by the c-*myc* oncogene fused with the immunoglobulin heavy chain enhancer. Proc Natl Acad Sci USA 1988; 85:3130–3134.

63. Knowles BB, McCarrick J, Fox N, et al. Osteosarcomas in transgenic mice expressing an α-Amylase-SV40 T-antigen hybrid gene. Am J Pathol 1990; 137:259–262.

64. Koike K, Jay G, Hartley JW, et al. Activation of retrovirus in transgenic mice: Association with development of olfactory neuroblastoma. J Virol 1990; 64:3988–3991.

65. Kollias G, Evans DJ, Ritter M, et al. Ectopic expression of Thy-1 in the kidneys of transgenic mice induces functional and proliferative abnormalities. Cell 1987; 51:21–31.

66. Korf H-W, Gotz W, Herken R, et al. S-antigen and rodopsin immunoreactions in midline brain neoplasms of transgenic mice: Similarities to pineal cell tumors and certain medulloblastomas in man. J Neuropathol & Exp Neurol 1990; 49:424–437.

67. Lang RA, Metcalf D, Cuthbertson RA, et al. Transgenic mice expressing a hemopoietic growth factor gene (GM-CSF) develop accumulations of macrophages, blindness, and fatal syndrome of tissue damage. Cell 1987; 51:675–686.

68. Lassam N, Feigenbaum L, Vogel J, et al. Transgenic approach for the study of pathogenesis induced by human viruses. Mol Biol Med 1989; 6:319–331.

69. Lavigueur A, Maltby V, Mock D, et al. High incidence of lung, bone and lymphoid tumors in transgenic mice overexpressing mutant alleles of the p53 oncogene. Mol Cell Biol 1989; 9:3982–3991.

70. Leder A, Kuo A, Cardiff RD, et al. v-Ha-*ras* transgene abrogates the initiation step in mouse skin tumorigenesis: Effects of phorbol esters and retinoic acid. Proc Natl Acad Sci USA 1990; 87:9178–9182.

71. Leder A, Pattengale PK, Kuo A, et al. Consequences of widespread deregulation of the c-*myc* gene in transgenic mice: Multiple neoplasms and normal development. Cell 1986; 45:485–495.

72. Lindgren V, Sippola-Thiele M, Skowronski J, et al. Specific chromosomal abnormalities characterize fibrosarcomas of bovine papillomavirus type 1 transgenic mice. Proc Natl Acad Sci USA 1989; 86:5025–5029.

73. Mahon KA, Chepelinsky AB, Khillan JS, et al. Oncogenesis of the lens in transgenic mice. Science 1987; 235:1622–1628.

74. Mangues R, Seidman I, Pellicer A, et al. Tumorigenesis and male sterility in transgenic mice expressing a MMTV/N-*ras* oncogene. Oncogene 1990; 5:1491–1497.

75. Marks JR, Lin J, Hinds P, et al. Cellular gene expression in papillomas of the choroid plexus from transgenic mice that express the simian virus 40 large T antigen. J Virol 1989; 63:790–797.

76. Matsui Y, Halter SA, Holt JT, et al. Development of mammary hyperplasia and neoplasia in MMTV-TGF transgenic mice. Cell 1990; 61:1147–1155.

77. Mayo KE, Hammer RE, Swanson LW, et al. Dramatic pituitary hyperplasia in transgenic mice expressing a human growth hormone-releasing factor gene. Mol Endocrinol 1988; 2:606–612.

78. McMahon AP, Moon RT. Ectopic expression of the proto-oncogene *int*-1 in *Xenopus* embryos leads to duplication of the embryonic axis. Cell 1989; 58:1075–1084.

79. Meckl K, Wagner EF. In situ analysis of c-*fos* expression in transgenic mice. In: Current Communications in Molecular Biology, Cysecchi MR, ed. New York, Cold Spring Harbor Press 1989; pp. 117–129.

80. Messing A, Chen HY, Palmiter RD, et al. Peripheral neuropathies, hepatocellular carcinomas and islet cell adenomas in transgenic mice. Nature 1985; 316:461–463.

81. Messing A, Pinkert CA, Palmiter RD, et al. Developmental study of SV40 large T antigen expression in transgenic mice with choroid plexus neoplasia. Oncogene Res 1988; 3:87–97.

82. Metcalf D, Moore JG. Divergent disease patterns in granulocyte-macrophage colony-stimulating factor transgenic mice associated with different transgene insertion sites. Proc Natl Acad Sci USA 1988; 85:7767–7771.

83. Mickisch GH, Merlino GT, Galski H, et al. Transgenic mice that express the human multidrug-resistance gene in bone marrow enable a rapid identification of agents that reverse drug resistance. Proc Natl Acad Sci USA 1991; 88:547–551.

84. Muller WJ, Lee FS, Dickson C, et al. The *int*-2 gene product acts as an epithelial growth factor in transgenic mice. EMBO J 1990; 9:907–913.

85. Muller WJ, Sinn E, Pattengale PK, et al. Single-step induction of mammary adenocarcinoma in transgenic mice bearing the activated c-*neu* oncogene. Cell 1988; 54:105–115.

86. Nakamura TKA, Mahon R, Muken A, et al. Differentiation and oncogene-

sis: Phenotypically distinct lens tumors in transgenic mice. New Biol 1989; 107:221–228.

87. Nocka K, Majumder S, Chabot B, et al. Expression of c-*kit* gene products in known cellular targets of W mutations in normal and W mutant mice—evidence for an impaired c-*kit* kinase in mutant mice. Genes & Dev 1989; 3:816–826.

88. O'Brien JM, Marcus DM, Bernards R, et al. A transgenic mouse model for trilateral retinoblastoma. Arch Opthalmol 1990; 108:1145–1151.

89. Ornitz DM, Hammer RE, Messing A, et al. Pancreatic neoplasia induced by SV40 T-antigen expression in acinar cells of transgenic mice. Science 1987; 238:188–193.

90. Palmiter RD, Brinster RL. Germ-line transformation of mice. Annu Rev Genet 1986; 20:465–499.

91. Palmiter RD, Chen HY, Messing A, et al. SV40 enhancer and large-T antigen are instrumental in development of choroid plexus tumors in transgenic mice. Nature 1985; 316:457–460.

92. Parada LF, Laud H, Weinberg RA, et al. Cooperation between genes encoding p53 tumor antigen and *ras* in cellular transformation. Nature 1984; 312:649–651.

93. Paul D, Hohne M, Pinkert C, et al. Immortalized differentiated hepatocyte lines derived from transgenic mice harboring SV40 T-antigen genes. Exp Cell Res 1988; 175:354–362.

94. Pavlakis GN, Felber BK, Kaplin G, et al. Regulation of expression of the HTLV family of retroviruses. In: The Control of Human Retrovirus Gene Expression, Banbury Conference, Cold Spring Harbor, NY, Cold Spring Harbor Press, 1988; pp. 281–289.

95. Propst F, Rosenberg MP. Unpublished observations.

96. Propst F, Rosenberg MP, Cork LC, et al. Neuropathological changes in transgenic mice carrying copies of a transcriptionally activated *mos* proto-oncogene. Proc Natl Acad Sci USA 1990; 87:9703–9707.

97. Quaife CJ, Pinkert CA, Ornitz DM, et al. Pancreatic neoplasia induced by *ras* expression in acinar cells of transgenic mice. Cell 1987; 48:1023–1034.

98. Reynolds RK, Hoekzema GS, Vogel J, et al. Multiple endocrine neoplasia induced by the promiscuous expression of a viral oncogene. Proc Natl Acad Sci USA 1988; 85:3135–3139.

99. Rindi G, Grant SGN, Yiangou Y, et al. Development of neuroendocrine tumors in the gastrointestinal tract of transgenic mice. Am J Pathol 1990; 136:1349–1363.

100. Rosenberg MP, Lehman JM. Murine tetracarcinomas. In: In Vitro Models for Cancer Research, Webber MM, Sekely LI, eds. Boca Raton, CRC Press 1988; pp. 225–250.

101. Russell ES. Review of the pleiotropic effects of W-series genes on growth and differentiation. In: Aspects of Synthesis and Order in Growth, Rudnick D, ed. Princeton, New Jersey, Princeton University Press 1955; p. 113.

102. Ruther U, Garber C, Komtowski D, et al. Deregulated *fos* expression interferes with normal bone development in transgenic mice. Nature 1987; 325:412–416.

103. Ruther U, Komtowski D, Schibert FR, et al. c-fos expression induces bone tumors in transgenic mice. Oncogene 1989; 4:861–865.
104. Ruther U, Muller W, Sumida T, et al. c-fos expression interferes with thymus development in transgenic mice. Cell 1988; 53:847–856.
105. Saitoh A, Kimura M, Takahashi R, et al. Most tumors in transgenic mice with human c-Ha-ras gene contained somatically activated transgenes. Oncogene 1990; 5:1195–1200.
106. Sandgren EP, Luetteke NC, Palmiter RD, et al. Overexpression of TGF in transgenic mice: Induction of epithelial hyperplasia, pancreatic metaplasia, and carcinoma of the breast. Cell 1990; 61:1121–1135.
107. Sandgren EP, Quaife CJ, Paulovich AG, et al. Pancreatic tumor pathogenesis reflects the causative genetic lesion. Proc Natl Acad Sci USA 1991; 88:93–97.
108. Sandgren EP, Quaife CJ, Pinkert CA, et al. Oncogene-induced liver neoplasia in transgenic mice. Oncogene 1989; 4:715–724.
109. Schmidt EV, Pattengale PK, Weir L, et al. Transgenic mice bearing the human c-myc gene activated by an immunoglobulin enhancer: A pre-B-cell lymphoma model. Proc Natl Acad Sci USA 1988; 85:6047–6051.
110. Schoenenberger C-A, Andres A-C, Groner B, et al. Targeted c-myc gene expression in mammary glands of transgenic mice induces mammary tumors with constitutive milk protein gene transcription. EMBO J 1988; 7:169–175.
111. Schuh AC, Keating SJ, Monteclaro FS, et al. Obligatory wounding requirement for tumorigenesis in v-jun transgenic mice. Nature 1991; 346:756–760.
112. Sidman CL, Marshall JD, Harris AW. Genetic studies on Eμ-myc transgenic mice. Curr Top Microbiol Immunol 1988; 141:94–99.
113. Sigmund CD, Jones CA, Fabian JR, et al. Tissue and cell specific expression of a renin promoter-reporter gene construct in transgenic mice. Biochem Biophys Res Commun 1990; 170:344–350.
114. Sinn E, Muller W, Pattengale P, et al. Coexpression of MMTV/V-H-ras and MMTV/c-myc genes in transgenic mice: Synergistic action of oncogenes in vivo. Cell 1987; 49:465–475.
115. Siracusa LD, Russell LB, Eicher EM, et al. Genetic organization of the agouti region of the mouse. Genetics 1987; 117:93–100.
116. Small JA, Khoury G, Jay G, et al. Early regions of JC virus and BK virus induce distinct and tissue-specific tumors in transgenic mice. Proc Natl Acad Sci USA 1986; 83:8288–8292.
117. Sola C, Tronik D, Dreyfus M, et al. Renin-promoter SV40 large T-antigen transgenes induce tumors irrespective of normal cellular expression of renin genes. Oncogene Res 1989; 5:149–153.
118. Stewart TA, Pattengale PK, Leder P. Spontaneous mammary adenocarcinomas in transgenic mice that carry and express MTV/myc fusion genes. Cell 1984; 38:627–637.
119. Suda Y, Aizawa S, Hirai S, et al. Driven by the same Ig enhancer and SV40 T promoter ras induced lung adenomatous tumors, myc induced pre-B cell lymphomas and SV40 large T gene a variety of tumors in transgenic mice. EMBO J 1987; 6:4055–4065.

120. Sutrave P, Kelly AM, Hughes SH. *ski* can cause selective growth of skeletal muscle in transgenic mice. Genes & Dev 1990; 4:1462–1472.

121. Tan JC, Nocka K, Ray P, et al. The dominant W^{42} spotting phenotype results from a missense mutation in the c-*kit* receptor kinase. Science 1990; 247:209–212.

122. Teitelman G, Alpert S, Hanahan D. Proliferation, senescence, and neoplastic progression of μ cells in hyperplastic pancreatic islets. Cell 1988; 52:97–105.

123. Theuring F, Gotz W, Balling R, et al. Tumorigenesis and eye abnormalities in transgenic mice expressing MSV-SV40 large T-antigen. Oncogene 1990; 5:225–232.

124. Tremblay PJ, Pothier F, Hoang T, et al. Transgenic mice carrying the mouse mammary tumor virus *ras* fusion gene: Distinct effects in various tissues. Mol Cell Biol 1989; 9:854–859.

125. Tsukamoto AS, Grosschedl R, Guzman RC, et al. Expression of the *int-1* gene in transgenic mice is associated with mammary gland hyperplasia and adenocarcinomas in male and female mice. Cell 1988; 55:619–625.

126. van Lohuizen M, Verbeek S, Krimpenfort P, et al. Predisposition to lymphomagenesis in pim-1 transgenic mice: Cooperation with c-*myc* and N-*myc* in murine leukemia virus-induced tumors. Cell 1989; 56:673–682.

127. Verbeek S, van Lahuixen M, van der Valk, et al. Mice bearing the Eμ-*myc* and Eμ-*pim*-1 transgenes develop pre-B-cell leukemia prenatally. Mol Cell Biol 1991: 11:1776–1779.

128. Vogel J, Hinrichs SH, Reynolds RK, et al. The HIV *tat* gene induces dermal lesions resembling Kaposi's sarcoma in transgenic mice. Nature 1988; 335:606–611.

129. Westphal H. Perturbations of lens development in the transgenic mouse. Cell Differ Dev 1988; 25:33–37.

130. Wettstein PJ, Jewet L, Faas S, et al. SV40 T-antigen is a histocompatibility antigen of SV40-transgenic mice. Immunogenetics 1988; 27:436–441.

131. Williams RL, Courneidge SA, Wagner EF. Embryonic lethalities and endothelial tumors in chimeric mice expressing polyoma virus middle T oncogene. Cell 1988; 52:121–131.

132. Witte ON. Steel locus defines new multipotent growth factor. Cell 1990; 63:5–6.

133. Woychic RP, Generoso WM, Russell LB, et al. Molecular and genetic characterization of a radiation-induced structural rearrangement in mouse chromosome 2 causing mutations at the limb deformity and *agouti* loci. Proc Natl Acad Sci USA 1990; 87:2588–2592.

134. Wundle JJ, Albert DM, O'Brien JM. Retinoblastoma in transgenic mice. Nature 1990; 343:665–669.

135. Yee S-P, Mock D, Greer P, et al. Lymphoid and mesenchymal tumors in transgenic mice expressing the v-*fps* protein-tyrosine kinase. Mol Cell Biol 1989; 9:5491–5499.

136. Yee S-P, Mock D, Maltby V, et al. Cardiac and neurological abnormalities in v-*fps* transgenic mice. Proc Natl Acad Sci USA 1989; 86:5873–5877.

Chapter 11

Molecular Diagnostics in Cancer

Ramesh Kumar

Rationale

Conventional methods of detecting cancer are based on physical examination or immunological assays for tumor-specific antigens. More recently, the use of diagnostic imaging aids such as radioactive probes and monoclonal antibodies has improved the specificity and speed of these methods.[10] The establishment of oncogenes and tumor-suppressor genes as causative factors in cancer combined with the refinements of nucleic acid and protein detection methodologies has ushered in the era of molecular diagnostics in cancer.[12] These molecular approaches offer several advantages over conventional methods:

1. Since oncogene activation precedes the onset of neoplasia, diagnostics based on the early events of oncogenesis do not depend on the appearance of the tumor mass. Indeed, altered oncogenes can be detected in the tumor precursor cell.[2] This can result in earlier detection of the threat of cancer.
2. The higher sensitivity and resolution of the DNA based approaches permit detection in very small samples and in samples where tumor material may be heavily contaminated by nontumor stromal component.[9]
3. These approaches are based on the actual identification of the etiologic genes and therefore may permit better classification of

From *The Molecular Basis of Human Cancer:* edited by B. Neel, M.D., Ph.D., R. Kumar, Ph.D. © 1993, Futura Publishing Co. Inc., Mount Kisco, NY.

tumor types and improve the understanding of the mechanisms of carcinogenesis.[27]

4. Once a gene defect is identified in a patient, molecular techniques can be used for the genetic analysis of the patient's family.[25]

5. Precise molecular definition of the mutation may be useful (in the future) for devising highly specific genetic therapies including the use of toxin linked monoclonal antibodies,[18] antisense nucleic acids, and ribozymes (Chapter 12).

6. Automation, easily usable kit formulations, and mass production promise a low-cost, reliable, and rapid way of monitoring populations at risk of developing cancer.

Early and accurate diagnosis of cancer is expected to offer several advantages to both the clinician and the patient. Molecular staging of the disease is of great prognostic value. The detection of inherited or early acquired gene alteration can be useful for monitoring patients at risk and can be of value in developing preventative dietary or exposure regimens for the affected individuals. Finally, molecular diagnostics can pinpoint the biochemical nature of the mutation, thus allowing the choice of the appropriate anticancer agent. At present, these advantages are yet to be realized in clinical practice. Currently, molecular diagnostics is contributing to epidemiologic and pathological studies, helping build a strong cause and effect relationship between oncogene activation and cancer incidence. In the not too distant future this emerging technology may be applied to clinical practice in oncology.

Methodology

Figure 1 depicts various approaches in molecular diagnostics of cancer. It is possible to analyze tumor-specific markers at the cellular or the subcellular levels. Either the tumor or the nontumor tissues carrying tumor precursor cells can be sampled. An immune response to the tumor antigens can be monitored by testing serum samples. Tumor material can be subjected to fractionation to derive proteins, RNA, and DNA for analysis. In some tests, tissue sections or dispersed cells can be directly utilized.

The number and type of diagnostic procedures applicable to any sample depend on the quantity and quality of the available material.

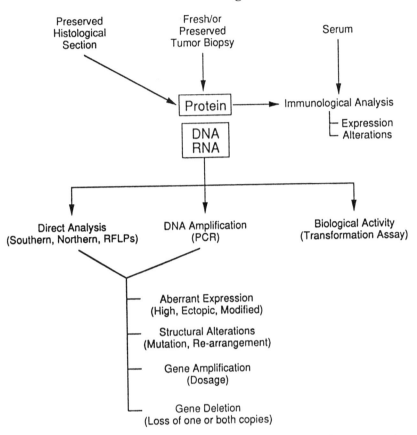

Figure 1. *Molecular approaches to the diagnosis of cancer. Samples from preserved or fresh tumor specimens can be used to derive protein, DNA, or RNA. Serum samples can be analyzed by immunological methods designed to detect the expression and alterations of oncogenic activity. Nucleic acids can be tested directly by hybridization or after amplification by the PCR technique. The genomic DNA can be tested for oncogenic activity by a transfection assay using NIH3T3 cells.*

In general, protein based detection methods require greater amount of the sample due to their lower sensitivity. Nucleic acid detection methods, in particular RNA analysis, may impose impractical restrictions on the quality of the tissue material, i.e., its collection, storage, and preparation. Since clinical and surgical procedures used for the collection of the tumor samples are heavily constrained in many ways, tests that will place stringent storage and collection requirements are unlikely to be useful for widespread applications.

A great deal of progress has been made in the development of protocols for the handling and processing of tumor biopsies. The ability to separate protein and nucleic acids allows parallel analysis of these materials by immunological and molecular methods. In particular, the recent emergence of high sensitivity Polymerase Chain Reaction (PCR) and sequencing based assays have greatly expanded the spectrum of tests that can be applied to a single tumor or biopsy specimen.[23] The following sections briefly describe immunological and DNA-based analytical methods.

Immunological Methods

The detection and assay of the biochemical activities of oncoproteins is usually accomplished by using immunological methods. Antibodies can be used for the detection of new antigenic specificities in tumor samples or for the detection of modified proteins in the tumor cell. In some patients, the presence of antitumor antibodies can also be of diagnostic value. The necessary reagents for these techniques, the antibodies, can be obtained in two different ways:

1. The immune system of patients carrying tumors is often provoked to generate specific antibodies to novel antigens. The supply and variety of these reagents is severely limited. Alternatively, biopsies of tumor material can be used to immunize laboratory animals for developing antisera. This was the earliest approach that was successfully applied to the detection and imaging of tumors.[10] Most of the tumor-specific antigens are expressed on the surface of the tumor cell. These include growth factor receptors, cell contact, adhesion and signaling molecules, or cell-specific markers such as histocompatibility antigens. Antibodies used before the 1980s were polyclonal antisera raised in rabbits. A recent refinement in this area has been the use of murine monoclonal antibodies. In the future, human monoclonal antibodies generated by various recombinant DNA approaches may be available. The technology of generating monoclonal antibodies in bacteria will expand the repertoire of useful antibodies for diagnostic applications.
2. In some cases, oncogenic conversion leads to a change in the properties of the protein, such as increased stability or altered specificity of action. These changes can be easily detected using

antibodies. Several conformation-specific antibodies to the p53 oncoproteins are currently being used in the analysis of cell-lines and tumors. Antibodies can be used for the quantitative detection of surface markers such as growth factor receptors. One possible clinical application involves the detection of the *neu* oncogene product in breast carcinoma.[14,24] Combined with the use of a Fluorescence Activated Cell Sorter (FACS), these antibodies can be useful for separating tumor cells from normal cells. Antibodies may also be used to determine the subcellular location of the oncoprotein (Fig. 2). In some instances, oncogenic activation can cause an alteration in the normal locale of the protein which can be detected using immunological methods.[11]

3. Identification and isolation of causative oncogenes, suppressor genes, and tumor-associated molecules such as cell-adhesion proteins have led the way to a new approach to obtaining antibodies specific to these proteins. The cloned gene can be

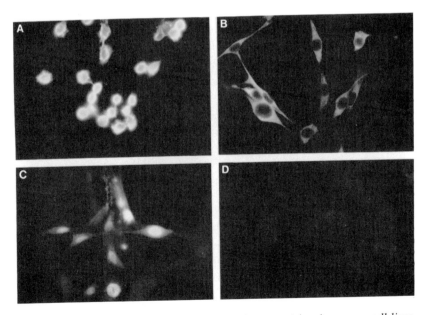

Figure 2. *Immunocytochemical localization of oncoproteins in cancer cell-lines. Monoclonal antibodies were employed for the immunofluorescent staining of Neu in A431 cells (A), Ras (B), and SV40 T-antigen (C) in NIH3T3 cells. Panel D depicts a negative control staining of nontransformed NIH3T3 cells. (Photo courtesy of Dr. X. Montano.)*

used to make appropriate recombinant DNA constructs and used for expression in *Escherichia coli*, yeast, baculoviruses, or mammalian cells in culture. The expressed protein can be purified and used as an antigen for making polyclonal and monoclonal antibodies. These technologies have vastly expanded the catalog of the available reagents.

DNA-Based Methods

The unique advantage offered by the modern molecular diagnostic approaches is the ability to detect oncogenes at the nucleic acid level. This has improved both the sensitivity and the speed of analysis. Quantitative as well as qualitative analytical methods can be applied for the analysis of DNA and mRNA. The latter is usually detected as cDNA after the enzymatic conversion of mRNA using reverse transcription. The following sections summarize various methods of detection and quantitation of the oncogenes and tumor-suppressor genes.

1. *Direct detection of DNA, RNA, or cDNA in tumor samples*: The detection of nucleic acids in the tumor samples is limited by the sensitivity of the hybridization techniques as well as the quality of the tumor samples. In general, both radioactive (usually ^{32}P) and nonradioactive labeling have been applied to the generation of probes for Northern and Southern blot analysis. Radioactively (usually ^{35}S) labeled single-stranded RNA probes are useful for the in situ detection of mRNA in thin sections of tissues.[26] This methodology is most useful for the localization of neoplastic cells in the tissue biopsies. Direct detection methods are applicable to the analysis of oncogene amplification,[1] such as in the *myc* gene, and for the detection of gene rearrangements and polymorphism.[8] These methods can also be applied to the detection of oncogenes in transfected tissue culture cells (see Chapter 1). However, the lower sensitivity and resolution of these methods and the complexity of these operations preclude their widespread use in clinical practice.

2. *Indirect detection*: These methods are based on the PCR. PCR is based on the principle of enzymatic synthesis of DNA on an existing template.[22] A prior knowledge of the DNA sequence of the target gene is required, thus limiting use to the detection of

previously described alterations or the variations of the known genetic aberrations. Since PCR permits 10^6-to 10^7-fold amplification of the template, tumor samples containing a mixture of normal and neoplastic cells can be used in this analysis. Various applications of PCR based diagnostic approaches, all applicable to DNA or RNA are outlined below.

i) Aberrant expression or rearrangements: PCR amplification of cDNA or genomic DNA can be used for the detection of the inappropriate expression of a tissue or development of stage-specific oncogene in a tumor. Many thyroid carcinomas express the proto-oncogene *trk* whose expression in normal tissues is restricted to the brain.[3] *trk* expression can be detected in the carcinomas by the amplification of a segment of the *trk* gene from cDNA templates prepared from the tumor samples. Several different types of leukemias are caused by oncogenes generated by the translocation of two different chromosomes.[13] Such rearrangements create novel oncogenes that can be detected by using PCR. Primers specific for the fusion gene created at the site of chromosomal rearrangement can be designed for these analyses. Such primer sets can only amplify the rearranged allele and therefore permit easy diagnosis. Examples of fusion oncogenes include the *bcr-abl* oncogene in leukemia and tropomyosin-*trk* fusion gene in a colon carcinoma.[19] The sensitivity of PCR detection can permit detection of these sequences even at the single cell level (Fig. 3A).

ii) Mutations: Both the protein coding and noncoding portions of proto-oncogenes and tumor-suppressor genes are subject to mutational alteration. Point mutations can be spread anywhere over a vast expanse of DNA, and in most of the cases preferred sites of mutagenesis cannot be defined. Mutations of the Rb and the p53 genes are dispersed over the entire gene including in all the exons and introns. Two simple approaches based on PCR have been applied to the detection of mutations in these genes. In the technique of multiplex PCR, several different segments of DNA are simultaneously amplified in a single reaction.[21] These multiple PCR primers are designed to generate amplified fragments of different sizes from each of the various targets. The lack of a DNA fragment or an alteration in the size of a specific fragment would then indicate the presence and type of an oncogene (Fig. 4A). Point mutations within a specific DNA fragment can be rapidly detected by the ingenious Single Strand Chain Polymorphism (SSCP) technique.[20] In this method, the ampli-

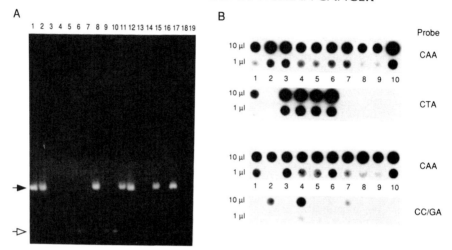

Figure 3. *A: Direct detection of specific oncogenes by PCR. In certain cases where the oncogene is a novel DNA molecule (often generated by the juxtaposition of two different sequences by DNA rearrangement) or when the oncogenic activity is manifested by inappropriate expression of the oncogene in specific tissues, the detection by PCR amplification of the DNA sequences is a direct indication of the presence of the oncogene. Lane 1 is amplified cloned oncogene as a positive control, lane 19 is a negative control (normal cells). Lanes 2 to 18 are different tumor samples where samples 2, 7, 10, 11, 15, and 17 are positive for the tested sequences. B: Mutant oncogenes can be detected by nucleic acid hybridization. PCR amplified DNA corresponding to the region surrounding the 61st codon of the H-ras gene was amplified by PCR. Oligonucleotide probes specific either for the normal allele (CAA at the 61st codon) or three different mutant alleles (CTA or CC/GA) were used for the detection of mutations in nine tumor samples (1–9) or a control normal tissue sample (lane 10) by a dot blot assay. The hybridization of the DNA samples to the CAA probe indicates that all samples carried the normal allele. Samples 1, 3, 5, and 6 also carried the CTA mutant allele. Samples 2 and 7 carried either a CCA or CGA mutation. Sample 4 carried more than one mutant allele.*

fied DNA, which typically contains a mixture of normal and mutant molecules, is denatured and single strands are separated by gel electrophoresis. Under appropriate conditions, the mutant and normal DNA strands migrate differentially and can be detected (Fig. 4B). This method permits rapid analysis of a large number of samples.

iii) Specific point mutations: The most frequent alterations found in oncogenes are single base changes causing miscoding, misregulating, or missplicing mutations. Two major types of methodologies have been applied to the detection of point mutations in PCR amplified DNA. In the simplest approach, single-stranded synthetic oligode-

A   B

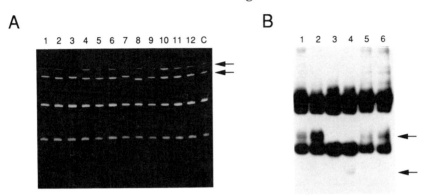

Figure 4. *A: Detection of gross abnormalities in oncogenes. Multiplex PCR for the detection of changes in multiple exons of the human p53 gene. Arrows point to specific bands of amplified DNA that vary among different tumor samples [compare lanes 7 and 9 with the control (C) lane]. The amplified aberrant band can be cloned and sequenced to determine the specific nature of the defect. (Photo courtesy of Drs. I. Runnebaum and S. Sukumar.) B: Single Strand Chain Polymorphism (SSCP) detection of mutations in a mixed sample of normal and mutant molecules. After PCR amplification, the DNA sample (which is radioactively labeled during PCR) is denatured and resolved by nondenaturing polyacrylamide gel electrophoresis. The appearance of new bands or disappearance of a band indicates the present of aberrant single strands. Compare lane 6 (control) with lane 3 (missing band) or lane 4 (novel band).*

oxy-nucleotide probes are employed.[15] PCR generated DNA is denatured and hybridized to mutation-specific labeled oligonucleotide probes. For each of the possible base changes in the DNA segment, a separate oligonucleotide is employed. Hybridization to an oligonucleotide corresponding to the proto-oncogene sequence is used as a control for amplification. However, certain tumor samples may lack the proto-oncogene sequences and *are* classified as hemizygous. Conditions can be defined to allow stringent hybridization of DNA to the cognate probe and the identification of a specific mutant allele. Two modifications have recently been incorporated into this method. These include the use of a mixture of different oligonucleotide probes, a "cocktail," to detect any of several different possible (or expected) point mutations (Fig. 3B) and the use of a mixture of a labeled probe specific for the mutation and an unlabeled probe corresponding to control proto-oncogene sequences in the hybridization mixture. Such mixtures of normal and mutant probes can permit the detection of mutation in samples containing only a minority of mutant molecules, such as in tumor biopsies.

Novel approaches to the detection of point mutations using RFLPs have been described recently.[16] These methods are based on the ability of restriction endonucleases to discriminate between two alleles. In many cases the target of mutation may contain an overlapping recognition sequence for the restriction enzyme. Mutations at the target site can abolish the enzyme recognition site and generate a diagnostic RFLP (Fig. 5). Less frequently, a specific point mutation can lead to the creation of a novel restriction site. In these instances, both the detection and the definition of the point mutation can be accomplished by an RFLP assay. A variation of PCR can be used to generate RFLPs specific for almost every possible mutation at any given locus. Applications described in the literature include the detection of mutations in the *ras* gene. Most of the known mutations in this gene are located in the 12th, 13th, or 61st codon.[4] However, any mutation involving the first and second nucleotide of these codons can activate the proto-oncogene. Therefore, a large number of different mutations can be responsible for the conversion of the gene to an oncogene. In this method, a PCR primer carrying a designed nucleotide change is coupled with a second primer for PCR amplification of the gene segment. The amplified DNA can carry either one or two nucleotide changes. The designed change in the primer in combination with the oncogenic mutation can create a restriction enzyme recognition site diagnostic of the mutation. The DNA amplified from the normal template carries only one of the changes (via the designed PCR primer) and does not create the restriction enzyme site. Examples of the use of this technique are shown in Table 1. The advantages of this method include its high resolution, sensitivity, simplicity, and the feasibility of nonradioactive methods of detection.[16,17] The major disadvantage is the need for multiple oligonucleotide primers and the limitations of the availability of restriction enzyme specificities that can exclude certain mutations from this application (Table 1). The combination of this method with automated electrophoresis and fluorescent DNA detection systems promises to simplify and speed up the analysis of large number of samples for screening of populations at risk.[7]

Assays Based on Activity

Oncogene and proto-oncogene products often have distinct biochemical and biological properties. These unique properties can be

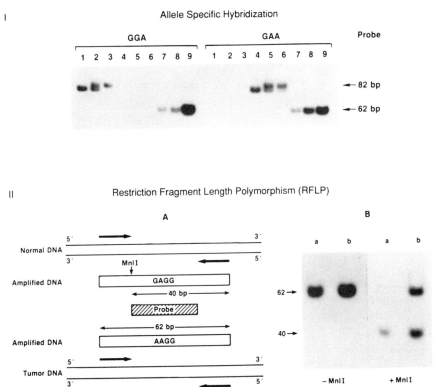

Figure 5. *Allele-specific detection of mutant oncogenes. I: Allele-specific oligonucleotide probes can be used in liquid hybridization analysis under conditions that permit only specific hybrids to form. In this illustration, the normal H-ras gene (GGA at the 12th codon) or the H-ras oncogene (GAA at the 12th codon) are distinguished by stringent hybridization. Samples 1–3 carry only the normal allele, samples 4–6 only the mutant allele, and the samples 7–9 are heterozygous for both alleles. The different sizes of the amplified DNA results from the choice of the PCR primers. II: The use of Restriction Fragment Length Polymorphisms (RFLPs) permits detection of mutations in samples that may carry a mutation at a very low frequency, such as in clinical biopsy tumor samples. In this approach, the sequence at the site of mutation must correspond to a restriction enzyme recognition site. Mutation, therefore, can alter the sequence and make the DNA an unsuitable substrate for the restriction enzyme. In the example shown (the 12th codon region of the rat H-ras gene) the normal amplified DNA can be digested with the restriction enzyme MnlI. Mutation at the 12th codon (GGA→GAA) abolishes the MnlI site. Resistance of the amplified DNA to MnlI digestion indicates the presence of the mutation in the sample. A. Schematic description of the approach. B. Analysis of normal (a) sample carrying MnlI sensitive DNA and tumor (b) sample carrying both MnlI sensitive and resistant DNA indicating the presence of the mutant allele. A variation of this approach, designed for situations where no normal RFLPs exist, is described in the text and Table 1.*

TABLE 1.
Detection of K-*ras* Mutations by Designed RFLPs

A. RFLPs

Codon	Created Site	Mismatch	Size (bp)
12 (GGT)	HphI	C-T	61,14
61 (CAA)	Tth111 III	CT-TG	47,10

B. Primers*
  1. 12th codon (Amplified DNA 75 bp)
       A. AGAGGCCTGCTGAAAATGACT
       B. CGTCAAGGCACTCTTGCCTACG<u>TC</u>
  2. 61st codon (Amplified DNA 57 bp)
       A. ACCTGTCTCTTGGATATTCTC
       B. GTCCCTCATTGCACTGTACTC<u>TGC</u>

*Mismatches are underlined.

exploited for the detection and quantitation of oncogenic activity. The ability of isolated oncogenes to cause morphological transformation when transferred into indicator cell-lines has been used to detect and isolate known and novel oncogenes (see Chapter 1). Although this method is too cumbersome and time-consuming for routine clinical applications, it is currently used in research and specialized laboratories.

Easy enzymatic assays for the detection of oncogenes have yet to be developed. The discovery of specific substrates and indicators for the detection of an oncogenic enzyme can be anticipated based on recent research on signal-transduction.[5] Oncogenes derived from tyrosine kinase receptors often exhibit qualitative changes in kinase activity which can be detected in sensitive assays (Chapter 6). Instances where an oncoprotein's enzymatic activity is abolished by mutation could be the easiest to detect but have not yet been described.

Mutations that alter the DNA-(or protein-) binding activity of transcription factor-derived oncoproteins can also be readily assayed when the targets of these proteins are well defined. Application of this method to the detection of viral oncogenes has been described and could be extended to the analysis of cellular oncoproteins in the future.[11] Many mutant oncoproteins exhibit an alteration of the protein conformation. These structural changes can be identified using conformation-specific antibodies. Many mutant forms of the p53 tumor-suppressor protein can be detected by using specific monoclonal antibodies that do not react with the normal p53 protein. Antibodies that detect the mutant but not the normal *ras* protein have also been described.[6] These reagents are also possibly conformation sensitive.

References

1. Alitalo K, Schwab M. Oncogene amplification in tumor cells. A review. Adv Cancer Res 1987; 47:235–281.
2. Bishop JM. Molecular themes in oncogenesis. Cell 1991; 64:235-248.
3. Bongarzone I, Pierotti MA, Mouzini N, et al. High frequency of activation of tyrosine kinase oncogenes in human papillary thyroid carcinoma. Oncogene 1989; 4:1457–1462.
4. Bos JL. The *ras* gene family and human carcinogenesis. Mutat Res 1988; 195:255–271.
5. Bourne HR, Defranco AL. Signal transduction and intracellular messengers. In: Oncogenes and the Molecular Origins of Cancer, Weinberg R, ed. New York, Cold Spring Harbor Press 1989; pp. 97–124.
6. Carney WP, Petit D, Hammer P, et al. Monoclonal antibody specific for an activated RAS protein. Proc Natl Acad Sci USA 1986; 83:7485–7490.
7. Chehab FF, Kan YW. Detection of specific DNA sequences by fluorescence amplification: A color complementation assay. Proc Natl Acad Sci USA 1989; 86:9178–9182.
8. Cory S. Activation of cellular oncogenes in hematopoietic cells by chromosome translocation. Adv Cancer Res 1986; 47:189-234.
9. Crescenzi M, Seto M, Herzig GL, et al. Thermostable DNA polymerase chain amplification of t (14:18) chromosome breakpoints and detection of minimal residual disease. Proc Natl Acad Sci USA 1988; 85:4869–4873.
10. Goldenberg DM, Goldenberg H, Sharkley RM, et al. Imaging of colorectal carcinoma with radiolabeled antibodies. Semin Nucl Med 1989; 19:262–282.
11. Harlow E, Crawford LZ, Pim DC, et al. Monoclonal antibodies specific for simian virus 40 tumor antigens. J Virol 1981; 39:861–869.
12. Harrison LC. The impact of molecular biology on the practice of medicine. Part 2. diagnostics, therapeutics and ethics. Med J Australia 1987; 147:81–89.
13. Kawasaki ES, Clark SS, Coyne MY, et al. Diagnosis of chronic myclosal and acute lymphocytic leukemias by detection of leukemia-specific mRNA sequences amplified in vitro. Proc Natl Acad Sci USA 1988; 85:5698–5702.
14. Kraus MH, Popescu NC, Ausbaugh SC, et al. Over-expression of the EGF receptor-related proto-oncogene *erb*-B2 in human mammary cell lines by different molecular mechanisms. EMBO J 1987; 6:605–610.
15. Kumar R, Barbacid M. Oncogene detection at the single cell level. Oncogene 1989; 3:647–651.

448   THE MOLECULAR BASIS OF HUMAN CANCER

16. Kumar R, Dunn LL. Designed diagnostic restriction fragment length polymorphisms for the detection of mutations in *ras* genes. Oncogene Res 1989; 4:235–241.
17. Kumar R, Sukumar S, Barbacid M. Activation of *ras* oncogenes precedes the onset of neoplasia. Science 1990; 248:1101–1104.
18. Ledbetter JA, Clark EA. Therapeutic uses of agonistic monoclonal antibodies to human lymphocyte cell-surface molecules. Adv Drug Delivery Rev 1988; 2:319–342.
19. Martin-Zanca D, Hughes SH, Barbacid M. A human oncogene formed by the fusion of truncated tropomyosin and protein tyrosine kinase sequences. Nature 1986; 319:743–748.
20. Orita M, Iwahana H, Kanazawa H, et al. Detection of polymorphisms of human DNA: Gel-electrophoresis of single strand conformation and polymorphism. Proc Natl Acad Sci USA 1989; 86:2766–2770.
21. Runnebaum IB, Nagarajan M, Bouman M, et al. Mutations in p53 as potential molecular markers for human breast cancer. Proc Natl Acad Sci USA 1991; 88:10657–10661.
22. Saiki RK, Scharf S, Faloona F, et al. Enzymatic amplification of beta-globin genomic sequences and restriction site analysis for diagnosis of sickle cell anemia. Science 1985; 230:1350-1354.
23. Shibata D, Martin WJ, Arnheim N. Analysis of DNA sequences in forty-year-old paraffin-embedded thin tissue sections: A bridge between molecular biology and classical histology. Cancer Res 1988; 48:4564–4566.
24. Slamon DJ, Clark GM, Wong SG, et al. Correlation of relapse and survival with amplification of the HER-2/*neu* oncogene. Science 1987; 235:177–182.
25. Stanbridge EJ, Norvell PC. Origins of human cancer revisited. Cell 1990; 63:867–874.
26. Tecott LH, Barchas JD, Eberwine JH. In situ transcription: Specific synthesis of complementary DNA in fixed tissue sections. Science 1988; 240:1661–1664.
27. Weinberg RA. Oncogenes, anti-oncogenes and the molecular bases of multistep carcinogenesis. Cancer Res 1989; 49:3713-3721.

Chapter 12

Molecular Therapeutic Approaches

Ximena Montano

The identification of oncogenes and antioncogenes and the establishment of the molecular basis of cancer were the first important steps in the search for rational therapies for human malignant diseases. The definition of molecular targets for drug development and the availability of biochemical assays for the activity of oncogenic proteins has ushered in the golden era of molecular therapy in cancer. Two different types of molecular treatments have been suggested:

1. therapeutic agents and vehicles for the elimination of the cancer cell, and
2. drugs that specifically block the activity of the oncogene or its product.

Drugs in the first category are typically based on the use of specific antibodies, either alone or in combination with nonspecific toxins or poisons. The second group includes both proteins such as lymphokines and nucleic acids such as antisense RNAs. This chapter will describe a selection of approaches utilized for molecular therapy of genetic diseases with emphasis on the treatment of cancer.

Antibodies as a Tool for Therapy

Antibodies have been shown to be very important tools to further our understanding of a variety of biological and molecular mecha-

From *The Molecular Basis of Human Cancer:* edited by B. Neel, M.D., Ph.D., R. Kumar, Ph.D. © 1993, Futura Publishing Co. Inc., Mount Kisco, NY.

nisms. Antibodies are very selective and specific agents which can be raised against a variety of substances, generally can bind specifically to their respective antigens with high affinity, and upon binding can mediate numerous effector functions which result in the immune response. For example, by taking advantage of the high specificity of antibodies, it has been possible to show association between the protein products of DNA tumor virus transforming genes and suppressor genes such as SV40 large T with p53,[55,60] and adenovirus Ela protein with the Retinoblastoma gene product.[102]

The development of monoclonal antibody technology based on the production of antibody secreting cell-lines[54] has been the first step to ensure abundant supply of homogeneous antibodies with a single specificity. This technology, together with the fact that all antibodies have the same basic structure, has made it possible to seek the redesign of these molecules for further biological studies at the molecular and clinical level.

Antibody Structure

Antibodies are Y shaped molecules (Fig. 1) composed of light and heavy chains linked through disulphide bridges. Both chains have variable (V) and constant (C) regions. However the heavy chain also has a hinge region (H), which confers flexibility to the "arms" of the molecule followed by two constant regions (CH_2 and CH_3). These three domains form the stem of the molecule.

The variable regions provide the specificity and are capable of binding to the antigen. The constant region is involved in triggering effector biological functions. Antibodies can mediate cytotoxicity by triggering the complement cascade which leads to cell lysis, or by binding to receptors on the surface of phagocytes or killer cells and triggering phagocytosis or antibody dependent cell-mediated cytolysis.[57]

In addition to the interchain bridge disulphide bond between light and heavy chains, each antibody protein has internal disulphide bridges or intrachain bonds which allow to form loops within the protein and hence to produce globular domains. Upon digestion of antibody molecules with enzymes such as pepsin and papain it is possible to detect three types of proteolytic products $F(ab)_2$, $F(ab)$, and Fc fragments (see Fig. 1). A pepsin $F(ab)_2$ fragment is a divalent molecule with regard to antigen recognition; whereas a papain F(ab)

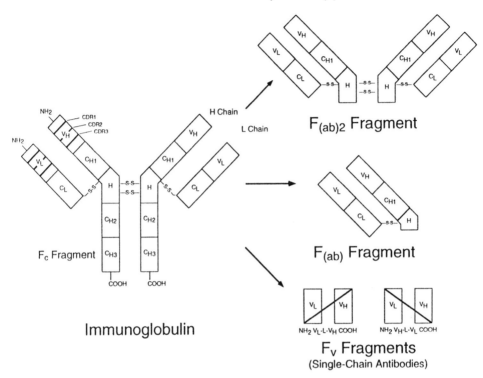

Figure 1. *Structure of the antibody molecule and antibody fragments. Antibodies contain two heavy and two light chains linked by disulphide bridges producing a bivalent entity capable of recognizing two antigen molecules. The F(ab)₂ fragment is also bivalent with regard to antibody binding. The F(ab) molecule is monovalent, recognizing a single antigen molecule. Both F(ab)₂ and F(ab) fragments contain the complete light chain but only a section of the heavy chain which does not include the CH₂ and CH₃ (constant) regions. Fᵥ fragments contain the heavy and light chains variable regions. This diagram shows Fᵥ in two configurations, with the linker running from the amino terminus of the light chain variable region or the amino terminus of the heavy chain variable region.*

fragment is monovalent. In both cases the Fc region fragment produced corresponds to the stem of the molecule.

Crystallographic studies[2,5,87,88] of fragments of antibodies has shown that the antigen-binding site contains hypervariable loops, or complementarity-determining regions (CDRs) enclosed within regions of β strands formed by the association of the V_H and V_L regions. Sequence comparison[50,51] revealed that each region has three hypervariable domains flanked by four conserved framework regions (FRs).

The specificity for a given antigen is conferred within the CDRs since these contain the greatest sequence variability. The rate of hypervariability or mutation has been described to approach 10^{-3} to 3×10^{-4} mutations per base pair per cell division.[23] This is the reason why it is possible to produce a large antibody repertoire with a variety of specificities. Similarly, the conformation of these loops has been shown to be the principal element in determining the three-dimensional configuration of the antigen combining site.

Antibody Engineering

Complete antibodies, F(ab)₂ and F(ab) fragments

Antibodies are very amenable to protein engineering. The functional domains are very well defined and the antigen binding moieties [F(ab)₂, F(ab)] and effector bindings moiety (Fc) can be used separately as fragments. For the past several years hybridoma cells producing antibodies of known specificity have provided the raw material to obtain the rearranged genes coding for the heavy and light chain proteins. Genomic and cDNA libraries have been obtained from these cells.[26,67,78] However more recently, degenerate primers containing desirable cloning restriction sites have been employed to rescue genes using polymerase chain reaction (PCR). The restriction sites permit the cloning of the amplified fragment into mammalian or bacterial expression vectors.[56,69]

Antibody genes have been expressed in myeloma and cell-lines of nonlymphoid origin such as fibroblasts and epithelial cells (NIH3T3 cells, Chinese Hamster Ovary Cells, HeLa cells).[10,20] This is still the preferred method for expression of whole functional antibodies. This system has been used to study different effector functions within the molecule such as glycosylation patterns which are known to be involved in protein stability, proteolytic degradation, secretion, as well as in protein folding and solubility.[40,44,68,92,93,96]

In the case of certain antibodies such as MOPC 603 it has been shown that glycosylation has no influence in its antigen/antibody-binding capacity.[76] The same results have been obtained with the antibody Y13–259 which recognizes the protein product of the *ras* oncogene.[35,65] However with certain antibodies there is evidence that lack of glycosylation reduces the capacity to activate complement and induce cellular cytotoxicity which is conferred through the Fc region.[57]

Although complete antibodies are large molecules (estimated molecular weight 150,000 daltons) smaller fragments have also been produced. In these cases, the heavy chain gene was modified to express a smaller protein fragment containing the V_H, C_H, and a section of the H region containing only cysteines which allow disulphide bridges between the heavy and light chain proteins F(ab), as well as disulphide bridges between the modified heavy chain proteins F(ab)$_2$. These smaller molecules have been shown to retain antigen-binding activity.[32,33]

There has been a strong emphasis on expressing antibodies in alternative eukaryotic systems such as yeast,[46,106] plants,[43] and Baculovirus[41,81]; however, the most versatile system for expression has proved to be *Escherichia coli*.[45,76,79] A prokaryotic system such as *E coli* allows large scale production (fermentation) of complete antibodies and antibody fragments.

When antibodies are expressed in *E coli* it is important to consider: 1) secretion; 2) correct folding; and 3) synthesis of stoichiometric quantities of heavy and light chains or corresponding components of the modified fragments. Several protocols for antibody expression in *E coli* have been designed that have dealt with these considerations with different degrees of success; these include:

1. Cytoplasmic expression which involves the direct expression of the antibody chains without the signal sequences.[4,18,32,33,53] In this case the yields of antibody chain or fragments varies and is dependent upon the design of the translation initiation region, the proteolytic stability of the protein, as well as the choice of bacterial strain. In most cases inclusion bodies are produced due to protein overexpression. The expressed polypeptides are denatured and reduced and can carry a methionine or formyl methionine at the amino terminus; therefore the protein has to be renatured in vitro and in many instances the optimal conditions for renaturation have not been found.[16,47]

2. Expression as a fusion protein. In this case antibody polypeptides are fused at the amino terminus with cleavable cytoplasmic proteins. The advantage of this method is that the translation initiation signal can be made more efficient and the choice of the amino-terminal protein might help protect antibodies from proteolytic degradation. In this system precise in vitro cleavage of the fused protein gives rise to a protein with the desired amino terminus.

3. Expression of secreted fusion proteins. The antibody chains or fragments have been fused at the amino or carboxy terminus to *Staphylococcus aureus* protein A or with hemolysin A.[76,77] With the former fusion, the hybrid proteins are secreted into the periplasm, and after lysis of the outer cellular membrane the protein can be purified. In the case of haemolysin A fusion, a hybrid protein is directly secreted into the medium. In this case purification is more difficult due to the hydrophobic nature conferred by haemolysin A.

4. Functional expression. This has proved to be the most efficient system. The goal in this strategy is to reproduce in *E coli* the normal folding and assembly pathway of antibodies observed in an eukaryotic cell. In this case the bacterial periplasm is assumed to be a functional equivalent of a protein transport system to the lumen of the endoplasmic reticulum. In order to express stoichiometric amounts of either chains or fragments an operon had to be modified (such as the case of the Lac promoter/operator[79]). Transport of both chains or fragments to the periplasm has been achieved by fusing to two different *E coli* signal sequences, OMP A (outer membrane protein A) and phoA (alkaline phosphatase).[67,78] However other signal sequences have also been used.[8] To obtain an active antibody, signal sequences have to be cleaved at the correct position to produce an amino terminus.

The coexpression of antibody chains or fragments leads to expression of an assembled functional molecule with correct disulphide bridges.[13,100] This product cannot be degraded as it is expressed in the periplasm. Antibodies and antibody fragments produced with this system have been shown to have the same binding capacity as those produced by hybridomas.[77]

F_v fragments and antibody heavy or light chain expression

The availability of efficient methods to obtain functional antibody molecules has made it possible to design: 1) F_v fragments; 2) expression of only the heavy or light chain of a given antibody molecule; and 3) catalytic antibodies which will not be discussed in this chapter (the reader should refer to other reviews[4,76,78,85,104]).

Single chain antibodies or F_v fragments are recombinant proteins composed of the variable regions from the light and heavy chains (V_L and V_H) linked to each other by a 15 to 25 amino acid peptide in such a way that a single molecule can be produced (see Fig. 1). The linker polypeptide is chosen so as not to interfere with correct folding of the variable domains[14] and therefore with antigen-binding.[11,12,39,49] It is not critical if V_H or V_L is at the amino terminus since F_v fragments of either configuration have been produced in which the affinity for their antigen has not been diminished.[11]

Single chain antibodies against a variety of antigens (haptens and proteins) have been produced.[11,12,49,95] F_v fragments have been expressed in E coli using promoters such as phage $\lambda O_L/P_R$, lac, Tac, or Phage T7. Also, there are reports of F_v fragments expressed in mouse NIH3T3 cells.[65] When binding affinities between F_v and F(ab) fragments produced in E coli have been compared, it has been possible to see that both have the same binding affinity[2,49,95]; in some instances higher affinities have been reported.[11]

When isolated whole or modified heavy or light chain genes have been expressed in E coli, V_H regions alone have been shown to have antigen-binding capacity.[101] However their expression and antigen-binding capacity needs to be examined further. These regions have an exposed hydrophobic surface which makes them very "sticky," and this characteristic is variable between different antibodies. It has been shown that not all V_H of a variety of antibodies can bind their target antigen.[78] The same results have been observed when expressed in mouse fibroblasts.[65] V_L regions can dimerize, and the association constant varies depending on the antibody; so far, there are no reports indicating V_L regions binding antigens.

Therapeutic Use of Antibodies

The most important aim of current antibody technology has been to design molecules that can be targeted to specific antigens in a variety of tumors or to major histocompatibility/human leukocyte antigen (MHC/HLA) products and related antigens. Although antibodies have been recognized as important tools in clinical diagnostics and treatment, there are still many factors that have to be controlled and improved in order to be used successfully.

The usefulness of antibodies is determined by the following characteristics:

1. Affinity/avidity which determines how easily their target is detected; cross-reactive antibodies should not be used; this is especially important in the case of cross reactivities with tumor-associated blood antigens.
2. Class/subclass (for example IgG_1, IgG_{2a}) determines how efficient it is in eliciting cytotoxicity as well as the biodistribution and in vivo stability.
3. Antibody structure, i.e., whole antibody, $F(ab)_2$, $F(ab)$, or F_v. Antibody fragments have shorter half-life than whole antibodies, therefore larger doses of these molecules are needed during therapy.[12]

Monoclonal antibodies have been used against tumor antigens for in vivo imaging of cancer by carrying the imaging agent, usually a radionucleotide.[101] They have also been used to deliver toxic agents (drugs, toxins, or isotopes), to target tumor or infected cells through cell-mediated cytolysis,[6] or to complement as well as to induce selective removal of tumor cells.[62]

The following problems have been encountered in these applications:

1. Complete antibody molecules enter and clear from the human body very slowly.
2. Only a fraction of the initial antibody injected will reach its target.
3. If murine antibodies are used for clinical diagnostics and therapy it is known that these will elicit an immune response.

Preliminary clinical trials with monoclonal antibodies were related to targeting hematopoietic malignancies utilizing anti-Leu-1 antibodies against T lymphocytes in patients with leukemia,[62] and with the T101 monoclonal antibody in patients with chronic lymphocytic leukemia and cutaneous T lymphomas.[7,80] Both trials showed a significant drop in T-cell count in blood and antibody-binding to circulating blasts and lymph nodes.

These studies were important to elucidate the level of toxicity and side effects during treatment (which included fever, chills, rash, nausea, and pulmonary or renal failure). In the case of acute lymphoblastic leukemia, monoclonal antibody treatment against differentiation antigens has caused the elimination of leukemia cells without the destruction of stem cells; therefore patients can be recipients of autologous donors (in the absence of HLA matched donors). Trials have also been carried out for solid tumors. These include melanoma, as well as gastric, lung, and urologic malignancies. The most promising result has been in melanoma treatment using antibodies against cell surface antigens: 30% partial response has been obtained[95]; however, further work is still in progress.

It has been shown that there is no need to use complete antibody molecules; it is possible to target tumors with antibody fragments, F(ab)$_2$ and F(ab), and demonstrate that the smaller the antigen-binding molecule the shorter the clearance time. Similarly, a smaller molecule has been seen to penetrate tumors more easily, to accumulate at a high concentration, and to provide low antigenicity.[101] The most successful molecules for treatment are potentially F_v fragments.

In cancer treatment, the aim is to deliver a toxic substance specifically to a tumor; any unbound material should be cleared from the body in such a way that the normal tissues are unharmed. This has been tested in animal systems. An example is the B6.2 F_v fragment that can target human tumor xenografts in mice.[11] The advantage of F_v fragments is that they can bind to the target and clear rapidly from the body, thereby reducing toxic side effects. These molecules can be used for in vivo diagnosis and treatment of diseases other than cancer.

In order to avoid the human antimouse response, there have been important developments in the modification of antibodies. Human antibodies have been increasingly difficult to produce. Preliminary reports indicate that the combinational approach to repertoire cloning[17,48,75] seems to be a more successful technique. F(ab) fragments have already been obtained in this way. Nevertheless there is still an emphasis on studying different approaches to overcome this issue.

As already discussed, antibody molecules contain, in the V_L and V_H hypervariable regions, CDRs separated by more conserved regions or FRs (see Fig. 1). These regions have been modified to create chimeric antibodies as follows:

1. By replacing the V_L and V_H regions from human antibodies with those of murine antibodies that carry the specificity for the antigen.[19,26,82]
2. By modifying the CDRs and therefore producing humanized antibodies.[26,99]

Both of these types of molecules would reduce the ability of the immune system to recognize the antibody as a foreign molecule. Chimeric antibodies are currently being clinically tested.

"Humanizing" antibodies has proven to be more challenging.

Preliminary reports indicate that both CDRs and FRs interact to convey specificity to the antibody, showing that any modification to this region has to be carefully analyzed. Structural studies have indicated that the hypervariable domains make close interactions with the framework of the molecule; therefore, mutations of single noncon-served amino acids in the CDRs can abolish completely its capacity for antigen recognition.[26] Humanized antibodies are still being analyzed and modifications are carefully being assessed.

Antibodies are also characterized by inducing an immunological response via their own antigenic determinants (idiotypes) which facilitate the regulation of the immune system in a predictable way. The sequence of events is as follows: "antigen" which is the idiotype which in turn induces an antiidiotype response. The immunogenic property of these molecules is present mostly within the CDRs of the variable regions. As already indicated, if these CDRs are changed by those obtained from another antibody molecule it is possible to maintain the specificity of the donor molecule. However, it is also possible to change these CDRs with functional domains that share the primary structure of the CDR of the antibody and the respective possible antigen.[105] This procedure has been taken one step further by expressing a foreign peptide within an integral site within the variable region in such a way that an immune response of predetermined specificity can be induced in vivo. An important result was obtained by introducing three copies of a tetrapeptide of malarial *Plasmodium falciparum circumporozoite* in the CDR3 of the heavy chain of a chimeric mouse/human antibody.[9] (The CDR3 loop of the heavy chain was chosen because it expresses an immunodominant idiotype.) Rabbits and mice immunized with this modified antibody induced an anti-body response specific for the peptide on the parasite's antigen. This strategy constitutes an important approach to produce antibody vaccines against pathogenic agents such as viruses and bacteria.

Recently a new technique has been developed, i.e., the intracellu-lar expression of monoclonal antibodies (Fig. 2).[10] The aim of this technique is to express an antibody in such a way that it can block the biological activity of a specific antigen.

Intracellular expression of antibodies in yeast has been carried out[104] with antibodies against yeast aldehyde dehydrogenase. How-ever, only partial blocking of the enzymatic activity was achieved. This is probably due to the fact that the yeast internal milieu is not favorable for proper folding and antigen recognition. This technique has also been carried out using mouse fibroblasts for expression (see

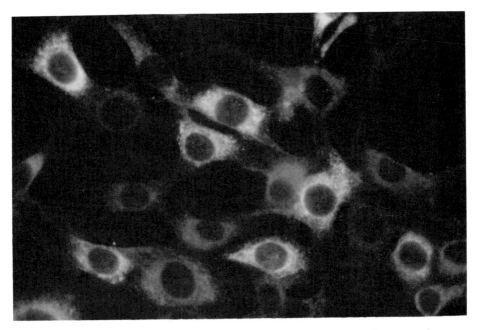

Figure 2. *Expression of antibody Y13–259 anti-p21 ras monoclonal, as seen by staining with Texas red conjugated antirat antibodies.*

Fig. 2).[65] These experiments used a monoclonal antibody against the *ras* activated oncogene[35] and showed that it can block its ability to transform as shown in a change from a transformed to a nontransformed phenotype. This technique needs to be developed further, and experiments are needed to show that intracellular expression can work in animal models before it can be used for human therapy.

Immunotoxins

Immunotoxins are hybrid immunoglobulin molecules or fragments that are cytotoxic. They can be used to target a receptor, growth factor, or any exposed epitope within a protein which has been shown to have a very high affinity for the immunoglobulin moiety within the immunotoxin.[74]

An immunotoxin consists of a whole antibody or antibody fragment linked to a toxin. There are several choices with respect to the molecular size of the components as well as with the chemical linkage.

An antibody can be used as a whole or as fragments such as $F(ab)_2$, $F(ab)$, or F_v.[22] Bacterial and plant toxins (which are some of the most efficient cytotoxic agents) act by obstructing protein synthesis in an irreversible fashion. The bacterial toxins that have been most widely used are *Pseudomonas* exotoxin and Diphtheria toxin. Both toxins inactivate elongation factor 2, which is an essential component of protein synthesis. In the case of plant toxins, ricin has been the choice; it cleaves a glycosidic bond in 28S ribosomal RNA which leads to the inability of ribosomes to synthesize proteins. Toxins enter the cells by endocytosis and become processed to produce an active fragment that has the ability to translocate across the plasma membrane into the cytoplasm where it can reach the components of the protein synthesis machinery.

Pseudomonas exotoxin and Diphtheria toxin are both simple polypeptides which have three major domains (Fig. 3). Domain I is the cell-binding domain. Domain II is required for translocation, and domain III is required for adenosine diphosphate ribosylation and inactivation of elongation factor 2. In the case of diphtheria toxin, the domains are positioned in reverse order when compared to *Pseudomonas* exotoxin. Similarly, in the case of *Pseudomonas* exotoxin there is a subdomain that has an unknown function, the toxin is still functional when this domain is deleted. Ricin is composed of two subunits that are linked by a disulfide bond. The A chain contains the enzymatic activity. The lectin B chain binds to galactose residues present in surface glycoproteins as well as glycolipids.

During the construction of immunotoxins, the toxin has to be modified so it cannot interact with its cellular receptors and, therefore, the entry of the immunotoxin can only be mediated through the binding of the immunoglobulin moiety. In the case of ricin this has been achieved through removal of the lectin B chain, blockage of galactose-binding sites,[98] or linkage of a galactose-rich carbohydrate to the B chain, and by removing the carbohydrate moiety contained in the A chain (see Fig. 3).[34]

In the case of *Pseudomonas* exotoxin the modification takes place at the time of coupling through domain I or when this domain is deleted and coupling takes place through domain II. Diphtheria toxin becomes modified by the mutation of an amino acid at the carboxy-terminal region of the binding domain or through its deletion (see Fig. 3).

In the case of ricin the linkage between IgG and the A chain is

A Ricin

B Pseudomonas Exotoxin

C Diphtheria Toxin

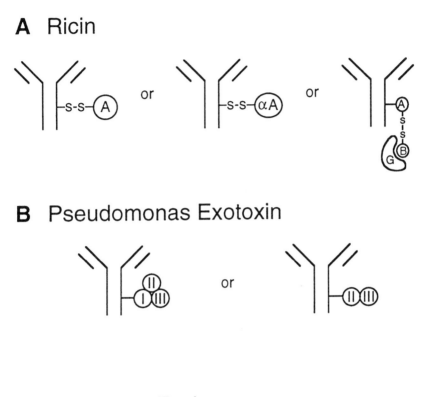

Figure 3. *Design of immunotoxins. Effective immunotoxins have been obtained by coupling antibodies to one of the following types of toxins: A. ricin modified by mutagenesis to eliminate the sites of glycosylation, deglycosated ricin A, and ricin A; B. Pseudomonas exotoxin or an exotoxin lacking domain I (which has been shown to be more efficient); and C. diphtheria toxin or its modified form.*

carried out by heterobifunctional crosslinkers which introduce a disulphide bond between both members.[36,37]

Therapeutic Effect

A variety of immunotoxins have been developed and approved for clinical trials. Two types of trials have been carried out: 1) the addition of immunotoxins to bone marrow (in order to eliminate contaminating cancerous cells) which is reinfused back into patients who are undergoing autologous bone marrow transplant[74] and 2) introduction (systematically or localized) of immunotoxins to patients with cancer. These drugs have been in phase I and II trials and a good response has been observed in the case of lymphomas,[91] but not much success has been observed in the case of carcinomas and other solid tumors. Therefore there is a need to improve the system[30] even at the level of lymphoma, especially when combined with other immunodeficiency diseases.

The anticancerous effect of a F(ab) or whole IgG molecule coupled to a deglycosylated ricin A chain was tested to treat combined immunodeficiency diseases by using the antibody raised against CD22 which is an antigen present in neoplastic B cells of patients with nonHodgkins lymphoma. These molecules were employed in the treatment of mice with severe combined immunodeficiency disease induced by human Daudi cell tumors. The mice developed extranodal disease including infiltration in vertebral column. After administration of the drugs it was possible to observe that both immunotoxins were equally as efficient in inhibiting the number and size of neoplastic foci.[38] The technique of using mice as the donor partner for injection of human tumor cells has been very successful in trying new molecules such as Fv.

There are a variety of antibodies that recognize carbohydrate moieties on the surface of tumors. One of these, B3, recognizes the carbohydrate antigen of LE[4] family. This antigen is found in carcinomas of the colon, stomach, ovaries, breast, and lungs. A single chain antibody (B3Fv) coupled to a deleted *Pseudomonas* exotoxin moiety has been shown to be effective in inducing regression of human carcinoma cell-lines which developed into solid tumors when administered to mice.[15]

More recently several laboratories have been emphasizing the humanization of immunotoxins. The heavy chain gene of a mouse/ human chimeric antibody that recognizes the human transferrin receptor has been fused to the gene for angiogenin, which is a human homolog of pancreatic RNAse. A $F(ab)_2$ antibody enzyme fusion was created and introduced into a transfectoma that expressed the light chain protein. The secreted molecules were capable of inhibiting the growth and protein synthesis of K562 cells that express the human transferrin receptor, but not VERO cells which lack the receptor. Similarly, the unmodified antibody did not induce inhibition of protein synthesis, and it was capable of blocking the activity of the antibody enzyme fusion.[84]

Antibodies are potentially important tools for clinical treatment, and molecular biology has opened up the possibility of manipulating this tool to make it amenable to therapeutics. There is still much development needed to produce a successful molecular entity.

Gene Therapy

Research on gene transfer into humans has mainly focused on recessive gene diseases. The aim has been to correct single gene hereditary disorders. In this case a functional gene is introduced that can restore the normal function. For example genes involved in blood clotting can be introduced in somatic cells, and their systematic expression/secretion has been shown to be needed to restore the process of coagulation.[3]

Research has been directed towards treatment of human infectious diseases as well as cancer. Among these the most relevant targets have been malignant melanoma, neuroblastoma, and more recently AIDS.[3,58,63] Within the context of gene treatment, gene transfer protocols have been divided in two groups: clinical gene marking and clinical gene therapy. In both cases, retroviral vectors have been used to introduce genes into cells.[28,29,61]

Clinical Gene Marking

Gene marking of tumor infiltrating lymphocytes (TILs) has been used for the treatment of malignant melanoma. During initial developmental stages of treatment for this malignancy, lymphocytes were directly isolated from the tumor and grown in large numbers in the presence of interleukin-2 (IL-2).[58,83] After expansion of the culture, these cells were reinfused back into the original patient in addition to high doses of IL-2 for several days. In clinical trials it was observed that 35% to 40% of patients did respond to this protocol. However this procedure was expensive and clinically difficult, and not all patients responded with similar ease. Similarly it was not known which subset of lymphocytes was the one acting against the tumor. A way to answer these questions was to use gene marking.[3,63]

The aim of gene marking is twofold: 1) to see if an exogenous gene can be transferred safely into a patient and 2) to be able to detect the expressed gene in cells obtained from patients after reinfusion in order to determine the length of time TILs stay in the patient.

Current protocols using TILs have established that an aliquot of cells has to be taken from a patient and cultured in vitro. When the cells are still in early culture a neomycin resistance gene is transferred through a retroviral vector. These marked cells are grown in parallel to unmarked cells and both populations are reintroduced back into the patient. At predetermined time intervals cells are withdrawn in order to detect how many marked cells are present in the tumor. During the treatment patients receive marked and unmarked TILs together with IL-2.[52]

Results of this procedure have shown that the marked TILs remained in the patient with an average life of three weeks, which related to the time in which the patient received IL-2. However, in one case it was possible to detect marked TILs in tumor samples for as long as nine weeks after infusion.

When neomycin marked TILs were obtained from tumor biopsies and grown in G418 selection, the T-cell receptor β chain heterogeneity was analyzed. The DNA pattern of the infused TILs and those obtained from a day 5 tumor biopsy showed that TIL DNA from the tumor had a subset of bands in common with the infused TILs; however, the G418 selected population had fewer subsets of bands when compared to the infused TILs. Based on these trials, two interpretations were obtained: 1) transduced TILs found in tumors were not a random subset of cells and 2) different populations of TILs grew during the process of selection; therefore it was not possible to establish during the treatment which specific TIL population was the one involved in the effector function. However, it was clear that the introduction of a gene into a patient did not produce any toxic effect.[3,52]

Clinical Gene Therapy

The first human gene therapy trial involved the transfer of the adenosine deaminase gene (ADA) into T cells. ADA deficiency induces high levels of 2'-deoxyadenosine in blood, which in turn is toxic to both T and B cells, resulting in combined immunodeficiency. This deficiency can be lethal, but it has been shown that it can be corrected upon bone marrow transplantation as well as by injections of pure bovine ADA conjugated to polyethylene glycol (PEG). Although injection of PEG-ADA can be partially successful, the consensus is to improve its efficiency and this has been achieved by producing ADA within T cells.[3,63]

In current gene therapy trials patients are treated with PEG-ADA as well as with infusion of their own transduced lymphocytes which can express ADA as well as the neomycin marker gene. With this procedure patients have improved their immunological response and the transduced T cells persist over six months after infusions have been finalized. Deficiency of purine nucleotide phosphorylase[70] as well as hypoxanthine guanine phosphoribosyl-transferase is being surveyed to establish a similar type of treatment.[58,83]

Animal models have been helpful to organize possible human gene trial protocols.[59] Preliminary results with low-density lipoprotein (LDL) receptor have been obtained by introducing the gene into hepatocytes. In this case, Watanabe hyperlipidemic rabbits have been used. Introduction of the LDL gene into rabbit hepatocytes which in turn are reintroduced into the liver has resulted in a 30% reduction of cholesterol levels for four months. These results are currently in consideration to set human LDL therapy trials.[64]

Cancer, as already indicated, is an area in which gene therapy is being emphasized. Tumor necrosis factor (TNF) or IL-2 genes have been transferred into tumor cells of patients with malignant melanoma.[3,58,63] It is expected that secretion of their products would stimulate a tumor-specific immune response which should result in tumor destruction, slow growth, or being able to recruit TILs from lymph nodes that are due to the site of the tumor. This approach has been based on animal studies. Mice immunized with tumor cells originally transduced with a given cytokine gene produced antitumor activity mediated by T cells.[58] TNF is a very powerful antitumor agent which can be highly toxic. Therefore patients are undergoing preliminary toxicity trials and are being tested with TNF transduced TILs; however, these results are still preliminary.

An initial attempt to introduce genes directly into somatic cells without removal of cells from patients has been carried out by transferring the Class I Human Major Histocompatiblity antigen (HLBA-7) into tumor cells that do not express this antigen. The aim is to induce antitumoral response. In this case the liposome-mediated DNA transfer technique has been employed.

Recently human gene therapy trials have been approved in the U.S.A. as well as in Italy, the Netherlands, and China. However, safety considerations are still being taken into account. One of the issues involves possible insertional mutagenesis which can potentially take place if retroviral vectors are the vehicle of choice to introduce genes. The development of in situ gene transfer techniques can allow the introduction of genes in nondividing cells and overcome possible recombination of retroviral sequences which can lead to the release of free virus which can produce widespread infection. Similarly, a better understanding of the effects on immunoserveillance after introduction of foreign genes is needed. It has been shown that not all genes have high levels of expression when introduced in somatic cells. Gene expression of transduced genes in keratinocytes has been shown to be low, and decreases after grown cells are used for grafting.[31,66,97] Therefore techniques for gene expression need to be improved.[70,72]

Ribozymes

Very recently, certain RNA molecules with catalytic activity have been identified. RNA molecules which can replicate in plants alone (viroid RNAs) or when dependent on a helper virus (satellite RNAs) have self-catalytic activity; these include Avocado Sunblotch viroid, Tobacco Ringspot virus (satellite), and Lucerne Transient Streak virus (satellite). Self-catalysis is an essential part in their life cycle. Self-catalysis of these molecules is an intramolecular reaction. A single RNA molecule contains all the functions required for cleavage. The most analyzed RNA molecule is the group I ribosomal RNA from *Tetrahymena thermophila*. The reader should refer to reviews.[1,21,71]

Origin, Structure, and Function of Ribozymes

The term ribozyme is used to describe RNA molecules with self-catalytic activity. Initial studies to determine the minimum infor-

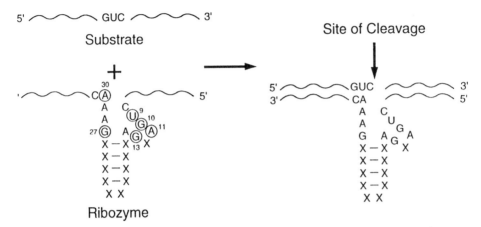

Figure 4. *Basic structure of a ribozyme. Hammerhead ribozyme showing the conserved nucleotides (circled and numbered) involved in substrate cleavage and in keeping the functional configuration of the molecule.*

mation necessary to produce an optimal ribozyme were based on Tobacco Ringspot virus.[42] A single self-cleaving domain from the (+) strand was obtained and its substrate and enzymatic activities were determined. Figure 4 shows the minimal structural requirements for ribozyme catalyzed RNA cleavage: 1) a region which contains the sequence GUC which is adjacent to the cleavage site; 2) a second region containing conserved nucleotides giving rise to a conserved structure also denominated hammerhead structure; and 3) flanking region 5' and 3' to the conserved region which can base pair with the substrate to stabilize interaction and to produce the desired cleavage. Substrates were initially chosen on the basis of possessing little conserved sequences and no defined secondary structure; however, more recently larger substrates with possible secondary structures have also been used.[107]

In naturally occurring self-cleaved RNA it has been shown that the sequence GUC is the one usually preceding the site of cleavage; however, there are exceptions. GUA has been seen to precede the cleavage site of the (−) strand of Lucerne Transient Streak virus. Similarly changes of GUC to GUA or GUU do not seem to alter the catalytic activity. Sequences giving rise to the hammerhead contain conserved nucleotides which cannot be modified.[24,103] The length of base paired stem and associated loops does not need to be conserved; the catalytic region and the RNA substrate are held together by base pairing. The extent and type of base pairing affects the specificity, affinity, and turnover of the enzyme.

Ribozymes can be very powerful tools not only to manipulate a variety of technical aspects within molecular biology, but also to study regulation of gene expression and even for possible therapeutic treatment. Currently the aim has been to see if these molecules are functional in vivo. Ribozymes have been tested in *Xenopus* oocytes. Transfer RNA genes transcribed by polymerase III have been shown to be suitable cassettes for the expression of the ribozymes. After microinjection, it has been possible to observe efficient cleavage of the 5' sequences of U7sn RNA.[25] A ribozyme against c-*fos* mRNA has been produced and its expression was directed by the mouse mammary tumor virus long terminal repeat (MMTV LTR) which is an inducible promoter. The expression of the ribozyme was assayed in cells transfected with c-*fos* which was also expressed by the MMTV LTR promoter. The cells of choice for this experiment were A2780 DDP which are resistant to the chemotherapeutic agent, cisplastin. It has been reported that the role of c-*fos* proto-oncogene is to induce resistance to anticancer agents, especially cisplastin, and it has also been proposed that c-*fos* regulates DNA synthesis and repair pathways. Upon ribozyme synthesis it was possible to observe a decrease in c-*fos* expression, which in turn gave rise to an increased sensitivity to cysplastin. A decrease in dTMP synthase, DNA polymerase β, and Topoisomerase I, was also observed.[89]

Preliminary studies using ribozymes as therapeutic agents have already been considered. Results with these molecules have been obtained with HIV-I. CD4+ HeLa cells expressing a ribozyme directed against HIV-I *gag* sequences were challenged with HIV-I. Seven days after infection it was possible to observe specific cleavage of HIV-I *gag* RNA sequences.[86] These experiments have given a clear indication that ribozyme can work in vivo. However two major problems have been encountered: the lack of RNA stability and the difficulty of targeting and delivering the molecules into the cells.

These problems have been addressed as follows. The role of the ribose-phosphate backbone is being studied. The backbone is very important in view of the fact that DNA molecules with similar base sequence do not have catalytic activities. Similarly, studying the backbone should give an indication of which nucleotides and chemical structures are critical for their activity. Replacement of nucleotides with 2'0-Allyl-and 2'0-methyl ribonucleotides has identified a set of six nucleotides in contiguous positions which have a strong effect on catalytic activity. These include U_9, C_{10}, A_{11}, G_{13}, G_{27}, and A_{30}. Ribozymes made of these synthetic polymers (but keeping the obligatory six unchanged nucleotides) have shown to be resistant to degradation and very stable in serum.[73]

In the case of *Tetrahymena thermophila* ribozyme, it has been shown that mutations in the nonconserved sequence region J½ that connects the RNA substrate-binding site to the catalytic core increases its catalytic activity and specificity by partitioning the RNA substrate to optimize tertiary interactions and therefore ensure correct cleavage.[107] Several laboratories are also studying the role of two hydroxyl groups in the conserved guanosines and their effect in catalysis. The role of Mg^{2+} and other metals in efficient polynucleotide strand scission is currently being determined.[27]

More detailed research is still needed to allow use of ribozymes in human therapy; this tool is potentially one of the most promising for the future.

References

1. Alman S. Ribonuclease P: An enzyme with a catalytic RNA subunit. Adv Enzymol 1989; 62: 1–36.
2. Alzari PM, Lascombe M-B, Poljak RJ. Three-dimensional structure of antibodies. Ann Rev Immunol 1988; 6:551–581.
3. Anderson WF. Human gene therapy. Science 1992; 256:808–813.
4. Baldwin E, Schultz PG. Generation of a catalytic antibody by site-directed mutagenesis. Science 1989; 245:1104–1107.
5. Bentle GA, Boulot G, Riottot MM, et al. Three-dimensional structure of an idiotope-anti-idiotope complex. Nature 1990; 348: 254–257.
6. Berg J, Lötscher E, Steimer KS, et al. Bispecific antibodies that mediate killing of cells infected with human immunodeficiency virus of any strain. Proc Natl Acad Sci USA 1991; 88:4723–4727.
7. Bertram JH, Gill PS, Levine AM, et al. Monoclonal antibody T101 in T cell malignancies: A clinical pharmacogenetic and immunologic correlation. Blood 1986; 68:752–761.
8. Better M, Chang CP, Robinson RR, et al. *Escherichia coli* secretion of an active chimeric antibody fragment. Science 1988; 240:1041–1043.
9. Billetta R, Hollingdale MR, Zanetti M. Immunogenicity of an engineered internal image antibody. Proc Natl Acad Sci USA 1991; 88:4713–4717.
10. Biocca S, Neuberger MS, Cattaneo A. Expression and targeting of intracellular antibodies in mammalian cells. EMBO J 1990; 9: 101–108.
11. Bird RE, Walker BW. Single chain antibody variable regions. TIB TECH 1991; 9:132–137.
12. Bird RE, Hardman KD, Jacobson JW, et al. Single-chain antigen-binding proteins. Science 1988; 242:423–426.

470   THE MOLECULAR BASIS OF HUMAN CANCER

13. Boss AM, Kenten JH, Wood CR, et al. Assembly of functional antibodies from immunoglobulin heavy and light chain synthesized in *E coli*. Nucleic Acids Res 1984; 12:3791–3806.
14. Boulot G, Eisele J-L, Bentley GA, et al. Crystallization and preliminary X-ray diffraction study of the bacterially expressed F_v from the monoclonal anti-lysozyme antibody D1.3 and of its complex with the antigen, lysozyme. J Molec Biol 1990; 213:617-619.
15. Brinkmann U, Pai LH, Fitzgerald DJ, et al. B3(Fv)-PE38KDEL, a single-chain immunotoxin that causes complete regression of a human carcinoma. Proc Natl Acad Sci USA 1991; 88: 8616–8620.
16. Buchner J, Rudolph R. Renaturation, purification and characterization of recombinant Fab fragments produced in *E coli*. Bio/technol 1991; 91:157–164.
17. Burton DR. Human and mouse monoclonal antibodies by repertoire cloning. TIB TECH 1991; 9:169–175.
18. Cabilly S, Riggs AD, Pande H, et al. Generation of antibody activity from immunoglobulin polypeptide chains produced in *Escherichia coli*. Proc Natl Acad Sci USA 1984; 81:3273-3277.
19. Carter P, Presta L, Gorman CM, et al. Humanization of an anti-p185[HER2] antibody for human cancer therapy. Proc Natl Acad Sci USA 1992; 89: 4285–4289.
20. Cattaneo A, Neuberger MS. Polymeric immunoglobulin M is secreted by transfectants of nonlymphoid cells in the absence of immunoglobulin J chain. EMBO J 1987; 6:2753–2758.
21. Cech TR. Self-splicing of group I introns. Annu Rev Biochem 1990; 59:543–568.
22. Chaudhary VK, Batra JK, Gallo MG, et al. Rapid method of cloning functional variable-region antibody genes in *Escherichia coli* as single-chain immunotoxins. Proc Natl Acad Sci USA 1990; 87:1066–1070.
23. Cheetham J. Reshaping the antibody combining site by CDR replacement-tailoring or tinkering to fit? Protein Eng 1988; 2:170–172.
24. Chowrira BM, Berzal-Herranz A, Burke JM. Novel guanosine requirement for catalysis by the hairpin ribozyme. Nature 1991; 354:320–322.
25. Cotten M, Birnsteil M. Ribozyme mediated destruction of RNA in vivo. EMBO J 1989; 8:3861–3866.
26. Cunningham C, Harris WJ. Antibody engineering—How to be human. TIB TECH 1992; 10:112–113.
27. Dange V, Van Atta RB, Hecht SM. A Mn^{2+}-dependent ribozyme. Science 1990; 248:585–588.
28. Danos O, Mulligan RC. Safe and efficient generation of recombinant retroviruses with amphotropic and ecotropic host ranges. Proc Natl Acad Sci USA 1988; 85:6460–6464.
29. Eglitis MA, Anderson WF. Retroviral vectors for introduction of genes into mammalian cells. BioTechniques 1988; 6:608–614.
30. Engert A, Martin G, Pfreundschuh M, et al. Anti-tumor effects of ricin A chain immunotoxins prepared from intact antibodies and Fab fragments on solid human Hodgkins disease tumors in mice. Cancer Res 1990; 50:2929–2935.
31. Fenjves ES, Gordon DA, Pershing LK, et al. Systemic distribution of apolipoprotein E. secreted by grafts of epidermal keratinocytes: Implica-

tions for epidermal function and gene therapy. Proc Natl Acad Sci USA 1989; 86:8803–8807.

32. Field H, Rees AR, Yarranton GT. A functional recombinant immunoglobulin variable domain from polypeptides produced in *Escherichia coli*. Vaccines 1988; 88:29–34.

33. Field H, Yarranton GT, Rees AR. Expression of mouse immunoglobulin light and heavy chain variable regions in *Escherichia coli* and reconstitution of antigen-binding activity. Protein Eng 1989; 3:641–647.

34. Fulton RJ, Uhr JW, Vitetta ES. In vivo therapy of the BCL tumor: Effect of immunotoxin valency and deglycosylation of the ricin A chain. Cancer Res 1988; 48:2626–2631.

35. Furth ME, Davis LJ, Fleurdelys B, et al. Monoclonal antibodies to the p21 products of the transforming gene of harvey murine sarcoma virus and of the cellular *ras* gene family. J Virol 1982; 43:294–304.

36. Ghetie V, Ghetie MA, Uhr JW, et al. Large scale preparation of immunotoxins constructed with the Fab^2 fragment of Ig G$_1$ murine monoclonal antibodies and chemically deglycosylated ricin A chain. J Immunol Methods 1988; 112:267–277.

37. Ghetie V, Thorpe P, Ghetie MA, et al. The G.L.P. large scale preparation of immunotoxins containing deglycosylated ricin A chain and a hindered disulfide bond. J Immunol Methods 1991; 142:223–230.

38. Ghetie MA, Richardson J, Tucker T, et al. Antitumor activity of Fab^1 and IgG-anti-CD22 immunotoxins in disseminated human B lymphoma grown in mice with severe combined immunodeficiency disease: Effect on tumor cells in extranodal sites. Cancer Res 1991; 51:5876–5880.

39. Glockshuber R, Malia M, Pfitziger I, et al. A comparison of strategies to stabilize immunoglobulin Fv-fragments. Biochemistry 1990; 29:1362–1367.

40. Granato DA, Neeser JR. Effect of trimming inhibitors on the secretion and biological activity of a murine IgE monoclonal antibody. Mol Immunol 1987; 24:849–855.

41. Hasesmann CA, Capra JD. High-level production of a functional immunoglobulin heterodimer in a baculovirus expression system. Proc Natl Acad Sci USA 1990; 87:3942–3946.

42. Haseloff J, Gerlach WL. Simple RNA enzymes with new and highly specific endoribonuclease activities. Nature 1988; 334: 585–591.

43. Hiatt A, Cafferkey R, Bowdish K. Production of antibodies in transgenic plants. Nature 1989; 342:76–78.

44. Hickman S, Kornfeld S. Effect of tunicamycin on IgM, IgA, and IgG secretion by mouse plasmacytoma cells. J Immunol 1978; 121:990–996.

45. Holland IB, Kenny B, Steipe B, et al. Secretion of heterologous proteins in *Escherichia coli*. Meth Enzymol 1990; 182:132–143.

46. Horwitz AH, Chang CP, Better M, et al. Secretion of functional antibody and Fab fragment from yeast cells. Proc Natl Acad Sci USA 1988; 85:8678–8682.

47. Horbett AT. Molecular origins of the surface activity of proteins. Protein Eng 1988; 2:172–174.

48. Huse WD, Sastry I, Iverson SA, et al. Generation of a large combinatorial library of the immunoglobulin repertoire in phage lambda. Science 1989; 246:1275–1281.

49. Huston JS, Levinson D, Mudgett-Hunter M, et al. Protein engineering of antibody binding sites: Recovery of specific activity in an anti-digoxin single-chain Fv analogue produced in *Escherichia coli*. Proc Natl Acad Sci USA 1988; 85:5879-5883.

50. Kabat EA, Wu TT, Bilofsky H, et al. Sequences of proteins of immunological interest. 3rd Ed., US 1983. Department of Health and Human Services.

51. Kabat EA, Wu TT, Reid-Miller M, et al. Sequences of proteins of immunological interest. 4th Edn, US, 1987. Department of Health and Human Services.

52. Kasid A, Morecki S, Aebersold P, et al. Human gene transfer: Characterization of human tumor-infiltrating lymphocytes as vehicles for retroviral mediated gene transfer in man. Proc Natl Acad Sci USA 1990; 87:473–477.

53. Kenten J, Helm B, Ishizaka T, et al. Properties of a human immunoglobulin E-chain fragment synthesized in *Escherichia coli*. Proc Natl Acad Sci USA 1984; 81:2955–2959.

54. Köhler G, Milstein C. Continuous cultures of fused cells secreting antibody of predefined specificity. Nature 1975; 256: 495–497.

55. Lane DP, Crawford LV. T antigen is bound to a host protein in SV40-transformed cells. Nature 1979; 278:261–263.

56. Larrick JW, Danielsson I, Brenner CA, et al. Polymerase chain reaction using mixed primers: Cloning of human monoclonal antibody variable region genes from single hybridoma cells. Biotechnology 1989; 7:934–938.

57. Leatherbarrow RJ, Rademacher TW, Dwek RA, et al. Effector functions of monoclonal aglycosylated mouse IgG_{2a}: Binding and activation of complement component C1 and interaction with human monocyte Fc receptor. Mol Immunol 1985; 22:407–415.

58. Lindahl A, Teumer J, Green H. Cellular aspects of gene therapy. In: Growth Factors in Health and Disease, Westermark B, Bersholtz G, Hokfelt B, eds. New York, Elsevier Science Publishers B.V.; 1990; pp. 383–392.

59. Lynch CM, Clowes MM, Osborne WRA, et al. Long-term expression of human adenosine deaminase in vascular smooth muscle cells of rats: A model for gene therapy. Proc Natl Acad Sci USA 1992; 89:1138–1142.

60. Linzer DIH, Levine A. Characterization of a 54K dalton cellular SV40 tumor antigen in SV40 transformed cells. Cell 1979; 17:43–52.

61. McGeady ML, Arthur PM, Seidman M. Development of a retroviral vector for inducible expression of transforming growth factor β1. J Virol 1990; 64:3527–3531.

62. Miller RA, Oseroff AR, Stratte PT, et al. Monoclonal antibody therapeutic trials in 7 patients with T cell lymphoma. Blood 1983; 62:988–995.

63. Miller AD. Human gene therapy comes of age. Nature 1992; 557: 455–460.

64. Miyanohara A, Sharkey MF, Witztum JL, et al. Efficient expression of retroviral vector-transduced human low density lipoprotein (LDL) receptor in LDL receptor-deficient rabbit fibroblasts in vitro. Proc Natl Acad Sci USA 1988; 85: 6538-6542.

65. Montano X, Jimenez A. Intracellular expression of the monoclonal antibody Y13–259 blocks the transforming activity of *ras* oncogenesis. Cell Growth and Differentiation. In Press.

66. Morgan JR, Barrandon Y, Green H, et al. Expression of an exogenous growth hormone gene by transplantable human epidermal cells. Science 1987; 237:1476–1479.

67. Morrison SL, Oi VT. Genetically engineered antibody molecules. Adv Immunol 1989; 44:65–92.

68. Nose M, Wigzell H. Biological significance of carbohydrate chains on monoclonal antibodies. Proc Natl Acad Sci USA 1983; 80: 6632–6636.

69. Orlandi R, Güssow DH, Jones PT, et al. Cloning immunoglobulin variable domains for expression by the polymerase chain reaction. Proc Natl Acad Sci USA 1989; 86:3833–3837.

70. Osborne WRA, Miller AD. Design of vectors for efficient expression of human purine nucleoside phosphorylase in skin fibroblasts from enzyme-deficient humans. Proc Natl Acad Sci USA 1988; 85:6851–6855.

71. Pace NR, Smith D. Ribonuclease P: Function and variation. J Biol Chem 1990; 265:3587–3590.

72. Palmer TD, Rosman GJ, Osborne WRA, et al. Genetically modified skin fibroblasts persist long after transplantation but gradually inactivate introduced genes. Proc Natl Acad Sci USA 1991; 88:1330–1334.

73. Paolella G, Sproat BS, Lamond AI. Nuclease resistant ribozymes with high catalytic activity. EMBO J 1992; 11:1913-1919.

74. Pastan I, Fitzgerald D. Recombinant toxins for cancer treatment. Science 1991; 254:1173–1177.

75. Perlmutter RM, Crews ST, Douglas R, et al. The generation of diversity in phosphorycholine-binding antibodies. Adv Immunol 1984; 35:1–37.

76. Plückthun A. Antibody engineering: Advances from the use of *Escherichia coli* expression systems. Biotechnology 1991; 9: 545–551.

77. Plückthun A, Skerra A. Expression of functional antibody F_V and Fab fragments in *Escherichia coli*. Methods Enzymol 1989; 178:497–515.

78. Plückthun A. Antibody engineering. Current Opinion in Biotechnology 1991; 2:238–246.

79. Plückthun A. Antibodies from *Escherichia coli*. Nature 1990; 347:497–498.

80. Press OW, Applebaum F, Ledbetter JA, et al. Monoclonal antibody IF5 (Anti-CD20) O therapy of human B cell lymphomas. Blood 1987; 69:584–591.

81. Putlitz J, Kubasek WL, Duchene M, et al. Antibody production in baculovirus infected insect cells. Biotechnology 1990; 8:651-654.

82. Riechmann L, Clark M, Waldmann H, et al. Reshaping human antibodies for therapy. Nature 1988; 332:323–327.

83. Russell SJ. Lymphokine gene therapy for cancer. Immunol Today 1990; 11:196–200.

84. Rybak SM, Hoogenboom HR, Meade HM, et al. Humanization of immunotoxins. Proc Natl Acad Sci USA 1992; 89:3165–3169.

85. Sastry L, Alting-Mees M, Huse WD, et al. Cloning of the immunological repertoire in *Escherichia coli* for generation of monoclonal catalytic antibodies: Construction of a heavy chain variable region-specific cDNA library. Proc Natl Acad Sci USA 1989; 86:5728–5732.

86. Sarver N, Cantin EM, Chang PS, et al. Ribozymes as potential anti-HIV-1 therapeutic agents. Science 1990; 247:1222–1225.

87. Saton Y, Cohen GH, Padlan EA, et al. Phosphocholine binding immunoglobulin Fab MCPc603. An X-ray diffraction study at 2.7Å. J Mol Biol 1986; 190:593–604.

88. Saul FA, Amzel LM, Poljak RJ. Preliminary refinement and structural analysis of the Fab fragment from human immunoglobulin new at 2.0Å resolution. J Biochem 1978; 253:585–595.

89. Scanlon KJ, Jiao L, Funato T, et al. Ribozyme-mediated cleavage of c-*fos* mRNA reduces gene expression of DNA synthesis enzymes and metallothionein. Proc Natl Acad Sci USA 1991; 88:10591–10595.

90. Scharfmann R, Axelrod JH, Verma IM. Long-term in vivo expression of retrovirus-mediated gene transfer in mouse fibroblast implants. Proc Natl Acad Sci USA 1991; 88:4626-4630.

91. Shen GL, Li JL, Ghetie MA, et al. Evaluation of four CD22 antibodies as ricin A chain containing immunotoxins for the in vivo therapy of human B-cell leukemias and lymphomas. Int J Cancer 1988; 42:792–797.

92. Sibley CH, Wagner RA. Glycosylation is not required for membrane localization or secretion of IgM in a mouse B cell lymphoma. J Immunol 1981; 126:1868–1873.

93. Sidman C. Differing requirements for glycosylation in the secretion of related glycoproteins is determined neither by the producing cell nor by the relative number of oligosaccharide units. J Biol Chem 1981; 256:9374–9376.

94. Sieger HF, Wallack NK, Vervaert CE, et al. Melanoma patient antibody responses to melanoma tumor associated antigens defined by murine monoclonal antibodies. J Biol Response Mod 1989; 8:37-52.

95. Skerra A, Plückthum A. Assembly of a functional immunoglobulin Fv fragment of *Escherichia coli*. Science 1988; 240:1038–1041.

96. Taylor AK, Wall R. Selective removal of μ-heavy-chain glycosylation sites causes immunoglobulin A degradation and reduced secretion. Mol Cell Biol 1988; 8:4197–4203.

97. Teumer J, Lindahl A, Green H. Human growth hormone in the blood of athymic mice grafted with cultures of hormone-secreting human keratinocytes. FASEB J 1990; 4:3245–3250.

98. Thorpe PE, Ross WCJ, Brown ANF, et al. Blockade of the galactose-binding sites of ricin by its linkage to antibody. J Biochem 1984; 140:63–71.

99. Verhoeyen M, Milstein C, Winter G. Reshaping human antibodies: Grafting an antilysozyme activity. Science 1988; 239: 1534–1535.

100. Ward ES, Güssow D, Griffiths AD, et al. Binding activities of a repertoire of single immunoglobulin variable domains secreted from *Escherichia coli*. Nature 1989; 341:544–546.

101. Wetzel R. Active immunoglobulin fragments synthesized in E coli from Fab to scantibodies. Protein Eng 1988; 2:169-176.

102. Whyte P, Buchkovich KJ, Horowitz JM, et al. Association between an oncogene and an anti-oncogene: The adenovirus E1A proteins bind to the retinoblastoma gene product. Nature 1988; 334:124–129.

103. Williams DM, Pieken WA, Eckstein F. Function of specific 2'-hydroxyl groups of guanosines in a hammerhead ribozyme probed by 2' modifications. Proc Natl Acad Sci USA 1992; 89: 918–921.

104. Winter E, Milstein C. Man-made antibodies. Nature 1991; 349: 293–299.
105. Wood CR, Boss MA, Patel TP, et al. The influence of messenger RNA secondary structure on expression of an immunoglobulin heavy chain in *Escherichi coli*. Nucl Acids Res 1984; 12:3937–3950.
106. Wood CR, Boss MA, Kenten JH, et al. The synthesis and in vivo assembly of functional antibodies in yeast. Nature 1985; 314:446–449.
107. Young B, Herschlag D, Cech TR. Mutations in a nonconserved sequence of the tetrahymena ribozyme increase activity and specificity. Cell 1991; 67:1007–1019.

Index

477